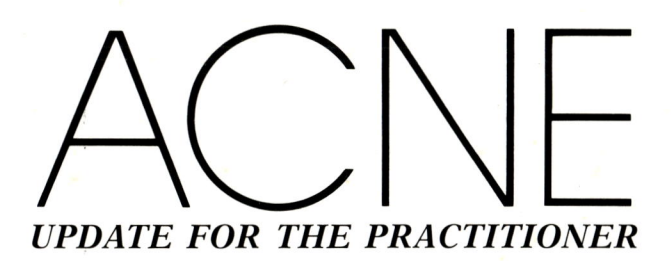

ACNE
UPDATE FOR THE PRACTITIONER

ACNE: Update for the Practitioner

Copyright © 1979 by Yorke Medical Books, Technical Publishing Company, a division of Dun-Donnelley Publishing Corporation, a Dun & Bradstreet Company.

All rights reserved. No part of this publication may be reproduced, stored in a retrieval system, or transmitted in any form or by any means, electronic, mechanical, photocopying, recording, or otherwise, without the prior written permission of the Publisher.

Printed in the United States of America

First Edition

Library of Congress Catalog Card Number: 79-63512

International Standard Book Number: 0-914316-16-8

ACNE
UPDATE FOR THE PRACTITIONER

EDITED BY
SAMUEL B. FRANK, MD
Professor of Clinical Dermatology
New York University School of Medicine

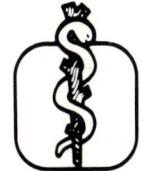

YORKE MEDICAL BOOKS
666 FIFTH AVENUE, NEW YORK, NEW YORK

To my wife,
Eleanor

Contents

Contributors	xi
Preface	xv

INTRODUCTION

1. **Enigmas and Hypotheses**   1
   Marion B. Sulzberger, MD

2. **History of Acne**   7
   Lawrence C. Parish, MD, Joseph A. Witkowski, MD

3. **Classification of Acne and Its Variants**   13
   Albert M. Kligman, MD, PhD, Gerd Plewig, MD

PATHOGENESIS

4. **Sebum: Lipogenesis**   27
   Victor R. Wheatley, PhD, DSc

5. **Bacteriology**   35
   Jack G. Voss, PhD

6. **Immunology**   47
   S. Madli Puhvel, PhD

7. **Hormones**   53
   F.J.G. Ebling, PhD, DSc

8. **Free Fatty Acid Hypothesis: Summarized**   67
   Robert E. Kellum, MD

9. **Other Pathogenic Factors**   74
   Ronald M. Reisner, MD

HISTOPATHOLOGY

10.	**Comedo Formation: Ultrastructure** Dennis D. Knutson, MD	81
11.	**Noninflammatory and Inflammatory Acne** Gerd Plewig, MD, Albert M. Kligman, MD, PhD	91

TREATMENT

12.	**An Overview of Acne Treatment** Ronald M. Reisner, MD	114
13.	**Vitamin A Acid Topical Therapy** Christopher M. Papa, MD	121
14.	**Vitamin A Acid Topical Therapy: Ultrastructural Effects** Helmut H. Wolff, MD, Gerd Plewig, MD	136
15.	**Benzoyl Peroxide Topical Therapy** James E. Fulton, Jr., MD, PhD, Antoinette Schenk	141
16.	**Combined Vitamin A Acid and Benzoyl Peroxide Topical Therapy** Sydney Hurwitz, MD	148
17.	**Topical Tetracycline Therapy** Harry L. Wechsler, MD, Jacquelyn Kirk, MD	156
18.	**Topical Erythromycin Therapy** Alan R. Shalita, MD	168
19.	**Topical Clindamycin Therapy** Richard B. Stoughton, MD, William Resh, MD	171
20.	**Oral Antibiotics** William A. Akers, MD, Howard I. Maibach, MD	179
21.	**Choice of Antibiotics: Management of Antibiotic-resistant Acne** James J. Leyden, MD	198

22.	**Treatment of Acne with Anovulatory Drugs** *Vincent P. Barranco, MD*	207
23.	**Physiotherapy** *Ervin Epstein, MD*	211
24.	**Other Therapies** *Joseph A. Witkowski, MD, Lawrence C. Parish, MD*	220
25.	**Surgery for Acne: Preventive, Therapeutic, and Rehabilitative** *Norman Orentreich, MD, Nancy Durr*	231

CONCLUSION

26.	**Summing Up** *Samuel B. Frank, MD*	243
	Index	267

Contributors

William A. Akers, MD Chief, Department of Dermatological Research, Letterman Army Institute of Research, San Francisco

Vincent P. Barranco, MD Associate Clinical Professor of Dermatology, University of Oklahoma Health Sciences, Tulsa

Nancy Durr New York City

F.J.G. Ebling, PhD, DSc Professor of Zoology, University of Sheffield, England

Ervin Epstein, MD Emeritus Associate Clinical Professor of Dermatology, University of California School of Medicine, San Francisco

Samuel B. Frank, MD Professor of Clinical Dermatology, New York University School of Medicine, New York City

James E. Fulton, MD, PhD Miami, Florida

Sidney Hurwitz, MD Associate Clinical Professor, Pediatrics and Dermatology, Yale University School of Medicine, New Haven, Connecticut

Robert E. Kellum, MD Associate Clinical Professor of Medicine (Dermatology), University of Washington School of Medicine, Seattle

Jacquelyn Kirk, MD Instructor of Medicine (Dermatology), University of Pittsburgh School of Medicine, Pennsylvania

Albert M. Kligman, MD, PhD Professor of Dermatology, Duhring Laboratories, University of Pennsylvania School of Medicine, Philadelphia

Dennis D. Knutson, MD Clinical Associate Professor of Dermatology, University of South Dakota School of Medicine, Sioux Falls

James J. Leyden, MD Associate Professor of Dermatology, Duhring Laboratories, University of Pennsylvania School of Medicine, Philadelphia

Howard I. Maibach, MD Professor and Vice Chairman, Department of Dermatology, University of California School of Medicine, San Francisco

Norman Orentreich, MD Clinical Associate Professor of Dermatology, New York University School of Medicine, New York City

Christopher M. Papa, MD Clinical Associate Professor of Medicine (Dermatology) and Acting Chief, Division of Dermatology, Rutgers Medical School, Piscataway, New Jersey

Lawrence C. Parish, MD Associate Clinical Professor of Dermatology and Comparative Dermatology, University of Pennsylvania School of Medicine, Philadelphia

Gerd Plewig, MD Privatdozent, Department of Dermatology, University of Munich, Germany

S. Madli Puhvel, PhD Adjunct Professor of Medicine (Dermatology), Department of Medicine, Center for Health Sciences, University of California, Los Angeles

Ronald M. Reisner, MD Professor and Chief, Division of Dermatology, Department of Medicine, Center for Health Sciences, University of California, Los Angeles

William Resh, MD Division of Dermatology, Department of Medicine, University of California, San Diego

Antoinette Schenk Miami, Florida

Alan R. Shalita, MD Associate Professor and Head, Division of Dermatology, SUNY Downstate Medical Center, Brooklyn, New York

Richard B. Stoughton, MD Professor and Chairman, Division of Dermatology, Department of Medicine, University of California, San Diego

Marion B. Sulzberger, MD Professor Emeritus of Dermatology, New York University School of Medicine, New York City; Clinical Professor of Dermatology, University of California School of Medicine, San Francisco

Jack G. Voss, PhD Sedona, Arizona

Harry L. Wechsler, MD Clinical Assistant Professor of Medicine (Dermatology), University of Pittsburgh School of Medicine, Pennsylvania

Victor R. Wheatley, PhD, DSc Associate Professor of Experimental Dermatology, New York University School of Medicine, New York City

Joseph A. Witkowski, MD Associate Professor of Dermatology, University of Pennsylvania School of Medicine, Philadelphia

Helmut H. Wolff, MD Privatdozent, Department of Dermatology, University of Munich, Germany

Preface

In recent years, the study of acne has aroused increased interest. Much clinical and academic work already has been done—and still is being conducted—making acne one of the more studied disorders of the skin. That this is so is justified by the fact that acne is one of the problems most frequently observed by the dermatologist, the pediatrician, the physician who specializes in adolescent medicine, the family physician, and the general practitioner. In addition, other medical specialists, such as the endocrinologist, the gynecologist, the plastic surgeon, and the psychiatrist, are called upon to aid in the management of the acne patient.

This book was written for those who demand to be kept abreast of the most current investigations and findings regarding the subject of acne. In the past few years, new observations have increased our knowledge of the pathogenesis of acne. Formerly held concepts have been further studied, enlarged, or altered; some have been discarded. The same is true in regard to the treatment of acne. An inspection of the charts of patients whom you treated just a few years ago will illustrate the changes that have since come about in acne therapy. The emphasis on prescribing tretinoin, topical antibiotics, and the benzoyl peroxide gel preparations, and the concomitant decrease in use of those old mainstays, sulfur and resorcinol, are examples of the changes that have taken place. Because of these and other changes, this update was written.

The reader will at once recognize that the authors of the various chapters represent the leaders in their respective subjects. I am proud and pleased that so many outstanding workers in the field of acne accepted my invitation to participate in this book. In a few instances, some of the writers present attitudes that may not be accepted by all. The choice of authors was based entirely on my desire to present the subject of acne as fully as possible, whether or not I was in agreement with the writers. I tried, in the final chapter, "Summing Up," to put the various thinkings in perspective; I hope I succeeded. Where my own thoughts were at variance with the thoughts of others, I presented my opinions as personal ones.

Every effort was made to prevent repetition. It was sometimes impossible for different authors to avoid presenting the same subject; but, where this occurred, different aspects of the subject were so well-presented that removal of any part was not warranted.

I thank all of the contributors for their efforts and their cooperation. I am grateful to them for having made this book possible. All of my colleagues agreed that the time had come to update the observations on acne. This book is the result.

Samuel B. Frank, MD

Chapter 1

Enigmas and Hypotheses
MARION B. SULZBERGER, MD

Acne is one of the most important of human diseases. Some may challenge this statement. True, acne doesn't kill, doesn't pain, and usually cures itself. But acne disfigures; attacks during the vulnerable and insecure adolescent period; affects sites that can't be hidden; interferes with the enjoyment of life and the attainment of social and occupational goals; produces morbidity totaling hundreds of millions of man-years; intensifies the teenager's instability and feelings of revolt; and often leaves permanent scars on the psyche and sometimes permanent scars on the cutaneous soma.

Small wonder, then, that so-called "acne remedies" are bought by the hundreds of millions, TV and radio commercials on "acne remedies" abound, continuing research is devoted to acne, and new textbooks on acne continue to appear. And, indeed, updated and authoritative texts on acne are needed at frequent intervals. Because of the continuing investigations conducted by dermatologists and other scientists, better understanding and improvements in management of acne become available in a steady stream.

This new book edited by Samuel Frank presents, in a useful, practical fashion, the most current knowledge concerning the various forms of acne, their pathogenesis, and management. Distinguished authorities from medical schools throughout the United States and Europe have contributed the latest findings and methods in their individual spheres of expertise, including endocrinology, microbiology, histopathology, chemotherapy, topical therapy, and surgery, to name a few.

The application of this new knowledge has vastly improved the management of acne during the past few years. But despite these extraordinary achievements, there still remain many controversial areas and unsolved riddles shrouding this common and important disease.

Let me remind you of a few of the unfathomed acne mysteries, and present some hypotheses regarding them.

Acne vulgaris almost always begins at puberty, at the time when skin structures such as the sebaceous glands, mammary glands, apocrine glands, and terminal hairs of the beard, axillae and pubes begin to increase in size and function. It is agreed that the biologic clock that starts all this can be traced to the hypothalamus, which sets off the hormonal chain reaction beginning in the anterior pituitary and affecting, in turn, the testes or ovaries, the adrenal cortex, and eventually the skin structures concerned. But what triggers the hypothalamus? Why does it begin to send stimuli to the anterior pituitary when the individual has already lived through eleven or so years?

Perhaps the simplest hypothesis to explain the awakening of the hypothalamus after a finite number of years is to postulate either a finite store or a continued production of hypothalamus-repressor substances—a store which becomes depleted, or a production which ceases, after a certain amount of time. One producer of such repressors could be a gland which regresses or undergoes involution within a fixed number of years. It is not difficult to infer that this concept points to a structure such as the thymus.

An even greater mystery is why most acne goes into remission in individuals sometime in their early twenties. I know that it is fashionable today to state that there are many patients, particularly women 30-40 or more years of age, who still have acne, or have acne again. Of course, this is true; no observant practitioner ever could have doubted it. But this in no way refutes the statement that most patients with adolescent acne get over their skin trouble sometime in their twenties. Why?

No longer tenable is the explanation that acne often stops being active in individuals in their twenties because there are, at that age, appreciable diminutions in the quantities, or significant changes in the ratios or composition, of the circulating sex or adrenocortical hormones. There are convincing modern biochemical assays to the contrary. Attention must then shift to the skin structures and end-organs of response: the pilosebaceous structures. Why do the sebaceous follicles in the usual acne sites fail to produce acne lesions after individuals have reached their twenties? More precisely, why do the follicles and sebaceous glands of the face, upper back, and chest usually respond to the acnegenic hormonal stimuli during the years between 11-20, and cease to respond to what are presumably identical hormonal stimuli sometime between 20-30 years of age and thereafter?

It seems to me that the process may well be so complex that any one, simple answer is not likely to be correct. Several hypotheses have been advanced as possible explanations. One of these, recently presented by Kligman, is that, after exposures to the hormones for a certain number of years, there is an accommodation or "hardening" of the pilosebaceous structures to the effects of these hormones. This would be akin to the well-known hardening and consequent cessation of reaction of the skin of some workers with occupational dermatitis who continue their uninterrupted exposure to allergenic or irritant chemicals, but finally cease to react with dermatitis.

Another hypothesis advanced by Kligman is that, as a result of maturation and aging, the follicle walls and immediately adjacent perifollicular tissue may thicken and become more resistant to the penetration, and exit into the surrounding tissues of the fatty acids and other irritating contents of the follicle. If the inflammation-producing irritants were prevented from entering the dermis, this in turn could prevent the inflammatory reaction which is at the basis of acne papules, pustules, and cysts.

Still another hypothesis is one which I proposed[1] shortly after studying the course and typical localizations of so-called "tropical acne" while in Guam. As is well known, this form of acne often affects men well over the usual acne age. In our series, 25 of the 51 patients were over 20 years old at the onset of their tropical acne. Moreover, it is clear that tropical acne in older patients often spares the common sites of adolescent acne while involving new areas not usually affected by the adolescent form. Because of this, the appearance of men with tropical acne is likely to be quite different from that of patients with ordinary adolescent acne or even those with cystic adolescent acne. In tropical acne, one often sees clear, unaffected skin areas on the face, sometimes with the oiliness and residual scars of a "burnt out" adolescent acne. In contrast, there are commonly many large, severe, cystic and undermining acne lesions on the front, sides, and back of the neck, on arms and forearms, buttocks, thighs, *etc*. My hypothesis to explain these findings is that certain selected pilosebaceous organs on the face, upper back, and chest have an exquisite sensitivity to the acnegenic effect of the early exposures to circulating acnegenic hormones. Once these highly sensitive structures have all been involved by acne lesions, they are either destroyed or scarred by the local inflammatory process, or they become hardened and desensitized to the hormonal stimuli. There are simply no acne-prone follicles left which are sensitive enough to respond to the usual level of adolescent hormonal stimuli. This leaves the follicles on other skin areas which are potentially the sites of acne but which, because of their higher threshold of response to acnegenic hormones, did not develop acne lesions during adolescence. If and when, later on, the constantly circulating hormonal acnegenic stimuli are reinforced and augmented by the heat, humidity, friction, and other possible stresses of tropical military service, some follicles which were spared during adolescence now react to the strong combination of stimuli. According to this hypothesis, adolescent acne "burns itself out" when the supply of follicles sensitive enough to respond to the ordinary hormonal and other stimuli of puberty have all become involved and destroyed, or have been altered and made more

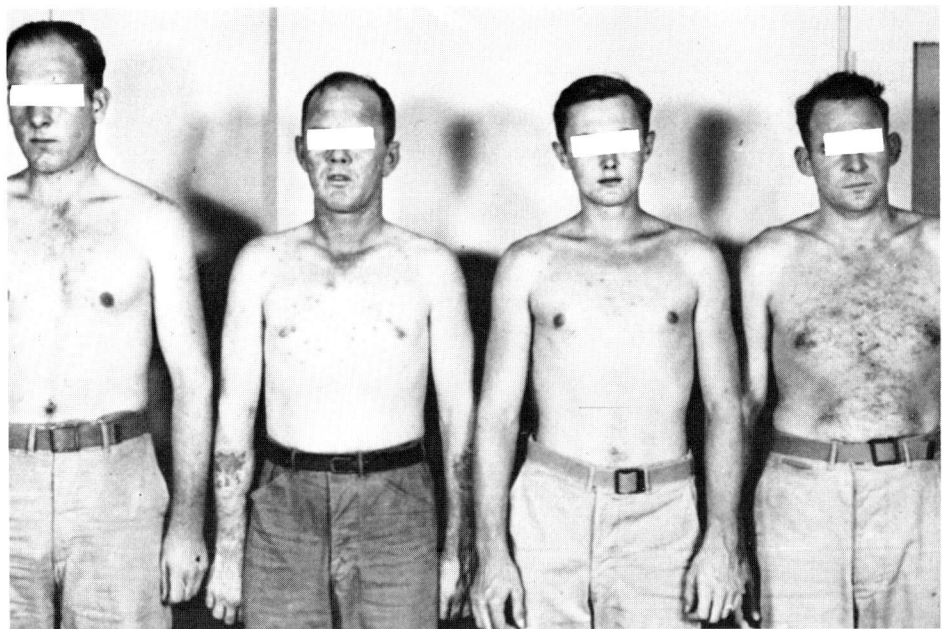

Figure 1. Front view of 4 of the 51 servicemen with tropical acne examined in Guam in 1945. Note that faces are quite clear.

Figure 2. Back view of the 4 patients in Figure 1. Note the severe involvement of backs, buttocks, thighs.

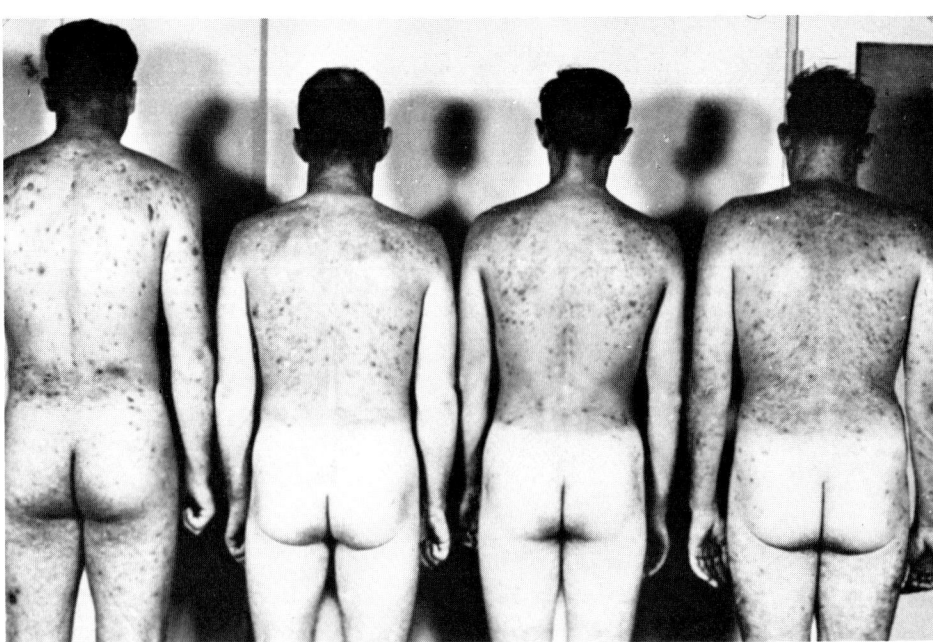

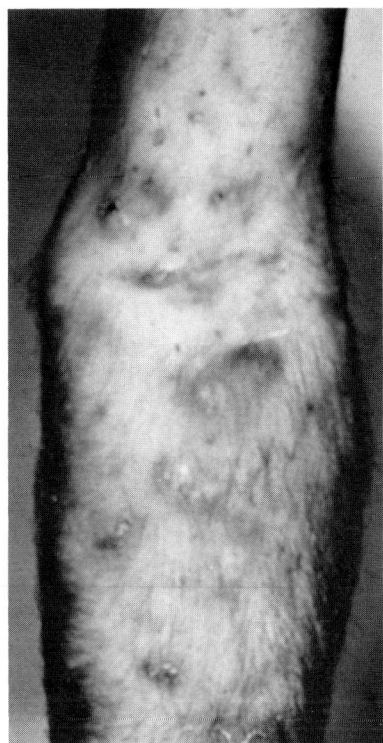
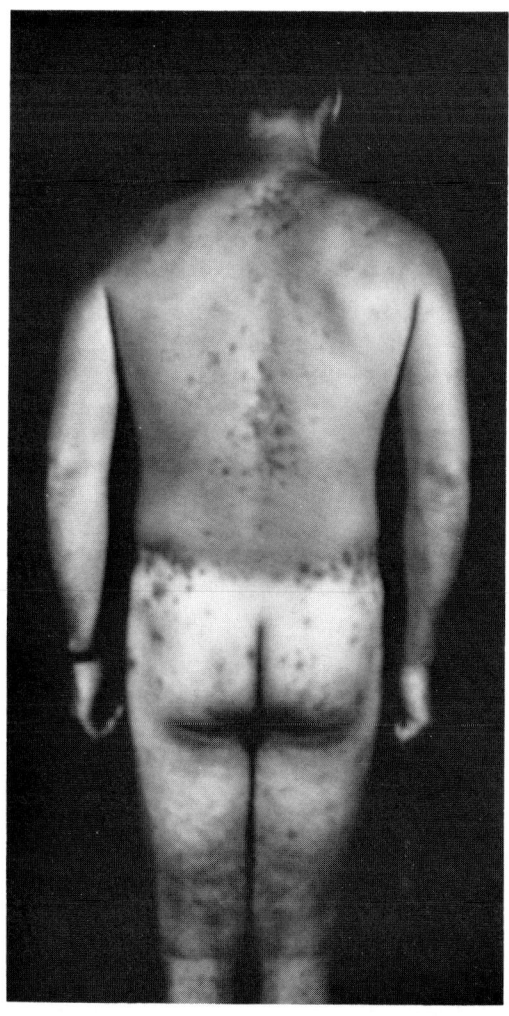

Figure 3. *above:* Arm of soldier with tropical acne. Note large cystic lesions in sites usually spared by adolescent acne. *right:* Back of another soldier with tropical acne. His face was clear. Note the deep cystic lesions on back, buttocks, and thighs, especially severe in areas subject to sweat and friction.

resistant to the usually affecting stimuli by their previous involvement.

Still another hypothesis to explain the usual cessation of appearance of new acne lesions on face, upper chest, and back is that, through some as yet unexplained mechanism, the natural development or spread of the disease is from head to tail. Pinkus[2] advanced this idea in his superb discussion of unsolved problems of the sebaceous glands and acne vulgaris. Pinkus based this hypothesis on the observations that, as acne conglobata patients get older, the eruptions leave the face and shoulders and progress cephalocaudad. Pinkus also mentioned that sebum becomes altered in its chemical composition as the individual grows older, and this may cause the contents of the follicles to become less acnegenic.

There are many more unanswered questions besides the enigmas of why and how acne starts and stops. I mention here only a few.

Why do many follicles with blackheads or whiteheads never develop acne papules, pustules, or cysts? Why do some patients develop many visible blackheads and whiteheads with practically no inflammatory lesions? Why do some patients develop cysts, while others do not? Why does the acne in women beyond the usual acne age so often localize on the chin or around the mouth? Why is there a lot of oil on the skin surface and little acne in some patients, while in others there is a lot of acne and little oil, and, in still others, a lot of both? Why do some acnes—even some mild, superficial ones—produce pitted scars, while others, sometimes equally or even more severe, produce little scarring?

And a last important series of questions: Knowing that a tendency to troublesome acne is familial, what is the nature of the cutaneous, genetically determined susceptibilities? Are there genetic peculiarities in the anatomic shape, size, and configuration of certain follicles, ducts, and orifices? Are there genetic chemical peculiarities of sebum? Of keratin? Are there peculiar susceptibilities to the irritancy of certain free fatty acids? Or do combinations of two or more of these factors account for the differences observed? Then again, perhaps other, entirely different genetically transmissible peculiarities are responsible for the different degrees and kinds of acne we see.

Through analogy, it seems possible that differences in either "stickiness" of sebum or composition of horny lamellae or their mixture may be genetically determined, as Petrakis et al[3] found to hold true of cerumen in different ethnic groups. The validity of this idea could be proved or disproved by rather simple research methods. And many of the other problems and hypotheses regarding acne are now becoming accessible to modern research methods.

In conclusion, let me say that the readers of this book will find the information on treatment of acne most effective and up-to-date. They will also become aware that acne vulgaris is a fascinating and complex disease which both requires and stimulates further scientific investigation.

REFERENCES

1. Sulzberger MB, Addenbrooke EF, Joyce SJ, et al: Tropical acne. *US Naval Bull* 46:1178, 1946.
2. Pinkus H: Sebaceous glands and acne vulgaris: unsolved problems. *J Invest Dermatol* 62:336, 1974.
3. Petrakis NL, Molohon KT, Tepper DJ: Cerumen in American Indians; genetic implications of sticky and dry types. *Science* 158:1192, 1967.

Chapter 2

History of Acne
LAWRENCE C. PARISH, MD
JOSEPH A. WITKOWSKI, MD

Acne, like psoriasis and scabies, has plagued mankind since antiquity. Even King Tut was found to have the scars of this disorder; his tomb contains a variety of medicaments for treating acne.

The word "acne" has a classical Greek background, although its exact derivation is somewhat obscured. The *Shorter Oxford English Dictionary*[1] defines acne as: "eruptions on the face . . . tumours, chiefly in the face." A more detailed discussion on the origin of the word "acne" can be found in two excellent papers on the history of the disease by Grant[2] and MacKenna.[3]

The designation of this disease entity has always been confused, as illustrated a century ago by George Henry Fox (1846–1937)[4] in his presentation to the American Dermatological Association, "On the Proper Use of the Term 'Acne'." Fox stated: *"The title of this paper implies that there is an improper use of the term 'acne.' This is evident to anyone who considers its variable signification, and admits that precision of statement must depend upon the use of definite terms. In a general sense, the term 'acne' is well understood, but as its strict definition has been slightly varied by nearly every writer since Willan, the term is now employed in such a careless way that it is a difficult matter to decide what is and what is not acne. Dr. Duhring, in his textbook, agrees with Hebra in defining acne as an inflammatory disease of the sebaceous glands, and classes seborrhoea and comedo as distinct affections. Dr. Piffard, in his book, like the majority of French writers, includes under the head of 'acne' nearly all affections of the sebaceous glands. The so-called 'acne-rosacea,' however, he regards as a separate affection."*[4]

Despite the prevalence of this disease, comparatively few textbooks have been devoted to the discussion of acne.[5-9] There is a hiatus of nearly 100 years between Bulkley's book and the more recent texts. Perhaps this is indicative of disinterest in this disease during that period.

Almost 250 years ago, Daniel Turner (1667–1741)[10] wrote the first textbook on dermatology in English and also received the first medical degree in America. He can be credited with first considering dietary restrictions in the treatment of acne. He believed that the pimple, or "varus," as he termed the lesion, arose as follows: *"[from the] alimentary Juices by some Accident lodged in the Pores of the Skin and growing, as it finds Liberty, into a little Tubercle, or unequal rising above the surface; which after some Time hardening, proves troublesome by disfiguring the Face."*[10] Regarding his recommendations for additional therapy, Turner wrote: *"If they [tubercles] give not Way, saith Johnstone, to Emollients and Discutients, they must be taken off by Ligature, rubbed down by Caustick or touched with Oil of Vitriol, Sulphur, or Tartar over Night, and washing in the Morning with an Infusion or Decoction of Bean-flower."*[10]

By the turn of the nineteenth century, therapy appeared to have changed little. Thomas Bateman (1778–1821),[11] Robert Willan's favorite student, followed the master's outline in classifying acne under "tubercles." He named 4 varieties—simplex, punctata, indurata, and rosacea—and described an eruption of distinct, hard, tubercles as characteristic of the disorder, sometimes persisting for a considerable length of time, often becoming suppurative. Stimulants, such as alcohol lotions, were favored, as was muriate of mercury. Whereas Willan was partial to oxymuriatic acid for acne punctata, Bateman preferred the ancient acetous acid or liquor ammoniae acitatii and sulfur.

Samuel Plumbe (1795?–1837?),[12] whose *Practical Treatise on Diseases of the Skin* (1829) was very popular, discussed acne in terms of obstruction of the sebaceous follicles due to disorders of the digestive system. He recommended frequent bathing with warm water, gentle friction with mild soap, and a good diet. Plumbe noted: *"It has been observed that these affections are usually of too trifling a character, except in females, to induce persons to take professional advice."*[12]

In 1845, Noah Worcester (1812–1847),[13] wrote the first American textbook of dermatology. He considered acne: *"a noncontagious eruption, characterized by small pustules, upon a conical inflamed base of greater or less size, usually of a dull red or livid, though sometimes of a natural colour, due to sedentary habits, dysmenorrhea, cold drinks, alcohol, masturbation, bilious or lymphatic temperments, with dark hair and smooth, pliable skin."*[13] He recommended cathartics, occasional blood-letting and stimulating washes, and ointments of ioduret of sulfur and nitrate of silver.

By the mid-nineteenth century, Erasmus Wilson (1809-1884),[14] a prominent London surgeon, author and dermatologist, discussed acne as a chronic inflammation of both the "sebiparous glands," as he called them, and their excretory hair follicles. Wilson wrote, *"The diagnostic characters of acne are: the conoidal form of the inflamed elevations; the suppuration of some of these elevations at their apices; the tardy growth and disappearance of others; the livid and indolent tubercle left behind by both; their evident seat in the sebiparous glands and the disorder of neighbouring glands evinced by the increased secretion of some; the concretion of the secretion of others; and, the presence of sebaceous miliary tubercles."*[14]

The leader of the Vienna School, Ferdinand von Hebra (1816–1880),[15] noted: *"No one has yet succeeded in discovering the exciting cause of acne. In fact, with the exception of a few cutaneous irritants, which appear to work only under certain conditions, and on certain persons, we know very little of what will produce it."*[15] Hebra recommended that acne pustules be scarified and rubbed with glycerine soap. He also used sulfur paste, in addition to douches and vapor baths, but admitted, "I know of no means internal or external for even retarding the formation of acne-nodules."[15]

Louis Duhring (1845–1913),[16] in *A Practical Treatise on Diseases of the Skin* (1877), divided treatment into constitutional and local, paying special attention to dyspepsia, constipation, and migraine. For local treatment, he recommended both soothing and stimulating medicaments. Sluggish papular lesions might be painted with carbolic acid. Among the several mechanical methods gaining in popularity at that time, he believed that sand rubbing was helpful in removing comedones.

In 1885, L. Duncan Bulkley (1845–1928),[5] the founder of the New York Skin and Cancer Hospital, wrote the first textbook specifically on acne. He commented: *"The aim . . . of general and constitutional treatment, is to modify the nutrition of the patient so that the functions of the sebaceous glands shall be properly performed; to this end the augmentation of the system must proceed perfectly, and assimilation and segregation must be properly carried out. To accomplish this, considerable attention should be given to the matter of diet and hygiene by the physician."*[5] Bulkley outlined a variety of popular topical preparations then in use, which included tannic acid ointment, zinc oxide ointment, and calamine. Candy, honey, ice cream, rich cheese, chocolate, and bananas were proscribed.

Other textbooks in vogue at that time offered little variation from those cited. Authors differed primarily on the subject of diet, and in their advocation of the use of lotions of varying formulations. The illustrations from the Jacobi and Pringle *Portfolio of Dermochromes*[17] are indicative of the interest of the clinician in the various manifestations of acne (Figure 1 and 2).

By the 1880's, dermatology had come to reflect the advances being made in other areas of medicine. Various instruments were perfected, including the ophthalmoscope and the otoscope. The Keyes punch, the Fox curette, and the acne instrument were all introduced into cutaneous medicine.[18] In 1876, Bulkley[19] wrote: *"The comedones, or clogged sebaceous glands, are best emptied by pressure upon them with the end of a small tube, with an aperture of about 1/16 of an inch, or a new watch key; the orifice is placed over the little black speck, and firm pressure is made perpendicular to the surface, when, in most cases, the worm-like mass will rise partly or completely from its gland, and may be readily removed."*[19]

Many inventive dermatologists also created their own comedo extractors. Henry Granger Piffard (1842-1910) of New York and Paul Gerson Unna (1850-1929)[20] of Hamburg perfected two of the more popular instruments which are used today.

In Paris, there was considerable interest in the manipulation of the acne lesion. A fine darning needle was inserted into the affected sebaceous gland, and was rotated until the gland was emptied. The needle was then reinserted to instill an alcoholic solution of iodine, resulting in a 24-hour orifice "cure."[21]

A major breakthrough in acne therapy occurred in 1901. William Allen Pusey (1865–1940)[22] of Chicago accidently discovered that acne lesions responded to the new roentgen rays: *"These 2 effects of x-rays, atrophy of the cutaneous follicles which they produce and the checking of pus formation, furnish good pathological grounds for suggesting* a priori *use of the agent in the treatment of acne. My observations upon this subject were first made in cases having slight acne, which were under treatment primarily for hypertrichosis."*[22]

Several other popular physical modalities at the time included electrosurgery, cryosurgery, and ultraviolet light. Phototherapy was so much a part of the armamentarium that, in 1929, Howard Fox (1873–1954)[23] of New York emphasized erythema and desquamation as integral therapeutic effects.

The major advance in the past generation has been the advent of antibiotics. Although penicillin and other antibiotics were tried in acne, Sulzberger et al[24] developed the present-day use of tetracycline, following the report of Andrews et al[25] in 1951.

Topical benzoyl peroxide has become a mainstay of acne therapy. This chemical has been known in medicine since 1905, and was used for many years as an antibacterial agent for a wide variety of skin diseases. In 1953, William Pace of London, Ontario began his work with benzoyl peroxide in acne therapy (personal communication, March 1977). During the next decade, he experimented with several different formulations, beginning with Quinolor® Ointment and eventuating with today's commercially available compounds.

Another important topical preparation is vitamin A acid. In 1959, Gunter Stüttgen of the Free University of Berlin recognized the pharmacological effects of retinoic acid (personal communication, March 1977). In 1963, at a staff conference at the University of Pennsylvania, Albert Kligman observed that the skin of a patient being treated for ichthyosis had turned red and was peeling. Thus, Kligman extrapolated that vitamin A acid would make a useful acne medicament.

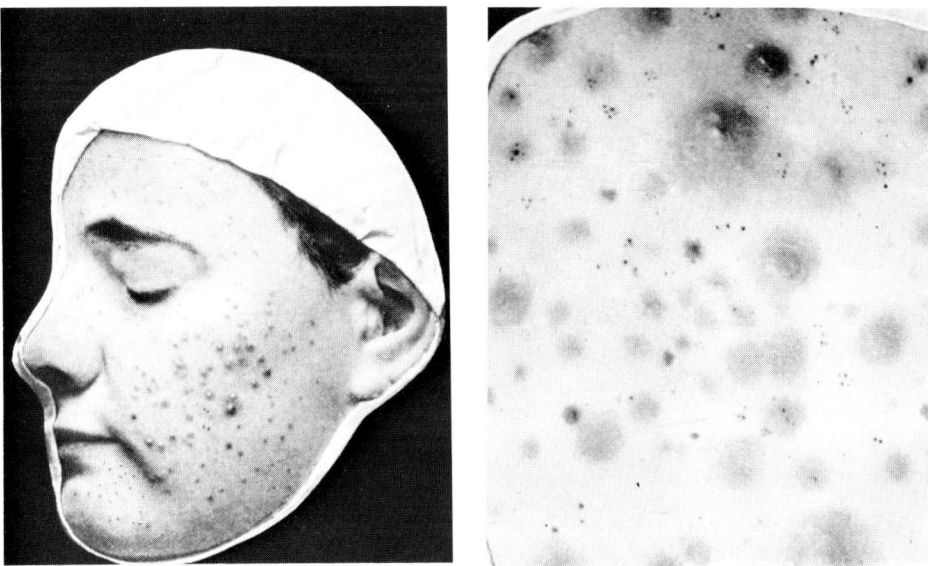

Figure 1 and 2. Illustrations of acne from the Jacobi and Pringle *Portfolio of Dermochromes*.[17]

As dermatologic research moves on in the last part of the twentieth century, laboratory and clinical investigations are underway for developing sebaceous gland antagonists. The age-old remedies of sulfur, salicylic acid, and resorcin, mainstays of treatment for decades, are still widely used, although occasionally maligned. Hormonal therapy, employing both estrogens and corticosteroids, has gained a certain amount of respectability in acne therapy, as has cryotherapy. Still, the final solution to the problem of acne is yet to be found.

REFERENCES

1. *The Shorter Oxford English Dictionary on Historical Principles*, p 17. Oxford: Clarendon Press, 1973.
2. Grant RNR: The history of acne. *Proc R Soc Med* 44:647, 1951.
3. MacKenna RMB: Acne vulgaris. *Lancet* 1:169, 1957.
4. Fox GH: On the proper use of the term "acne." *Arch Dermatol* 4:300, 1879.
5. Bulkley LD: *Acne: Its Etiology, Pathology and Treatment*. New York: GP Putnam, 1885.
6. Bobroff A: *Acne and Related Disorders of Complexion and Scalp*. Springfield: Charles C Thomas, 1964.
7. Frank SB: *Acne Vulgaris*. Springfield: Charles C Thomas, 1971.
8. Cunliffe WJ, Cotterill JA: *The Acnes: Clinical Features, Pathogenesis and Treatment*. Philadelphia: WB Saunders, 1975.
9. Plewig G, Kligman AM: *Acne: Morphogenesis and Treatment*. New York: Springer-Verlag, 1975.

10. Turner D: *De Morbis Cutaneis. A Treatise of Diseases Incident to the Skin*, ed 4, pp 237-267. London: J Walthoe, 1731.
11. Bateman T: *A Practical Synopsis of Cutaneous Diseases*, ed 8, Thomas AT (Ed), pp 333-345. London: Longman, Hurst, Rees, et al, 1836.
12. Plumbe S: *A Practical Treatise on Diseases of the Skin*, ed 3, pp 17-40. London: Nimmo, 1829.
13. Worcester N: *A Synopsis of Diseases of the Skin*, pp 102-119. Philadelphia: T Cowperthwait, 1845.
14. Wilson E: *On Diseases of the Skin*, pp 554-557. Philadelphia: Blanchard & Lea, 1857.
15. von Hebra F: *On Diseases of the Skin Including Exanthemata*, Fagge CH, Pye-Smith PH (Trs-Eds), pp 278-299. London: New Sydenham Society, 1868.
16. Duhring LA: *A Practical Treatise on Diseases of the Skin*, pp 257-268. Philadelphia: JB Lippincott, 1877.
17. Jacobi E, Pringle JJ: *Portfolio of Dermochromes*, vol 2. New York-London: Rebman, 1904.
18. Parish LC: "Highlights in the History of Skin Surgery," in Epstein E, Epstein E Jr (Eds): *Skin Surgery*, ed 4, pp 9-13. Springfield: Charles C Thomas, 1977.
19. Bulkley LD: Notes on the local treatment of certain diseases of the skin. *Arch Dermatol* 2:307, 1876.
20. Unna PG: Komedonenquetscher Komedonengusten. *Monatsschr Prakt Dermatol* 3:332, 1884.
21. Morin: Selections: treatment of acne simplex and acne rosacea. *J Cutan Vener Dis* 1:378, 1883.
22. Pusey WA: Acne and sycosis treated by exposures to roentgen rays. *J Cutan GU Dis* 20:204, 1902.
23. Fox H: Ultraviolet rays in dermatology. *Med J Rec* 130:645, 1929.
24. Sulzberger MB, Witten VH, Steagall RW Jr: Treatment of acne vulgaris. *JAMA* 173:1911, 1960.
25. Andrews GC, Domonkos AN, Post CF: Treatment of acne vulgaris. *JAMA* 146:1107, 1951.

Chapter 3

Classification of Acne and its Variants

ALBERT M. KLIGMAN, MD, PhD
GERD PLEWIG, MD

Acne vulgaris is but one species of a genus of disorders.[1] The denominations of these various eruptions are often careless and imprecise. Confused classification generally leads to misdiagnosis and improper treatment.[2-7] To further cloud the issue, some disorders have names which suggest a kinship to acne when, in fact, no such relationships exist (*eg*, acne keloidalis, acne rosacea, acne necrotica miliaris). The term "acneform" is used too loosely; the word evokes images which are, in many cases, inappropriate and misleading.

The morphologic criteria for including a disorder in the genus acne are: restriction to sebaceous follicles (these are usually found only on the face and trunk, and accordingly determine the pattern of distribution); and intrafollicular hyperkeratosis (comedones) and subsequent inflammation (pustules, papules).

It is useful at the outset to separate true acne from the acne-like, or acneform, eruptions. The former begins with a comedo which may rupture to give rise to pustules and papules. The reverse sequence occurs in the acneform disorders. The process starts with intrafollicular inflammation; comedones later develop and are usually not prominent. True acne encompasses 3 species, each of which includes a number of varieties: 1) *acne vulgaris*, the adolescent disease which exceeds all others in importance and prevalence; 2) *acne venenata*, provoked by external contactants; and 3) *physical acne* due to ultraviolet light and ionizing radiation (x-rays, *etc*).

Acneform eruptions are invariably provoked by drugs. They are readily distinguished from acne vulgaris by the following features: 1) sudden onset with a crop of papules or pustules; 2) not restricted to the adolescent period, but usually in adult life; 3) extension beyond the usual acne areas, onto the buttocks and arms; and 4) other signs of an adverse reaction to drugs (fever, *etc*).

True Acne

ACNE VULGARIS

Tropical Acne—If one were to envision a disease worse than acne conglobata, tropical acne[8-10] would be the appropriate image. It blows up with the suddenness and violence of a tropical tempest, sweeping over the entire integument. The victims are young men who had earlier brushes with acne vulgaris in adolescence, but whose disease is inactive until the following conditions simultaneously occur: 1) relocation to the tropics for an extended period—the condition generally appears in about 3 months; 2) vigorous physical activity while more or less fully-clothed; 3) intense perspiring, leading to continuous overhydration and maceration of the skin; 4) mechanical trauma which activates the disease (friction from tight, wet clothing; pressure from back packs, straps, belts, *etc*); and 5) inability to observe the daily regimen of good skin hygiene (hence, the frequency of the disease in soldiers living under stressful conditions).

Fortunately, only a small percentage of past acne sufferers will be later afflicted, but there is no way to predict who will get the disease. Once started, the process cannot be aborted or contained. Treatment is futile even with such powerful combinations as antibiotics, sulfones, and retinoic acid. The only remedy is to leave the tropics, after which the disease rapidly dissipates without benefit of specialized care.

We know as little or as much about this condition as we do of acne conglobata. Tropical acne is, in fact, an explosive form of acne conglobata. Bacteriologic, endocrinologic, and physiologic studies have not disclosed unique or unusual features which would explain susceptibility.

Pyoderma Faciale—This terrible disease is misnamed, misunderstood, and usually misdiagnosed. It is not a pyoderma, and it is not infectious. Pyoderma faciale is a kind of sister disease to tropical acne, *ie*, a malevolent variant of acne conglobata which occurs suddenly in women well past adolescence. It is confined to the face and seriously afflicts that area, covering most of the surface with innumerable fluctuant inflammatory nodules and papules which frequently fuse and form monstrosities.[11]

These acne sufferers have usually not been seriously troubled by acne in the past. While we are far from understanding how this process begins, or who will be afflicted, there is one important etiologic clue. All the women with this disease (the condition is not so rare) were observed by the authors to have suffered intense, prolonged, psychological trauma. Anxiety and distress are

CLASSIFICATION OF ACNE

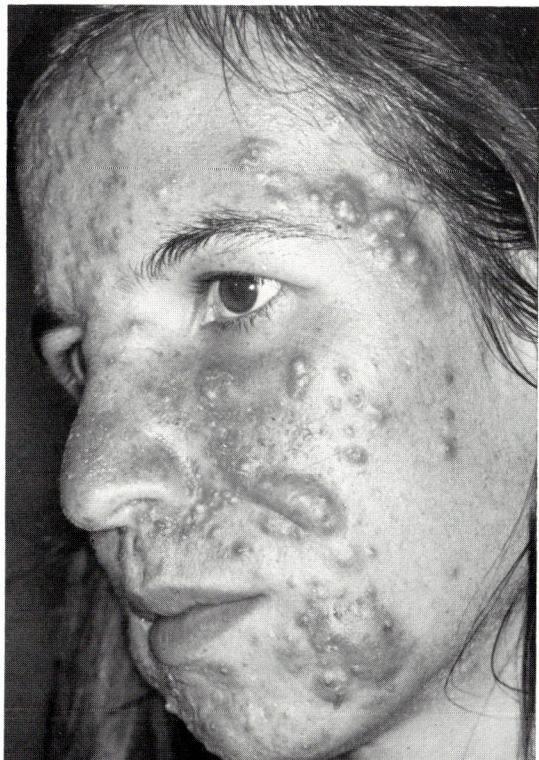

Figure 1. Pyoderma Faciale. Severe emotional trauma usually precedes this devastating eruption resembling the worst form of acne conglobata. It occurs exclusively in females and is misnamed; it is not a pyoderma.

extreme and continuous, and are precipitated by circumstances which are easily identified without deep psychiatric probings. Close questioning will elicit a spate of personal misery relative to recent emotional injuries, *eg*, a death, loss of job, marital discord, *etc*.

One very important clue to pathogenesis is that these acne sufferers are almost always aware of increased facial oiliness prior to onset. One is not likely to experience seborrhea without noticing it. It may be necessary to shampoo more frequently to counter scalp oiliness. Cosmetics and cleansers are used to minimize the disagreeable effects produced by excessive sebum.

The authors postulate that intense emotional stress somehow stimulates the pituitary-adrenal axis, resulting in increased androgen production; hence, the seborrhea. Accordingly, pyoderma faciale is viewed by the authors as a psychosomatic condition. Treatment is the same as that for acne conglobata. In addition, measures should be taken to moderate anxiety, *eg*, tranquilizers and psychiatric investigation.

Acne Fulminans—This is another disastrous skin disease which helps to maintain the reputation of acne as one of the most savage of human afflictions. The condition may be taken for acne conglobata at first glance, but acne fulminans is actually a distinctive disease.[12-15] The important differentiating feature of acne fulminans is the presence of systemic signs, notably, arthralgia, fever, and leukocytosis. Anemia and asthenia are common. While the nodular lesions resemble acne conglobata, they act in a very distinctive and destructive way, collapsing into painful ulcers with overhanging edges. The base of the ulcer is a soft, gelatinous mass into which a probe may be pushed without resistance. The trunk is extensively involved with large ulcerative plaques. The misery of the patients is beyond description. Little is known about the joint disease, except that rheumatoid arthritis can be ruled out; it is the larger joints that tend to be involved.

The candidates for this disease are those, usually males, who already have mild to moderate acne. Inflammatory lesions suddenly begin to behave differently, spreading and ravaging the surrounding tissue. No abnormality has been detected which can account for the inability of the skin to confine the inflammatory process. Massive tissue destruction by neutrophils is characteristic of all the malicious varieties of acne conglobata; some basic aberration of the leukocytes is probably common to all these disorders.

Treatment must be vigorous, and is best carried out in the hospital. Bed rest and high salicylates are indicated for the arthralgia and fever. The skin lesions slowly but surely regress, with the entire spectrum of anti-acne drugs, sulfones, and antibiotics being the mainstay. Benzoyl peroxide promotes healing of ulcers, and 40% urea compresses are useful for debridement.

Masculinizing Syndromes—An excessive production of androgens underlies a variety of syndromes which produce masculinization in female patients. Acne, often severe, is but one expression of a distressing assemblage of changes which include, among others, hirsutism, baldness, and clitoral enlargement.[16-20] Tumors and hyperplasias of the adrenals and ovaries are the principal sources of the excess androgen production.

It is worth noting the difference between Cushing's syndrome, due to cortisol, and masculinizing disorders, due principally to testosterone. Acne is common to both, but little else is shared. The differentiating features of Cushing's syndrome are striae, buffalo fat, and hypertension; hirsutism or baldness generally do not occur. The experienced physician should be able to easily differentiate corticosteroid acne from the acne vulgaris which accompanies masculinization.

Medical centers today have the technical resources to make accurate diagnoses, especially with the aid of sophisticated endocrinologic investigation. It is surprising, in view of the startling change in appearance, that the diagnosis of masculinizing disorders is often delayed until a late stage. This is unfortunate, since the great majority of such cases can be cured surgically with early intervention. Hirsutism and baldness, if advanced, regress very slowly; the return to normal is frequently incomplete.

It is important to remember that while acne is an androgen-dependent disease, it is not typically accompanied by excessive facial hair. So, suspicion should be aroused when a woman between the age of 30-50 states that her facial hairs are darker, thicker, and longer, and that acne has reappeared. Other clues are increased oiliness and menstrual irregularities.

Acne Neonatorum—This is a skin disease which often goes undetected;[21-23] fortunately, it is so mild and transient that its failure to be recognized is of little account. Pediatricians are so familiar with the sebaceous hyperplasia exhibited by so many neonates that they overlook the milia-like, closed comedones which stud the cheeks. Perhaps 20% of neonates have comedonal acne. An occasional inflammatory papule is interspersed. Maternal androgens are responsible for the enlarged sebaceous glands which most newborn babies exhibit, and it is doubtless the excess sebum produced that induces the comedones. Usually the hyperplasia regresses in a month or so; however, the closed comedones may persist for many months, and some may grow to the stage of open comedones or blackheads. In a few patients, mild comedonal and papulopustular acne may last for the first few years of life. There is evidence, at least in boys, that the gonads are capable of secreting testosterone for many months in early infancy.

If closed comedones are so numerous as to merit the attention of the mother, they are usually worthy of treatment with retinoic acid. In any case, the condition should not be shrugged off with the glib prediction that the skin will be normal in a month or two. Cautious follow-up is indicated; some of these patients will further develop moderate inflammatory acne which may last well into childhood. Very few of these babies have endocrinologic abnormalities. Childhood acne is more likely when both parents have had fairly severe acne. Family history is important in explaining neonatal acne and the likelihood of its persistence. Although no longitudinal studies have been done, it is the assumption of the authors that neonatal acne is the precursor of acne vulgaris later on. These infants should be watched carefully after age 5, since we now realize that acne vulgaris, especially in girls, often has its onset in childhood well before the customary signs of puberty appear.

Acne Mechanica—Trauma is an important factor in the aggravation of lesions in acne-prone individuals.[24] Various types of manipulations and physical force can intensify pre-existing acne, or can exacerbate acne vulgaris after it has gone into remission. Perhaps the most common of these manipulations is the habit of resting the chin on the hands, causing the so-called "chin acne." The more inflammatory the acne, the more readily will trauma precipitate inflammatory lesions. While physical force does not induce comedones, it easily causes rupture of the fragile microcomedones which are so characteristic of patients with serious acne. Subclinical inflammation already exists in these fragile microcomedones. Friction and pressure of all kinds facilitate rupture. These may be generated by sporting gear (eg,

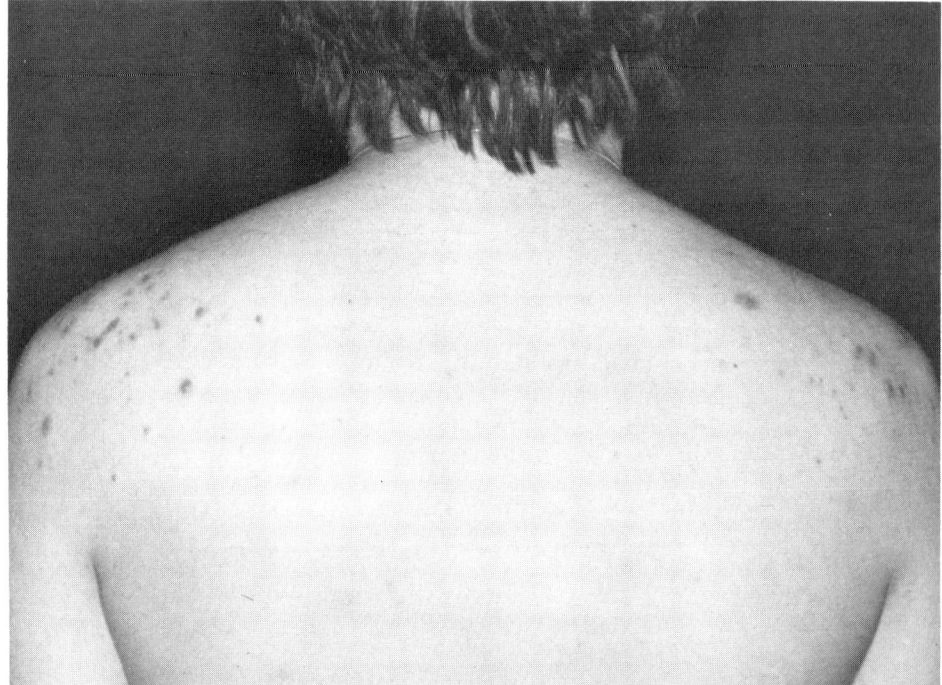

Figure 2. Acne Mechanica. This follicular eruption was provoked by tight-fitting clothing which continuously rubbed over the shoulders.

helmets, straps, *etc*), tight clothing or sweaters, tapes, straps, or casts. Rubbing and kneading facial skin with the fingers can give rise to large, numerous, inflammatory papules and nodules. Pressure from beds, seats and chairs can aggravate acne in individuals who stay in one position for long periods. Perspiration worsens the effect of the trauma.

Lesional distribution is a key to diagnosis. An intensification of acne in an unusual pattern or as a circumscribed patch calls attention to external forces. Facial acne is often asymmetric because one side is more traumatized by the hands and fingers. Acne over the forehead suggests pressure from a headband. Students often manipulate facial skin while studying.

It is important to understand that trauma does not induce acne; it merely exacerbates the appearance of the disease by inflaming or rupturing comedones. Nonetheless, patients generally know too little about the harm that trauma can produce.[24] Excessive scrubbing of the face with harsh, soapy cloths aggravates acne (detergent acne).[25] This practice, especially common among teenagers, is one which patients are reluctant to give up, so strong is their belief that the lesions can be scoured out by conscientious washing. Proprietary abrasives satisfy this same irrational belief, but they are ineffective in removing comedones and can do much harm when strongly applied.

Acne patients must be made to understand that they have vulnerable skin which has to be protected from the total environment with a good deal more care. Being kind to acne-bearing skin is an important way to moderate the disease.

Comedonal Acne, Papulopustular Acne, and Acne Conglobata—The lesions in comedonal acne are predominantly open and closed comedones. Some inflammatory lesions are usually present, but are not impressive in size or number. The severity of comedonal acne can be roughly assessed on a 4-point scale in which the comedones on one side of the face are counted, *ie*, Grade I: less than 10; Grade II: 10-25; Grade III: 25-50; Grade IV: over 50.

In papulopustular acne, there are myriads of papules and pustules with an admixture of comedones. The inflammatory lesions are dominant. Acne conglobata is the most violent expression of this disease, extending to other areas of the body such as the lower back, buttocks, lower arms, and intertriginous regions. The lesions are larger and include nodules, draining sinuses, and cysts.

Gram-negative Folliculitis—This is a new disease created by long-term antibiotic treatment of acne.[1] The diagnosis is made by collating history with observation. Initially, antibiotics provide adequate control. Later on, the drug not only becomes ineffective, but actually makes the condition worse. Two types of gram-negative folliculitis, Type I and Type II, are recognized. In Type I, which is more common, crowds of pustules fan out onto the face from the anterior nares. The organisms are usually species of *Enterobacter* and *Klebsiella*. Fluctuant, deep-seated, scattered nodules are characteristic of Type II. *Proteus* is responsible for this variety.

ACNE VENENATA (CONTACT ACNE)

Long-term inappropriate use of topical agents, or exposure to comedogenic chemicals, especially in acne-prone individuals, can lead to this type of acne. Patients are usually beyond the typical acne age.

Acne Cosmetica—This is a very common condition among adult and middle-aged women who, as a rule, are more aware of the cause than many physicians.[26] The disease is comparatively mild, consisting of a sprinkling of papulopustules and comedones. Nonetheless, cosmetic acne causes much distress because of its exceptional persistence—commonly over 20-30 years. These acne sufferers feel frustrated and angry that physicians often fail to make a correct diagnosis, or else advise waiting until the acne disappears, in accordance with the erroneous universal belief that the disease will ultimately involute spontaneously (see Chapter 12).

Many of these women experienced acne earlier, and therefore initially believe that they have had a relapse in their mid-twenties or early thirties. While this can occur spontaneously with the changing stresses of early adulthood, cosmetics and toiletries are chiefly responsible for sustaining a smouldering, low-grade acne which sometimes disappears for months, only to

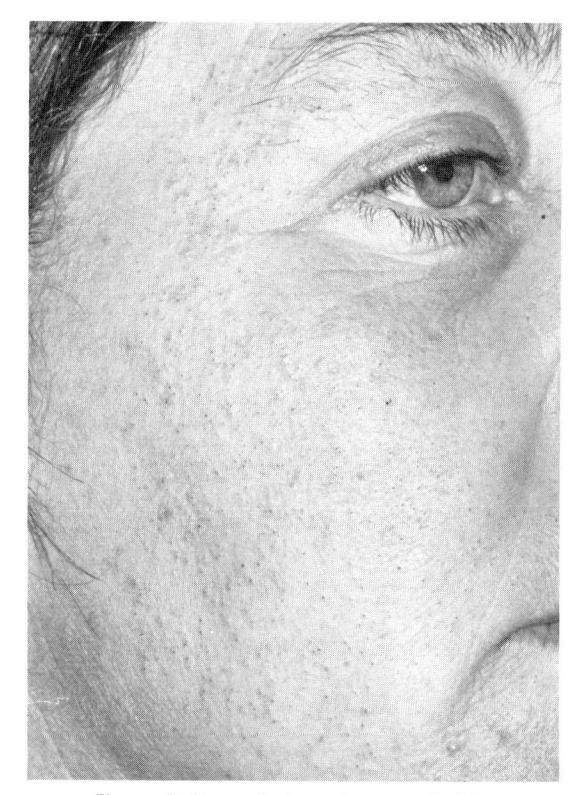

Figure 3. Cosmetic Acne. Low-grade follicular papulopustules in a middle-aged woman, invariably due to cosmetics.

flare up again later. Usually these women switch from one cosmetic to another and, on request, can bring in a suitcase full of moisturizers, cleansers, night-creams, and exotic formulations designed for a problem skin.

Cosmetic creams are complex mixtures, and certain ingredients may be acnegenic, especially esters of fatty acids. Greases and oils are not necessarily acnegenic. Lanolin, for example, is generally not comedogenic, but certain of its derivatives are. Red veterinary petrolatum is acnegenic, but ordinary petrolatum generally is not. Each material must be tested individually by the rabbit ear technique, keeping in mind that its composition may vary with the source. Moreover, a given cosmetic may be acnegenic at one time but not at another, as a result of reformulation or use of raw ingredients from a different supplier. Lists of nonacnegenic cosmetics are therefore not dependable, unless one can ascertain that no changes have been made in composition.

Cosmetics are used every day, year in and year out, and this is why they become troublesome. Even mild materials used indefinitely by susceptible persons can provoke the marginal but exasperating disease, cosmetic acne.

The cost of a cosmetic or the purity of its ingredients have nothing to do with whether it will be comedogenic or not. Indeed, some of the most expensive "moisturizers" have the greatest adverse activity.

It is important to realize that acne cosmetica is identical with acne vulgaris, the lesions being indistinguishable. The two may even be admixed in teenagers. In adults, persistent, low-grade acne is presumed to be cosmetic acne until proved otherwise.

One should inquire about everything that is repeatedly applied to the face. Even soaps may be acnegenic, especially "medicated" varieties. Moreover, a surprising number of sunscreens are comedogenic. Interestingly, it is the vehicle, not the ultraviolet absorbing compound, which is responsible for producing cosmetic acne.

Women with cosmetic acne cannot be expected to forego cosmetics altogether. Their use, however, might well be restricted to "occasions." Foundation lotions are safer than creams. Retinoic acid is quite effective and, used daily, will enable many women to continue using their favorite cosmetic. The condition must first be brought into remission, a process that takes months and should be so described to avoid disappointment.

Pomade Acne—Pomade acne is almost exclusively a problem of Black adults, especially men, who apply various greases and oils to the scalp as hair grooming aids. Some rub the pomade over the face as well. The incidence of the disease is very high. The lesions consist mainly of closely set, small, uniform, closed comedones, chiefly concentrated on the forehead and temples.[1]

Pomade acne is easily recognized in Blacks well past the acne age. Pomades, like cosmetics, are weak acnegens. They become significant only after prolonged daily use.

Occupational Acne Due to Chlorinated Hydrocarbons—Many diverse industrial chemicals are acnegens. These usually evoke lesions by contact, but ingestion or inhalation of the chemicals can produce widespread, devastating acne.

"Chloracne" is a term suitable only for those eruptions which are due to chlorinated hydrocarbons, such as chloronaphthalenes. Some occupational acnegens are highly toxic materials; they can produce serious systemic disease and even death when the mode of entry is not the skin. Extensive acne deserves thorough testing, with emphasis placed on liver function tests.

The archetypal lesion in occupational acne is either the open or closed comedo, which is often present in staggering numbers. These may reach enormous sizes, and are sometimes called "cysts." In acne-prone, light-skinned individuals, the lesions can become inflammatory and accompanied by numerous papules, pustules, and even nodules.

The patients are typically men. Epidemiologic inquiry is revealing: other workers may have the disorder, or the risk may be well-known to the manager. The disease may extend well beyond the usual territory of acne;

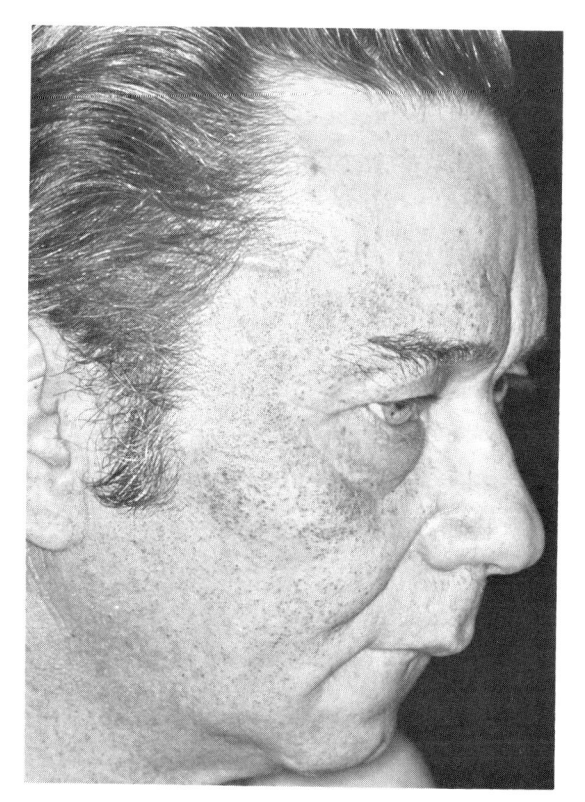

Figure 4. Occupational Acne. This worker was in daily contact with cutting oils. Telltale feature here is myriads of comedones.

indeed, any area bearing follicles can become involved. Even when the patient is removed from the damaging source, occupational acne may persist for years in a very active and disturbing form until the causative chemicals have been cleared from the body.

The drug of choice for clearing the comedones is retinoic acid. This must be used vigorously 2-3 times a day for many months.

Occupational Acne Due to Oils and Tars—Oils and tars are among the most common causes of occupational acne. Areas in contact with these agents show conspicuous comedones. Contaminated clothing produces highly inflammatory eruptions at pressure points such as the shoulders, thighs, buttocks, and lower arms. Tars and pitches lead to extensive eruptions in road workers, roofers, *etc*. Phototoxic reactions can complicate the picture.

ACNE DUE TO PHYSICAL AGENTS

Senile (Solar) Comedones (Favre-Racouchot)—Excessive exposure to sunlight causes open and closed comedones to appear around the eyes and cheeks of aging white individuals. In the elderly, these comedones become large enough to look like cysts situated on a yellowish, thickened, elastotic skin. The lesions are never inflamed.

Acne Due to Ionizing Radiation (Cobalt, X-Rays)—Treatment of skin tumors or internal malignancies with ionizing radiation induces hyperkeratotic follicular reactions.[1]

Mallorca Acne (Acne Aestivalis)—The lesions characteristic of this disease are small, uniform, follicular papules, mainly on the upper arm, shoulders, or upper trunk, which bloom in the summer and regress in winter. Their appearance and evolution are similar to those of corticosteroid acne, but the cause is still mysterious.[27]

Acneform Eruptions due to Drugs

While almost any drug can precipitate an acneform eruption, the most common ones responsible are iodides and bromides; isonicotinic acid hydrazide (isoniazid); corticosteroids; diphenylhydantoin; and phenobarbital.[28-34] (see Chapter 9, 24, and 26).

A mixture of true acne and an acneform eruption is not infrequent. The use of the aforementioned drugs is especially likely to worsen the conditions of acne patients with their highly reactive follicles. A sudden worsening of acne vulgaris should instantly arouse suspicion of a superimposed drug eruption. In their quest for relief, acne patients are willing to try a variety of drugs which are usually of questionable value and sometimes downright harmful. Topical corticosteroids are the most frequent offenders, and are often obtained without the advice or consent of a physician because of their great reputation for suppressing all inflammatory disorders.

Iodides and Bromides—Long-term ingestion of an iodide or bromide hidden in vitamin and mineral preparations, sedatives, asthma and cold remedies, thyroid preparations, analgesics, *etc*, can precipitate an eruption in the typical acne areas (face and upper trunk) as well as in other regions, commonly in an asymmetrical distribution pattern. At first, lesions are often follicular pustules. Later, comedones can emerge as a hyperkeratotic reaction to chronic inflammation.

Isonicotinic Acid Hydrazide (Isoniazid)—A variety of tuberculostatic drugs can lead to the sudden development of acneform eruptions which spread from face to trunk and even beyond. The lesions are reddish-brown papulopustules, sometimes resembling those of corticosteroid acne.

Corticosteroid Acne—Physicians are well-aware that an acneform eruption occurs in patients with chronic, health-destroying diseases who must be maintained on oral or parenteral corticosteroids. On the other hand, it is shocking how often topical corticosteroids are responsible for the eruption. These are frequently obtained without a prescription, owing to the popular belief in the miraculous powers of the corticosteroids to cure blem-

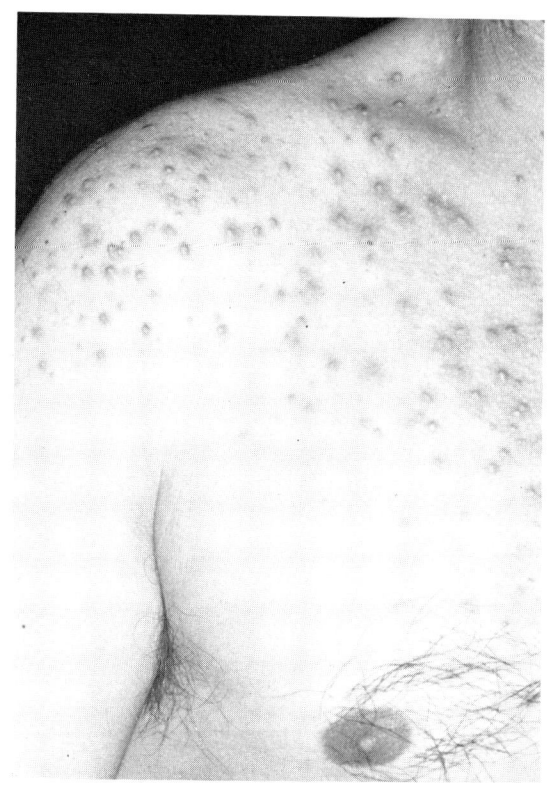

Figure 5. Corticosteroid Acne. Monomorphous eruption of papules appeared on the chest of a patient receiving oral corticosteroids. Lesions are all at the same stage; many will later evolve into comedones.

ishes and rashes of all kinds, including the common changes of advancing age. All too often, corticosteroids are ineptly prescribed by physicians who might have used another drug to treat some banal condition, or who at least might have used a weak corticosteroid-like hydrocortisone, in view of the high responsiveness of dermatoses on the face. Once corticosteroids are introduced for conditions such as rosacea or seborrheic dermatoses, it is very hard to discontinue their use. The original condition rebounds with unusual vigor; patients then get corticosteroid-addicted, for they soon find that the relapse can be suppressed by reapplication of the drug [35-37] (see Chapter 24).

To the experienced physician, corticosteroid acne is recognizable at a glance. The untutored observer rarely even considers that he is dealing with an acneform eruption, and may even prescribe corticosteroids! It is true enough that severe corticosteroid acne hardly looks like acne vulgaris, but even the most casual questioning will elicit the information that the patient has been applying fluorinated corticosteroids for months, and sometimes for years. The characteristic features of corticosteroid acne are: 1) abrupt onset of numerous lesions in a wave-like pattern, all at the same stage of development; 2) the lesions are all alike, consisting at first of dull red, dome-shaped papules which, months later, become closed and then open comedones; 3) most patients are women beyond the acne age; many have had some degree of adolescent acne and are thus acne-prone; and 4) whereas seborrhea is typical of true acne, corticosteroids do not increase sebum secretion, and the face is likely to be dry, rather than oily.

It is essential that laymen and physicians understand that potent corticosteroids should never, *but never,* be used for long periods on the face. As for treatment, corticosteroid acne responds very well to retinoic acid.

REFERENCES

1. Plewig G, Kligman AM: *Acne: Morphogenesis and Treatment.* New York: Springer-Verlag, 1975.
2. Kligman AM, Mills OH, McGinley KJ, et al: Acne therapy with tretinoin in combination with antibiotics. *Acta Derm Venereol [Suppl] (Stockh)* 74:111, 1975.
3. Kligman AM, Plewig G: Classification of acne. *Cutis* 17:520, 1976.
4. Kligman AM: Pathogenesis of acne vulgaris. *Mod Probl Paediatr* 17:153, 1975.
5. Kligman AM, Plewig G: Vitamin A acid in acneiform dermatoses. *Acta Derm Venereol [Suppl] (Stockh)* 74:119, 1975.
6. Leyden JJ, Kligman AM: Acne vulgaris: new concepts in pathogenesis and treatment. *Drugs* 12:292, 1976.
7. Leyden JJ, Kligman AM: The case for topical antibiotics. *Prog Dermatol* 10:13, 1976.
8. Lamberg SI: The course of acne vulgaris in military personnel stationed in Southeast Asia. *Cutis* 7:655, 1971.
9. Lewis CW, Griffin TB, Henning DR, et al: *Tropical Acne: Clinical and Laboratory Investigations,* report 16. Letterman Army Institute of Research, 1973.
10. Novy FG Jr: A severe form of acne developing in the tropics. *Arch Dermatol Syphilol* 60:206, 1949.
11. O'Leary PA, Kierland RR: Pyoderma faciale. *Arch Dermatol Syphilol* 41:451, 1940.
12. Goldschmidt H, Leyden JJ, Stein KH: Acne fulminans: investigation of acute febrile ulcerative acne. *Arch Dermatol* 113:444, 1977.
13. Kelly AP, Burns RE: Acute febrile ulcerative conglobate acne with polyarthralgia. *Arch Dermatol* 104:182, 1971.
14. Ström S, Thyresson N, Boström H: Acute febrile ulcerative conglobate acne with leukemoid reaction. *Acta Derm Venereol (Stockh)* 53:306, 1973.
15. Windom RE, Sanford JP, Ziff M: Acne conglobata and arthritis. *Arthritis Rheum* 4:632, 1961.
16. Freinkel RK, Freinkel N: "Dermatologic Manifestations of Endocrine Disorders," in Fitzgerald TB, et al (Eds): *Dermatology in General Medicine,* pp 1434-1459. New York: McGraw-Hill, 1971.
17. Janovski NA, Paramanandhan TL: "Ovarian Tumors of Sex-differentiated (Sex Cord) Mesenchymal Origin (Potentially Steroid-producing Ovarian Tumors)," in *Ovarian Tumors,* pp 61-65. Philadelphia: WB Saunders, 1973.
18. Meinhof W, Kaiser E, Loch EG: Die androgenetische Acne der Frau. *Hautarzt* 25:34, 1974.
19. Segre EJ: *Androgens, Virilization and the Hirsute Female.* Springfield: Charles C Thomas, 1967.

20. Stein IF, Leventhal ML: Amenorrhea associated with bilateral polycystic ovaries. *Am J Obstet Gynecol* 29:181, 1935.
21. Berlin C: Acne comedo in children due to paraffin oil applied on the head. *Arch Dermatol Syphilol* 69:683, 1954.
22. Forest MG, Cathiard AM, Bertrand JA: Evidence of testicular activity in early infancy. *J Clin Endocrinol Metab* 37:148, 1973.
23. Scheibenreiter S: Acne infantum. *Z Kinderheilkd* 99:195, 1967.
24. Mills OH, Kligman AM: Acne mechanica. *Arch Dermatol* 111:481, 1975.
25. Mills OH Jr, Kligman AM: Acne detergens. *Arch Dermatol* 111:65, 1975.
26. Kligman AM, Mills OH Jr: "Acne cosmetica." *Arch Dermatol* 106:843, 1972.
27. Mills OH, Kligman AM: Acne aestivalis. *Arch Dermatol* 111:891, 1975.
28. Fegeler F: Acneiforme Arzneiexantheme. *Arch Klin Exp Dermatol* 219:335, 1964.
29. Hesse PG: Die antituberkulöse Therapie und das akneiforme Exanthem. *Dermatol Monatsschr* 152:305, 1966.
30. Hitch JM: Acneform eruptions induced by drugs and chemicals. *JAMA* 200:879, 1967.
31. Lantis SH: Acneform eruptions. *J Am Med Wom Assoc* 24:305, 1969.
32. Cohen LK, George W, Smith R: Isoniazid-induced acne and pellagra: occurrence in slow inactivators of isoniazid. *Arch Dermatol* 109:377, 1974.
33. Jenkins RB, Ratner AC: Diphenylhydantoin and acne. *N Engl J Med* 287:148, 1972.
34. Puissant A, Vanbremeersch F, Monfort J, et al: Une nouvelle dermatose iatrogene: l'acne provoquée par la vitamine B_{12}. *Bull Soc Fr Dermatol Syphiligr* 74:813, 1967.
35. Kaidbey KH, Kligman AM: The pathogenesis of topical steroid acne. *J Invest Dermatol* 62:31, 1974.
36. Plewig G, Kligman AM: Induction of acne by topical steroids. *Arch Dermatol Forsch* 247:29, 1973.
37. Schöpf E: Nebebwirkungen externer Corticosteroidtherapie. *Hautarzt* 23:295, 1972.

Chapter 4

Sebum: Lipogenesis
VICTOR R. WHEATLEY, PhD, DSc

The characteristic lesion of acne vulgaris is the comedo, which results from ductal plugging of the pilosebaceous follicle. The cause of this plugging is unknown; however, the early developments in comedo formation were recently clarified. Knutson[1] described the formation of a compact horny layer of lipid-engorged cells in the infundibular region of the gland and, at the same time, the colonization of large masses of bacteria in the follicular lumen.

It has long been thought that acne is the result of an abnormality in sebum or sebaceous gland function,[2] and these latest observations are not inconsistent with this hypothesis. The changes in the horny layer of the infundibulum could thus be the result of an alteration in the composition or physical properties of sebum so that it becomes "comedogenic." The proliferation of bacteria could be the result of a change in sebum composition so that it either provides a richer milieu for bacterial growth or no longer contains an inhibitory factor. This Chapter reviews the possible role of sebum in acnegenesis.

Nature of Sebum

The sebaceous gland is an holocrine organ, the cells of which become its secretion, sebum. During differentiation of the sebaceous cell, a complex mixture of lipids accumulate in the cell until, at maturity, the cell disintegrates to liberate its contents into the sebaceous duct. Ultrastructural studies of the sebaceous gland reveal that the cell, at maturity, still contains recognizable nuclear and cytoplasmic components, the fate of which is uncertain. There is some evidence that the sebaceous secretion is pure lipid;[3] this would imply that extracellular, ductular processing of the liberated cell contents is required to remove all nonlipid components. While certain sebaceous glands probably secrete pure lipids, the material secreted by the large sebaceous glands of the face, which can be expressed by mild presure, is not oily in nature, but has a cheese-like consistency, and certainly contains appreciable amounts of nonlipid substances. Kligman[3,4] has repeatedly referred to the material as an "amalgam of bacteria, sebum, and horny cells," but this is probably an oversimplification; the role of the proteins of this secretion in the etiology of acne should not be overlooked.

Unfortunately, it is not feasible to collect pure, uncontaminated sebum in quantities sufficient for chemical analysis; therefore, the true nature of sebum is not yet resolved. Furthermore, it has become common practice to collect and study the skin surface lipids in an effort to elucidate disease processes. This has several disadvantages. The surface lipids are apparently derived from two sources: the sebaceous glands and the epidermis. The relative contribution from each source cannot, however, be accurately determined. Attempts to determine epidermal lipid secretion rates by direct measurements on palmar and plantar skin indicated negligible secretion,[5] but the stratum corneum on these areas is not comparable with that in other areas of the body. Indirect estimates, made by extrapolating the concentration of a certain surface lipid component to zero secretion rates,[6,7] assumed that sebum composition for a given individual is constant for all sebaceous glands. Recent evidence[8] suggested that different types of sebaceous glands may be secreting sebum with different chemical composition; hence, such estimates of epidermal contribution may not be valid. There is thus no way to determine the composition of the sebum secreted by the glands in a given area of skin from the composition of surface lipids of that area. Furthermore, in acne, the involved glands become blocked and the sebum they produce never reaches the skin surface. Hence, for one reason or another, the composition of the skin surface lipids may not reflect changes in sebum composition that are taking place as the result of a disease process.

Types of Sebaceous Glands

The wide variation in types of sebaceous glands has long been realized,[9] such that the larger glands are one thousand times the size of the smallest ones. The size, shape, and position of the gland in relation to the hair follicle vary considerably; despite these differences, however, the cellular morphology and sequence of differentiation are similar, although not necessarily identical. Not all sebaceous glands are involved in acne. A very large, somewhat specialized type of sebaceous gland, common only in certain areas of skin, has been termed the "sebaceous follicle."[3,10] This gland has a tiny hair follicle and a wide, deep, funnel-shaped orifice. It is only in this type of sebaceous gland that comedogenesis occurs,[11] although the reason for this is not clearly established. The characteristic morphological features of this gland have naturally led to speculation that these features favor acnegenesis.[12] It is also possible that the follicular epithelium of the wide canal differs from that of other types of sebaceous glands in its response to a component of sebum or to a product of bacterial origin. Another recent observation is worth noting here. Tosti[13] observed that the size of the terminal sebaceous cells in the sebaceous follicle is more than double the size of those of normal sebaceous glands. The sebaceous cell is a differentiating cell, and the larger cell size would imply a longer process of differentiation. Current work in this author's laboratory has shown that, for at least one type of animal sebaceous gland, the lipids accumulating in the sebaceous cell change in composition as the cell differentiates. Hence, the composition of the lipids secreted by the sebaceous follicle could be very different from that of other types of sebaceous glands. Unfortunately, we still have no reliable biochemical data regarding individual sebaceous glands.

Possible Changes in Acne

SEBUM SECRETION RATES

It has been repeatedly shown[14-16] that sebaceous gland activity on the forehead of the acne patient is significantly increased, and that the rate of secretion bears a direct relationship to the severity of acne.[16] On other areas, the sebaceous activity may be lower than normal,[17] presumably because of failure of the sebum to gain passage to the surface due to the blocked ducts of the involved follicles. The cause of the seborrhea is unknown, and, while it is a consistent finding in acne, seborrhea of the same magnitude is frequently found in acne-free individuals.[3,17] Since the sebaceous follicle is both the major producer of sebum[3] and the involved follicle[11] in acne, it is probable that the seborrhea is related to an increased number of sebaceous follicles in these individuals. Unfortunately, no quantitative observations concerning this have yet been made.

LIPOLYSIS OF SEBUM

The surface lipids of man contain appreciable amounts of free fatty acids, formed by the action of bacterial lipases on the triglycerides of sebum.[18,19] Since these free fatty acids are very irritating when injected intracutaneously,[20] they were thought to be implicated in acnegenesis, and a major hypothesis of comedogenesis has evolved concerning their role.[21] This role has been further emphasized by the fact that tetracycline, one of the few drugs effective in acne, reduces both the free fatty acids of the surface lipids and the bacterial flora of the skin, and also inhibits lipase.[22] Fulton et al[23] made an extensive study of bacterial lipases and recently developed drugs which act specifically by inhibiting these lipases. Such drugs, when administered to acne patients, reduce the free fatty acid level in the surface lipids, but fail to affect the clinical severity of acne. Thus, the role of the free fatty acids in comedogenesis remains obscure. It appears unlikely that the free fatty acids are responsible for the initiation of comedogenesis.

SURFACE LIPID COMPOSITION

Examination of the surface lipid fatty acids in 1959 showed no significant differences between normal individuals and acne patients.[24] Subsequent work[25] claimed that a minor component was increased, but current work has failed to substantiate this claim.[26] Studies of the overall composition of the skin surface lipids yielded somewhat conflicting results, and the observations were summarized in tabular form by Strauss et al.[27] While no consistent trend was observed by other investigators for waxes, triglycerides, and free fatty acids, claims for an increase in the squalene content were confirmed in three different laboratories.[26] Squalene was shown to be comedogenic,[28] and recent work indicated a high squalene content in the lipids of the larger sebaceous glands.[8] Hence, if comedogenesis is due to a lipid component of sebum, the most likely candidate at this time is squalene.

SEBUM RHEOLOGY

In a review of the pathogenesis of acne, Cunliffe and Shuster[29] considered that seborrhea and a second factor were implicated, and that "increase in sebum viscosity" was this second factor. Others[30] have emphasized the importance of "resistance to outflow of sebum". Burton,[31] however, failed to demonstrate any difference in the viscosity of the surface lipids in acne patients as compared with that in normal individuals. Other factors, such as the presence of abnormal amounts of nonlipid materials, could also increase sebum viscosity, but it is difficult to see how increased viscosity *per se* could initiate comedogenesis. The normal funnel-shaped orifice of the sebaceous follicle[3] would offer little resistance to sebum flow, and would not be affected by moderate changes in sebum viscosity. The duct would have to be partially obstructed before high hydrostatic pressure on the wall, resulting from increased viscosity, could cause abnormal cornification. Recently, however, Cunliffe et al[32] demonstrated that there is obstruction to the outflow of sebum due to keratin hydration at the mouth of the duct after polythene occlusion of the skin. It is thus possible that a combination of environmental factors (or even local hormonal action), and an increase in sebum viscosity, could create the climate in the follicle necessary to induce comedogenesis.

COMEDO LIPIDS

Nicolaides et al,[33] Nazzaro Porro et al,[34] and Wheatley (unpublished observations, November 1969) studied the composition of lipids extracted from expressed contents of comedones. The major difference between these lipids and the surface lipids of the same patient is a marked increase in free fatty acids. This is not an unexpected finding, since comedones contain appreciable amounts of bacterial and other lipases. Thus, the increase in free fatty acids reflects changes in the developing lesion as bacteria proliferate. They are gross changes, however; any small initial change would be obscured. It is unlikely that analysis of comedo lipids will shed light on the factors responsible for the initiation of comedogenesis.

Lipogenesis in the Sebaceous Gland

Many studies were made of the lipid metabolism of whole skin,[35] isolated epidermis,[36] and isolated sebaceous glands;[37] but, while there are certain minor differences as compared with other tissues, the basic mechanisms are the same.[38] Yet skin appears unable, except under extreme conditions,[39] to respond to the homeostatic mechanisms of regulation of lipogenesis observed in other tissues.[40] In order for it to perform its natural functions, it is important that skin be able to bypass such homeostatic mechanisms. No explanation of this phenomenon is forthcoming. Yet, as mentioned above, both the sebaceous gland and the epidermis are differentiating systems, and it is feasible that the gene regulation of this activity is able to override homeostatic regulation. The sebaceous cell differs from other lipogenic cells such as the adipocyte in that the lipids of the former are of a much more complex formation, and the diverse pathways of lipid synthesis appear to be closely linked to the process of cytodifferentiation. Only recently has this aspect of the sebaceous gland attracted the attention of investigators.

Extensive studies[41] established the marked dependence of the sebaceous glands on hormonal action. Androgens cause the glands to become larger and more highly differentiated; there is an increase in mitotic activity and secretion rate. It was recently established[42] that steroid hormones act by regulating protein synthesis in the target tissue. Appropriate receptor proteins transport the hormone to the cell nucleus. There it acts directly on the genome, thereby initiating transcription followed by new protein synthesis, altered cell function, and cytodifferentiation in the given tissue. Since lipogenesis appears to be linked to cytodifferentiation in the sebaceous cell, alterations are anticipated in response to these hormones. Sansone-Bazzano et al[43] presented evidence suggesting that these hormones actually initiate the synthesis of certain classes of lipids in the sebaceous gland. Not only does the sebaceous cell respond to hormonal action, but there is evidence[44] that steroid hormones (eg, dihydrotestosterone) are present in the sebaceous secretion. Furthermore, it was shown that there is active metabolism of steroid hormones in the sebaceous gland so that the gland has the ability to convert testosterone to dihydrotestosterone[45] (the active androgenic hormone). In addition to steroid hormones, other hormones, such as the bovine growth hormone[46] and the melanocyte-stimulating hormone,[47] appear to be able to stimulate the sebaceous gland. Such peptide hormones also have a direct action on the genome.

While extensive studies have been made of cutaneous lipogenesis, relatively few studies have been directed to the problem of acne. Sansone and Reisner[48] demonstrated an increase in the *in vitro* conversion of testosterone to dihydrotestosterone in the skin in acne. More recently, Cooper et al[49] initiated a detailed study of sebaceous lipogenesis in acne. It is hoped that extensive new data will be forthcoming from studies such as these.

Summary

The primary lesion in acne involves abnormal epithelial development of the pilosebaceous follicle,[1] rather than the gland itself. To date, extensive studies have been unsuccessful in pin-pointing a change in the sebaceous secretion as the cause of this lesion; yet there is very convincing evidence that the glands are involved in the acne process.[27] Hence, there is still need for more research on the sebaceous glands before the etiology of acne can be fully resolved.

REFERENCES

1. Knutson DD: Ultrastructural observations in acne vulgaris: the normal sebaceous follicle and acne lesions. *J Invest Dermatol* 62:288, 1974.
2. Strauss JS, Pochi PE, Downing DT: Skin lipids and acne. *Annu Rev Med* 26:27, 1975.
3. Kligman AM, Shelley WB: An investigation of the biology of the human sebaceous gland. *J Invest Dermatol* 30:99, 1958.
4. Kligman AM: An overview of acne. *J Invest Dermatol* 62:268, 1974.
5. Hodgson-Jones IS: The origin of sebum. *Trans St John Hosp Dermatol Soc* 36:26, 1956.
6. Boughton B, MacKenna RMB, Wheatley VR, et al: Studies of sebum. 8. Observations on the squalene and cholesterol content and possible functions of squalene in human sebum. *Biochem J* 66:32, 1957.
7. Greene RS, Downing DT, Pochi PE, et al: Anatomical variation in the amount and composition of human skin surface lipid. *J Invest Dermatol* 54:240, 1970.
8. Summerly R, Yardley HJ, Raymond M, et al: The lipid composition of sebaceous glands as a reflection of gland size. *Br J Dermatol* 94:45, 1976.
9. Sappey PC, cited by Bulkley LD: *Acne: Its Etiology, Pathology and Treatment*, p 3. New York: GP Putnam, 1885.
10. Horner WE: On the odoriferous glands of the Negro. *Am J Med Sci* 21:13, 1846.
11. Strauss JS, Kligman AM: Pathologic dynamics of acne vulgaris. *Arch Dermatol* 82:779, 1960.
12. Kligman AM, Plewig G: *Acne: Morphology and Treatment*, p 3. New York: Springer-Verlag, 1975.
13. Tosti A: A comparison of the histodynamics of sebaceous glands and epidermis in

man: a microanatomic and morphometric study. *J Invest Dermatol* 62:147, 1974.
14. Pachur R: Die Talgabsonderung auf der menschlichen Hautoberfläche. *Arch Dermatol Syphilol* 162:253, 1930.
15. Pochi PE, Strauss JS: Sebum production, casual sebum level, titratable acidity of sebum, and urinary fractional 17-ketosteroid excretion in males with acne. *J Invest Dermatol* 43:383, 1964.
16. Cunliffe WJ, Shuster S: The rate of sebum secretion in man. *Br J Dermatol* 81:697, 1969.
17. Hodgson-Jones IS, MacKenna RMB, Wheatley VR: The study of human sebaceous activity. *Acta Derm Venereol (Stockh)* 32 (suppl 29):155, 1952.
18. Scheimann LG, Knox G, Sher D, et al: The role of bacteria in the formation of free fatty acids on the human skin surface. *J Invest Dermatol* 34:171, 1960.
19. Shalita A: Genesis of free fatty acids. *J Invest Dermatol* 62:332, 1974.
20. Strauss JS, Pochi PE: Intracutaneous injection of sebum and comedones: histological observations. *Arch Dermatol* 92:443, 1965.
21. Freinkel RK: Acne vulgaris: follicles, fats and flora. *Cutis* 7:409, 1971.
22. Shalita A, Wheatley VR: Inhibition of pancreatic lipase by tetracycline. *J Invest Dermatol* 54:413, 1970.
23. Fulton JE Jr, Weeks JG, McCarty L: The inability of a bacterial lipase inhibitor to control acne vulgaris. *J Invest Dermatol* 64:281, 1975.
24. Boughton B, MacKenna RMB, Wheatley VR, et al: The fatty acid composition of the surface skin fats ('sebum') in acne vulgaris and seborrhoeic dermititis. *J Invest Dermatol* 33:57, 1959.
25. Kellum RE, Strangfeld K: Acne vulgaris: studies in pathogenesis: fatty acids of human surface triglycerides from patients with and without acne. *J Invest Dermatol* 58:315, 1972.
26. Morello AM, Downing DT, Strauss JS: Octadecadienoic acid in human skin surface lipid. *J Invest Dermatol* 64:207, 1975.
27. Strauss JS, Pochi PE, Downing DT: Acne: perspectives. *J Invest Dermatol* 62:321, 1974.
28. Kligman AM, Wheatley VR, Mills OH: Comedogenicity of human sebum. *Arch Dermatol* 102:267, 1970.
29. Cunliffe WJ, Shuster S: Pathogenesis of acne. *Lancet* 1:685, 1969.
30. Holmes RL, Williams M, Cunliffe, WJ: Pilo-sebaceous duct obstruction and acne. *Br J Dermatol* 87:327, 1972.
31. Burton JL: The physical properties of sebum in acne vulgaris. *Clin Sci* 39:757, 1970.
32. Cunliffe WJ, Perera WD, Tan SG, et al: Pilo-sebaceous duct physiology. 2. The effect of keratin hydration on sebum excretion rate. *Br J Dermatol* 94:431, 1976.
33. Nicolaides N, Ansari MN, Fu HC, et al: Lipid composition of comedones as compared with that of human skin surface in acne patients. *J Invest Dermatol* 54:487, 1970.
34. Nazzaro Porro M, Passi S, Caprilli F, et al: Gli acidi grassi dei lipidi del comedone e della superficie cutanea in pazienti di acne. *Boll Ist Dermatol Soc Gallicano* 8:191, 1973.
35. Hsia SL, Sofer G, Lane, B: Lipid metabolism in human skin. I. Lipogenesis from acetate-1-^{14}C. *J Invest Dermatol* 47:437, 1966.
36. Wilkinson DI: Incorporation of acetate-1-C^{14} into fatty acids of isolated epidermal cells. *J Invest Dermatol* 54:132, 1970.
37. Summerly R, Woodbury S: The *in vitro* incorporation of ^{14}C-acetate into the isolated sebaceous glands and appendage-freed epidermis of human skin: a technique for the study of lipid synthesis in the isolated sebaceous gland. *Br J Dermatol* 85:424, 1971.
38. Wheatley VR: Cutaneous lipogenesis: major pathways of carbon flow and possible

interrelationships between the epidermis and sebaceous glands. *J Invest Dermatol* 62:245, 1974.
39. Pochi PE, Downing DT, Strauss JS: Sebaceous gland response in man to prolonged total caloric deprivation. *J Invest Dermatol* 55:303, 1970.
40. Masoro EJ: Biochemical mechanisms related to the homeostatic regulation of lipogenesis in animals. *J Lipid Res* 3:149, 1962.
41. Ebling FJ: The effect of steroid hormones on the skin of experimental animals. *Symp Dtsch Gesamte Endokrinol* 17:19, 1971.
42. Chan L, O'Malley BW: Mechanism of action of sex steroid hormones. *N Engl J Med* 24:1322, 1976.
43. Sansone-Bazzano G, Bazzano G, Reisner RM, et al: The hormonal induction of alkyl glycerol, wax and alkyl acetate synthesis in the preputial gland of the mouse. *Biochim Biophys Acta* 260:35, 1972.
44. Karunakaran ME, Pochi PE, Strauss JS, et al: Androgens in skin surface lipids. *J Invest Dermatol* 60:121, 1973.
45. Gomez EC, Hsia SL: *In vitro* metabolism of testosterone-4-^{14}C and delta^{4}-androstene-3,17-dione-4-^{14}C in human skin. *Biochemistry* 7:24, 1968.
46. Ebling FJ, Ebling E, Randall V, et al: The sebotrophic action of growth hormone (BGH) in the rat. *Br J Dermatol* 92:325, 1975.
47. Thody AJ, Shuster S: Possible role of MSH in the mammal. *Nature* 245:207, 1973.
48. Sansone G, Reisner RM: Differential rates of conversion of testosterone to dihydrotestosterone in acne and in normal skin—a possible pathogenic factor in acne. *J Invest Dermatol* 56:366, 1971.
49. Cooper MF, McGrath H, Shuster S: Sebaceous lipogenesis in human skin; variability with age and with severity of acne. *Br J Dermatol* 94:165, 1976.

Chapter 5

Bacteriology
JACK G. VOSS, PhD

There is a broad spectrum of views concerning the etiology of acne vulgaris, ranging from sole consideration of the hormonal and other metabolic changes occurring in the patient to consideration of the microflora of the lesion as the all-important precipitating factor. Logically, the choice of therapy for the disease will be strongly influenced by the view taken as to its etiology. Thus, for example, the association of acne with increased production of sebum at puberty has led to many attempts to treat the disease by reducing the rate of sebum production. Other therapeutic efforts (*eg*, the use of retinoic acid) have been directed more toward the cosmetic benefits to be had by eliminating the highly visible comedones, without explicitly basing the treatment on assumptions regarding the etiology of the disease.

This Chapter emphasizes the probable significance of the microflora of the follicle as a causative factor in the development of the acne lesion. It is suggested here that this view is directly supported by the clearly beneficial effect achieved in acne patients through the use of both a number of antibiotics and the topical antibacterial, benzoyl peroxide, in treatment of the disease.

Since the demonstration by Unna in 1893 of the presence of gram-positive, diphtheroid organisms in acne lesions and the cultivation by Sabouraud in 1897 of such organisms,[1] the organism now known as *Propionibacterium acnes* has been regarded as a possible or probable causative agent of acne vulgaris. By 1903, it was stated[2] that this organism had been proved to be the cause of acne; staphylococci commonly found in the lesions were regarded as either contaminants or secondary invaders. Fleming,[3] in 1909, claimed successful treatment of acne with vaccines containing the acne bacillus and staphylococci. Subsequently, the growing realization that *P. acnes* occurs in large numbers on the normal skin[4] cast doubt on its significance in the etiology of acne.

More recently, Strauss and Kligman[5] proposed that free fatty acids liberated within the sebaceous follicle, probably by *P. acnes* lipase, are important in producing inflammatory reactions. It was shown[5,6] that the injection of living cells of the organism into keratinous cysts or sterile steatocystomas is followed by severe inflammation. Most of the recent studies on the pathogenesis of acne have been devoted to the hypothesis that free fatty acids play a central role in this disease, and it was demonstrated[7] that lipolysis by *P. acnes* is indeed the major source of free fatty acids on the face and scalp. However, it must be remembered that, although the anaerobic diphtheroids are most numerous in acne lesions, staphylococci and yeasts are almost uniformly present as well.[8]

The predominant role of free fatty acids, the products of bacterial lipolysis in the follicle, as a key factor in the pathogenesis of acne was recently questioned,[9,10] and a more general hypothesis of a microbial etiology of acne was mentioned.[9] Such a hypothesis is here discussed in greater detail, from a microbiologist's viewpoint and with the advantages and disadvantages of the parochial approach.

Sebum as Substrate for Microbial Growth

Strauss and Pochi[11] said that "acne is a disease for which there is a specific fuel; namely, sebum." This statement is undoubtedly correct, but perhaps in a manner somewhat different from the authors' intent. Sebum might better be regarded not solely as a mixture of lipids synthesized by the sebaceous gland, but as a conglomerate of lipids, proteins and their breakdown products, nucleic acids and nucleotides, and other materials resulting from the differentiation and degeneration of the sebaceous cells. Thus, native sebum could provide an excellent substrate for those microorganisms able to use the nonlipid components for growth. Inevitably, the result of the growth of masses of organisms within the follicle, using sebum as the primary substrate, would be that the materials reaching the skin surface would be: 1) products of bacterial metabolism; 2) those compounds resistant to microbial breakdown; and 3) the bacterial cells themselves. Free fatty acids are the most obvious by-products of bacterial metabolism, resulting from lipolysis of the triglyceride fraction of the sebaceous lipids. These free fatty acids, as well as hydrocarbons and wax esters, are evidently resistant to the action of the microorganisms, and therefore persist to reach the skin surface. Thus, it may be expected that those compounds important to bacterial growth and activity are consumed, and are not found on the skin surface, whereas the lipids, which have been studied so intensively, are those compounds which have little or no importance with respect to growth of the microflora. It might be said that the studies on sebum have been governed more by the abilities of the analytical chemist than by consideration of the probable properties of native sebum and its importance in providing a selective milieu for the growth of the few species of microorganisms which are found in the selective environment of the follicle.

It has been amply documented[12-14] that severity of acne is directly related to sebum excretion rate, as measured by lipid levels on the skin surface. Plewig and Christophers[15] showed that the proliferative activity of different sebaceous glands in the same area may vary considerably, with the average rate of renewal of lobules of normal size being about 20-25 days. Differences in size, number, and renewal rates of functioning glands must account for the differences seen in rates of excretion of sebaceous lipids; these differences between functioning glands must also be important in determining the size and nature of the bacterial flora.

Because of the relation between sebum excretion rate and severity of acne, much effort has been devoted to decreasing the production of sebum through the use of x-ray therapy, hormones, and other measures. It is likely that the general reason for the success which has attended these efforts, to the extent that they have been successful, has been the limitation of production of a selective substrate for the growth of microorganisms in the follicle and the consequent restriction of their potentially deleterious activity, rather than because of the limitation of sebum production *per se.*

Microbial Population of the Follicle and the Acne Lesion

In 1946, Douglas and Gunter[16] proposed the reclassification of *Corynebacterium acnes* as *Propionibacterium acnes,* largely on the basis of the organism's production of propionic acid. This view has been upheld by more recent work,[17,18] and has been adopted in the latest edition of *Bergey's Manual of Determinative Bacteriology.*[19]

Recent work[20] demonstrated the presence on the skin of not one but two species of anaerobic coryneform bacteria. These were described as *C. acnes* group I and II, but have more recently been designated *P. acnes* and *Propionibacterium granulosum,* respectively,[21] in accordance with recent opinion.[17-19] Biotypes and serotypes within these species were also described,[22] and may lead to further useful characterization of these organisms. In addition, various phage types of *P. acnes* were shown to exist;[23] no phages active against *P. granulosum* have yet been reported. Marples et al[8] observed the frequent presence of *P. acnes* phage on the skin surface and in acne lesions; it is thus deduced that phage must play a significant role in the ecology of the follicle.

Almost 30 years ago, Evans et al[4] suggested that the sebaceous glands (including follicles) were the primary habitat of skin bacteria, and found that the anaerobic diphtheroids were the most abundant part of the flora. Since then, a number of investigators have studied these organisms as a part of the normal skin flora and in relation to acne. Somerville[24,25] showed the anaerobic diphtheroids to be resident on most skin sites of most individuals, with great variation in numbers between sites and between individuals. They occur on the skin in microcolonies, which are generally composed of several hundred to several thousand cells each.

In 80 patients, examination of the contents of the large sebaceous follicles of the nose showed these follicles to generally consist of essentially pure cultures of *P. acnes* and/or *P. granulosum*.[21] Gram's stains of squeezings from the follicles showed enormous numbers of gram-positive diphtheroids, without the obvious presence of other organisms. Plate counts on the follicular contents showed about $20\text{-}100 \times 10^6$ anaerobic diphtheroids per mg of wet weight. Thus, in the lumen of the follicle these organisms attain a density comparable to that which they achieve through cultivation on favorable media in the laboratory.

The microbiology of acne lesions has been studied intensively in recent years by Marples et al. It was early emphasized[26] that both *P. acnes* (this must be understood to include *P. granulosum* in many of the reported studies) and coagulase-negative staphylococci are regularly found in large numbers in acne lesions; both types of organisms were thought to contribute to the pathogenesis of acne. More recently,[27] anaerobic diphtheroids were found to be of greater prevalence than cocci in acne pustules, with a much lower prevalence of aerobic diphtheroids and gram-negative species. Comedones contain larger numbers of anaerobic diphtheroids than they do cocci, with the largest numbers of both types occurring in closed comedones.[28] Yeast-like organisms *(Pityrosporon)* also occur regularly in open comedones;[8,28,29] larger numbers of yeasts and aerobic bacteria are found in open comedones than in closed comedones. The microflora of comedones thus consists regularly of *P. acnes* and/or *P. granulosum,* cocci (primarily Baird-Parker subgroup SII, or *Staphylococcus epidermidis* biotype 1),[19,28] *Pityrosporon* and *P. acnes* phage.[8,29] *Pityrosporon* has not been reported to occur so frequently in inflamed lesions. Of these organisms, the anaerobic diphtheroids are quantitatively the most significant.

The regular involvement of anaerobic diphtheroids and staphylococci in open and closed comedones strongly suggests a causal role for one or both. Unfortunately, the nature and size of the flora of inflammatory lesions has not been so thoroughly investigated. However, both groups of organisms are known to be present frequently in pustules, although such lesions sometimes appear to be sterile because of the self-sterilizing action of the inflammatory process. It is tempting to associate pus formation with the response to the staphylococci.

On the assumption that the anaerobic diphtheroids are most likely to be causally involved in acne lesions, it must be asked whether P. acnes or P. granulosum is more likely to be significant. Whiteside and Voss[21] observed that the ratio of prevalence of P. acnes to that of P. granulosum was greater in pustules and comedones than on normal skin and in normal sebaceous follicles of the nose. They concluded that P. acnes was therefore more likely to be associated with the development of acne lesions. On the other hand, Marples et al[29] counted the numbers of each of these two species in small open and closed comedones considered to be of recent origin and therefore more likely to reflect the flora involved in pathogenesis, and found that prevalence and density of P. granulosum were greater in the more severe lesions. Further study of the relation of these species to the development of acne lesions is needed.

As has been mentioned in an earlier review,[9] methods for study of individual follicles and their flora are urgently needed. Kligman[10] aptly emphasized that only an indeterminate proportion of the follicles harbors large populations of P. acnes. Recent developments suggest an approach to this problem which might make it possible to determine what proportion of follicles—and which ones—harbor large populations of anaerobic diphtheroids. The orifices of some follicles on the face show an orange-red fluorescence under ultraviolet light[30] which was attributed[31] to porphyrins produced by bacteria. P. acnes was shown[32] to produce coproporphyrin and protoporphyrin which are responsible for the orange-red fluorescence of comedones. It was recently observed[33] that tetracyclines and clindamycin reduce the fluorescence of follicles in acne patients and in control individuals. An orange-red fluorescence has been observed at the orifices of some follicles on the face, and a bluish-white fluorescence at other follicular orifices (JG Voss, unpublished observations, 1972). It is possible that those follicles showing a reddish fluorescence are heavily infested with P. acnes and/or P. granulosum, whereas the other follicles do not harbor large populations of these organisms. Under ultraviolet light, it may be possible to determine the proportion of follicles which is at risk of developing pathologic changes. Shifts in the proportion of follicles with large anaerobic populations could be traced during antibiotic therapy. Because surface collections of skin bacteria may be misleading in regard to the interpretation of changes occurring within the follicle,[9] it should be more instructive to follow changes in the proportion of infested follicles than changes in the numbers of organisms collected from an area of skin containing hundreds of follicles. It seems likely that a 50% reduction in the number of infested follicles would be more beneficial to the patient than would a 50% reduction in the population of the average follicle.

Possibly Harmful Products of Microorganisms

The idea that microorganisms, and particularly the anaerobic diphtheroids, play a role in initiating and maintaining the acne process is not a new one. Kligman[10] stated: "I rather think that *C. acnes* somehow induces the transformation into coherent horn formation, after which anaerobiosis is guaranteed and the multiplication of *C. acnes* becomes very brisk." He also believed that the rupture of comedones and formation of inflammatory lesions is largely due to *P. acnes*.

A variety of mechanisms whereby the pathogenesis of acne might take its course can be invoked. The role of free fatty acids has previously been discussed at some length.[9] It is well-recognized that free fatty acids, especially those of intermediate chain length, may show comedogenic and irritant activity in varying degrees. However, it has not yet been established that the free fatty acids are produced in the follicle in concentrations sufficient to display these activities to a significant extent. Indeed, Puhvel[34] adduced evidence that free fatty acid concentrations in the follicle do not reach inflammatory levels.

Marples et al[7] showed clearly that *P. acnes* is more important than is the aerobic flora in releasing the free fatty acids found in the surface lipids of the scalp and forehead. It is probable that *P. granulosum* is more active than *P. acnes* in lipolysis of the triglyceride in sebaceous lipid.[21] However, it should be remembered that levels of the free fatty acids found in lipids collected from the skin surface are not necessarily the same as those found in the individual follicles; comedones and the contents of the large sebaceous follicles of the nose show a more complete hydrolysis of the triglycerides than is usually to be found in surface lipids.[35-37]

It was suggested[7] that the action of tetracycline in reducing free fatty acid levels in surface lipids is due to inhibition of *P. acnes* lipase by the antibiotic, and it was shown[38] that the characteristics of the lipase found in comedones more nearly resemble the properties of *P. acnes* lipase than those of a staphylococcal lipase. However, it was also shown[39-41] that the concentration of tetracycline required for inhibition of *P. acnes* or *P. granulosum* lipase *in vitro* is at least several times that to be expected in the acne lesion.[42] Therefore, it seems probable that any improvement of acne through lowering of free fatty acid release by tetracycline would be attributable more to inhibition of bacterial growth or of enzyme synthesis than to inhibition of the activity of preformed lipase.[9]

It is possible to postulate other pathogenetic mechanisms of the microflora of the skin, and particularly of the masses of diphtheroids growing in at least a proportion of the follicles. Certainly, immunologic mechanisms might be expected to play a role in development of inflammatory reactions following release of bacterial antigens into the dermis. Imamura et al,[43] using immunofluorescent techniques, showed the presence of *P. acnes* antigen in follicles and comedones, and particularly in inflammatory lesions of acne, as well as in dermal infiltrates and macrophages. Puhvel et al[44] demonstrated a relation between severity of acne and levels of antibody production or of immediate dermal hypersensitivity to *P. acnes*. There are scattered reports which have suggested hypersensitivity to *P. acnes*[45] or a deficiency of circulating antibodies[46-48] as significant factors in the disease. It might be suggested that the antibody response found in most individuals to *P. acnes* and *P. granulosum* could affect the course of the disease by controlling the growth of the organisms in the follicle or, perhaps more likely, by inhibiting the activity of bacterial products which are important in pathogenesis. Preliminary experiments (JG Voss, unpublished observations, 1972) using immunofluorescent techniques have suggested the presence of antibody on the cell walls of *P. acnes* or *P. granulosum* in the follicle.

Important bacterial products, other than lipase and antigens, might include protease,[20,49] neuraminidase,[50] hyaluronidase[51,52] and lecithinase[53] among the enzymes produced by the anaerobic diphtheroids. The inflammation produced by intradermal injection of defatted comedones[54] may reflect, at least in part, a prior production of toxins or irritants by the microbial flora. This author has seen evidence of irritant activity of purified cell walls of *P. acnes* (JG Voss, unpublished observations, 1966). It is significant that Hägele et al[55] showed that patch tests with culture filtrates of *P. acnes* grown in defatted media as well as in the presence of added triglycerides produce inflammatory reactions on human skin. These investigators therefore cast doubt on the exclusive significance of free fatty acids as irritating products of bacterial metabolism, and concluded that *P. acnes* produces toxins, allergens, and/or irritants by metabolism of compounds other than triglycerides.

A recent observation of interest is that of Azuma et al,[56] who showed that cell walls of *P. acnes* and *P. granulosum* (as well as those of some other species) stimulate mitosis of mouse spleen cells and thymocytes. The investigators suggested that the cell walls serve as mitogens for both thymus-derived and bone marrow-derived lymphocytes. It is interesting to speculate that a similar mitogenic activity in the follicle might stimulate the overproduction of horny cells by the keratinizing epithelium, leading to comedo formation.

Thus, it seems quite likely that *P. acnes* and *P. granulosum* (and possibly staphylococci and yeasts as well) may contribute to the pathogenesis of acne lesions through mechanisms other than, or in addition to, the release of free fatty acids. If bacterial activity is indeed important in the pathogenesis of acne, a clear understanding of the biochemical process involved is not necessary for treatment of the disease, as long as the pertinent members of the flora can be controlled.

It is worthy of note that Maibach[57] considered *P. acnes* to be the cause of pustules on the scalp because the organism occurred in large numbers in the lesions, and because the condition was successfully treated with tetracycline. Similarly, the gram-negative folliculitis occasionally seen in acne patients treated with antibiotics has been clearly considered to be a disease resulting from infection of the follicles with gram-negative species.[58,59] If we can accept the probability that the bacteria are causally associated with the disease processes in these circumstances, we should also be able to accept the probability that large numbers of bacteria in the follicle are significant in the pathogenesis of acne, and to then recognize that these bacteria may be important in ways other than solely as producers of lipase.

Antibacterial Agents and Acne

That oral tetracycline, lincomycin, and erythromycin reach the skin surface in concentrations sufficient to affect the bacterial flora, and especially to cause reductions in the numbers of *P. acnes,* is well-recognized.[60-62] The presence of tetracycline has been demonstrated in comedones and other lesions,[63] and in the skin surface film.[64] Oral tetracycline is widely used and is well-known to be beneficial in the treatment of acne,[65] and effective in reducing the bacterial flora[60,62] and free fatty acids[7] on the surface of the skin. Topical tetracycline also reduces free fatty acids.[66] Although the reduction in free fatty acids has often been regarded as an end in itself, it is surely an important indicator of inhibition of growth and activity of *P. acnes* and *P. granulosum* within the follicle. Occasional observations that oral tetracycline did not significantly affect the flora of the face[67] may be due, as in the case of lipid composition,[35-37] to the fact that surface collections do not accurately reflect events occurring within the depths of those follicles harboring large populations of microorganisms.

The fact that not only tetracyclines but other antibiotics such as lincomycin,[68,69] oleandomycin,[70] and rifampin[71] as well are reported to be effective in treatment of acne strongly suggests that they act through their effect on the microflora and not, as suggested by Beveridge and Powell,[72] through their direct effects on the host. This conclusion is supported by the reported effectiveness of topical therapy with tetracycline,[73] chloramphenicol,[74] erythromycin,[75] and a mixture containing the antibacterials benzoyl peroxide and chlorhydroxyquinoline.[76] It is significant that all or nearly all of 16 freshly isolated strains of *P. acnes* were inhibited by 1.6 µg/ml or less of each of the aforementioned antibiotics.[77]

Resolution of Disease

The fact that acne finally resolves in essentially all cases, despite continued production of sebum and presence of large numbers of bacteria in the follicles, would seem to argue against a bacterial etiology. However, it is conceivable that the immune response which is commonly observed to *P. acnes* and *P. granulosum* may serve eventually to inhibit the function of biologically active bacterial products within the follicle, and thus to limit the development of pathological changes. Alternatively, long-term exposure to irritants may result in accommodation or "hardening" of the follicular epithelium,[78] so that it no longer responds to the damaging effects of the bacterial products in spite of their continued presence.

Summary

The view is here advanced that sebum as originally produced must contain materials, other than lipids, which may serve as a selective substrate for growth of bacteria and yeasts. Growth of large numbers of *P. acnes* and *P. granulosum* in some follicles is considered to place those follicles at risk of undergoing pathologic changes. Deleterious products of bacterial growth thus implicated could be, in addition to lipase and free fatty acids, other enzymes, as well as bacterial antigens and unspecified toxins or irritants. The possibility is suggested that follicles heavily infested with *P. acnes* and *P. granulosum* may be identified by their reddish fluorescence under ultraviolet light, thus permitting identification and study of those which are at risk. Antibiotics may be helpful in reducing the formation of harmful bacterial products during continued growth of the organisms. The eventually self-limiting nature of the disease may be due to the immune response to bacterial products, or to an accommodation of the follicular epithelium to the continued presence of irritant materials within the follicle.

REFERENCES

1. Frank SB: *Acne Vulgaris*, p 60. Springfield: Charles C Thomas, 1971.
2. Gilchrist TC: The etiology of acne vulgaris. *J Cutan Dis* 21:107, 1903.
3. Fleming A: On the etiology of acne vulgaris and its treatment by vaccines. *Lancet* 1:1035, 1909.
4. Evans CA, Smith WM, Johnston EA, et al: Bacterial flora of the normal human skin. *J Invest Dermatol* 15:305, 1950.
5. Strauss JS, Kligman AM: The pathologic dynamics of acne vulgaris. *Arch Dermatol* 82:779, 1960.
6. Kirschbaum JO, Kligman AM: The pathogenic role of *Corynebacterium acnes* in acne vulgaris. *Arch Dermatol* 88:832, 1963.
7. Marples RR, Downing DT, Kligman AM: Control of free fatty acids in human surface lipids by *Corynebacterium acnes*. *J Invest Dermatol* 56:127, 1971.
8. Marples RR, Leyden JJ, Stewart RN, et al: The skin microflora in acne vulgaris. *J Invest Dermatol* 62:37, 1974.
9. Voss JG: Acne vulgaris and free fatty acids: a review and criticism. *Arch Dermatol* 109:894, 1974.
10. Kligman AM: An overview of acne. *J Invest Dermatol* 62:268, 1974.
11. Strauss JS, Pochi PE: The pathogenesis of acne vulgaris. *J Soc Cosmet Chem* 19:644, 1968.
12. Pochi PE, Strauss JS: Sebum production, casual sebum levels, titratable acidity of sebum, and urinary fractional 17-ketosteroid excretion in males with acne. *J Invest Dermatol* 43:383, 1964.
13. Cotterill JA, Cunliffe WJ, Williamson B: Severity of acne and sebum excretion rate. *Br J Dermatol* 85:93, 1971.
14. Burton JL, Shuster S: The relation between seborrhoea and acne vulgaris. *Br J Dermatol* 85:197, 1971.
15. Plewig G, Christophers E: Renewal rate of human sebaceous glands. *Acta Derm Venereol (Stockh)* 54:177, 1974.

16. Douglas HC, Gunter SE: The taxonomic position of *Corynebacterium acnes*. *J Bacteriol* 52:15, 1946.
17. Moore WE, Cato EP: Validity of *Propionibacterium acnes* (Gilchrist) Douglas and Gunter comb. nov. *J Bacteriol* 85:870, 1963.
18. Johnson JL, Cummins CS: Cell wall composition and deoxyribonucleic acid similarities among the anaerobic coryneforms, classical propionibacteria, and strains of *Arachnia propionica*. *J Bacteriol* 109:1047, 1972.
19. Buchanan RE, Gibbons NE (Eds): *Bergey's Manual of Determinative Bacteriology*, ed 8, p 639. Baltimore: Williams and Wilkins, 1974.
20. Voss JG: Differentiation of two groups of *Corynebacterium acnes*. *J Bacteriol* 101:392, 1970.
21. Whiteside JA, Voss JG: Incidence and lipolytic activity of *Propionibacterium acnes* (*Corynebacterium acnes* group I) and *P. granulosum* (*C. acnes* group II) in acne and in normal skin. *J Invest Dermatol* 60:94, 1973.
22. Pulverer G, Ko HL: Fermentative and serological studies on *Propionibacterium acnes*. *Appl Microbiol* 25:222, 1973.
23. Pulverer G, Sorgo W, Ko HL: Bakteriophagen von *Propionibacterium acnes*. *Zentralbl Bakteriol [Orig A]* 225:353, 1973.
24. Somerville DA, Murphy CT: Quantitation of *Corynebacterium acnes* on healthy human skin. *J Invest Dermatol* 60:231, 1973.
25. Somerville DA, Noble WC: Microcolony size of microbes on human skin. *J Med Microbiol* 6:323, 1973.
26. Shehadeh NH, Kligman AM: The bacteriology of acne. *Arch Dermatol* 88:829, 1963.
27. Marples RR, Izumi AK: Bacteriology of pustular acne. *J Invest Dermatol* 54:252, 1970.
28. Izumi AK, Marples RR, Kligman AM: Bacteriology of acne comedones. *Arch Dermatol* 102:397, 1970.
29. Marples RR, McGinley KJ, Mills OH: Microbiology of comedones in acne vulgaris. *J Invest Dermatol* 60:80, 1973.
30. Bommer S: Hautuntersuchungen im gefilterten quarzlicht. *Klin Wochenschr* 6:1142, 1927.
31. Carrié C: Die Ursache der Porphyrin-Fluoreszenz in der Mundhöhle und auf der Haut. *Dermatol Z* 70:189, 1934.
32. Cornelius CE III, Ludwig GD: Red fluorescence of comedones: production of porphyrins by *Corynebacterium acnes*. *J Invest Dermatol* 49:368, 1967.
33. Martin RJ, Kahn G, Gooding JW, et al: Cutaneous porphyrin fluorescence as an indicator of antibiotic absorption and effectiveness. *Cutis* 12:758, 1973.
34. Puhvel SM, Sakamoto M: A re-evaluation of fatty acids as inflammatory agents in acne. *J Invest Dermatol* 68:93, 1977.
35. Nicolaides N: Skin lipids. IV. Biochemistry and function. *J Am Oil Chem Soc* 42:708, 1965.
36. Nicolaides N, Ansari MN, Fu HC, et al: Lipid composition of comedones compared with that of human skin surface in acne patients. *J Invest Dermatol* 54:487, 1970.
37. Anderson RL, Bozeman MA, Voss JG, et al: Individual and site variation in composition of facial surface lipids. *J Invest Dermatol* 58:369, 1972.
38. Pablo G, Hammons A, Bradley S, et al: Characteristics of the extracellular lipases from *Corynebacterium acnes* and *Staphylococcus epidermidis*. *J Invest Dermatol* 63:231, 1974.
39. Hassing GS: Inhibition of *Corynebacterium acnes* lipase by tetracycline. *J Invest Dermatol* 56:189, 1971.
40. Puhvel SM, Reisner RM: Effect of antibiotics on the lipases of *Corynebacterium acnes* in vitro. *Arch Dermatol* 106:45, 1972.
41. Weaber K, Freedman R, Eudy WW: Tetracycline inhibition of a lipase from

Corynebacterium acnes. Appl Microbiol 21:639, 1971.
42. Cullen SI, Crounse RG: Cutaneous pharmacology of the tetracyclines. *J Invest Dermatol* 45:263, 1965.
43. Imamura S, Pochi PE, Strauss JS, et al: The localization and distribution of *Corynebacterium acnes* and its antigens in normal skin and in lesions of acne vulgaris. *J Invest Dermatol* 53:143, 1969.
44. Puhvel SM, Hoffman IK, Reisner RM, et al: Dermal hypersensitivity of patients with acne vulgaris to *Corynebacterium acnes. J Invest Dermatol* 49:154, 1967.
45. Olansky S, Tully HT Jr: Hypersensitivity to *Corynebacterium acnes. Med Times* 89:72, 1961.
46. Shaffer LW, Schwimmer B, Staricco RJ: The effect of gamma globulin in pustular acne. *J Invest Dermatol* 30:97, 1958.
47. Sutton RL Jr, Asel ND: Treatment of acne vulgaris: adjunctive use of gamma globulin in severe cases. *South Med J* 52:515, 1959.
48. Warshaw T: Conglobate acne vulgaris associated with low levels of serum gamma globulin. *J Med Soc NJ* 64:218, 1974.
49. Steigleder GK, Blomeyer U: Talgdrüsen-artige Strukturen im Comedo. *Arch Klin Exp Dermatol* 218:496, 1964.
50. Müller HE: Über das Vorkommen von Neuraminidase bei *Corynebacterium acnes. Z Med Mikrobiol Immunol* 156:240, 1971.
51. Puhvel SM, Reisner RM: The production of hyaluronidase (hyaluronate lyase) by *Corynebacterium acnes. J Invest Dermatol* 58:66, 1972.
52. Smith RF, Willett NP: Rapid plate method for screening hyaluronidase and chondroitin sulfatase-producing microorganisms. *Appl Microbiol* 16:1434, 1968.
53. Werner H: Untersuchungen über die Lipase- und Lecithinase-Aktivität von aeroben und anaeroben *Corynebacterium-* und von *Propionibacterium*-Arten. *Zentralbl Bakteriol [Orig A]* 204:127, 1967.
54. Smith MA: The role of comedones in acne vulgaris. *Br J Dermatol* 74:337, 1962.
55. Hägele E, Schaefer H, Stüttgen G: Über die Bedeutung der Triglycerid-Spaltung durch *Corynebacterium acnes* für die Acne vulgaris. *Arch Dermatol Forsch* 246:328, 1973.
56. Azuma I, Taniyama T, Sugimura K, et al: Mitogenic activity of the cell walls of mycobacteria, nocardia, corynebacteria and anaerobic coryneforms. *Jpn J Microbiol* 20:263, 1976.
57. Maibach HI: Scalp pustules due to *Corynebacterium acnes. Arch Dermatol* 96:453, 1967.
58. Fulton JE Jr, McGinley K, Leyden J, et al: Gram-negative folliculitis in acne vulgaris. *Arch Dermatol* 98:349, 1968.
59. Leyden JJ, Marples RR, Mills OH Jr, et al: Gram-negative folliculitis—a complication of antibiotic therapy in acne vulgaris. *Br J Dermatol* 88:533, 1973.
60. Goltz RW, Kjartansson S: Oral tetracycline treatment on bacterial flora in acne vulgaris. *Arch Dermatol* 93:92, 1966.
61. Marples RR, Williamson P: Effects of systemic demethylchlortetracycline on human cutaneous microflora. *Appl Microbiol* 18:228, 1969.
62. Marples RR, Kligman AM: Ecological effects of oral antibiotics on the microflora of the skin. *Arch Dermatol* 103:148, 1971.
63. Faget H, Landes E: Untersuchungen über die Wirkung der Tetracycline bei der Acne vulgaris. *Hautarzt* 19:469, 1968.
64. Rashleigh PL, Rife E, Goltz RW: Tetracycline levels in skin surface film after oral administration of tetracycline to normal adults and to patients with acne vulgaris. *J Invest Dermatol* 49:611, 1967.
65. Smith EL, Mortimer PR: Tetracycline in acne vulgaris. *Br J Dermatol* 79:78, 1967.
66. Kraus SJ: Reduction in skin surface free fatty acids with topical tetracycline. *J*

Invest Dermatol 51:431, 1968.
67. Cunliffe WJ, Forster RA, Williams M, et al: Tetracycline and acne vulgaris: a clinical and laboratory investigation. *Br Med J* 4:332, 1973.
68. Moss HV: Acne vulgaris: treatment with newer antibiotics. *Cutis* 10:375, 1972.
69. Cunliffe WJ, Cotterill JA, Williamson B: The effect of clindamycin in acne: a clinical and laboratory investigation. *Br J Dermatol* 87:37, 1972.
70. Stitzler C, Frank L: Long-term oleandomycin therapy for acne. *Arch Dermatol* 81:958, 1960.
71. Tomasini C, Tagliavini R, Riboldi A: Ricerche clinico-microbiologiche e biometriche nell' acne trattata con rifampicina. *G Ital Dermatol* 45:613, 1970.
72. Beveridge GW, Powell EW: Sebum changes in acne vulgaris treated with tetracycline. *Br J Dermatol* 81:525, 1969.
73. Blaney DJ, Cook CH: Topical use of tetracycline in the treatment of acne. *Arch Dermatol* 112:971, 1976.
74. Miroliubov VI: Chloramphenicol in the treatment of folliculitis, acne vulgaris, and rosacea. *Vestn Dermatol Venereol* 37:68, 1963.
75. Fulton JE Jr, Pablo G: Topical antibacterial therapy for acne: study of the family of erythromycins. *Arch Dermatol* 110:83, 1974.
76. Frank L, Petrou P: Active oxygen plus chlorhydroxyquinoline in acne and pyodermas—including *in vitro* and *in vivo* bacteriological studies. *Cutis* 3:256, 1967.
77. Martin WJ, Gardner M, Washington JA II: *In vitro* antimicrobial susceptibility of anaerobic bacteria isolated from clinical specimens. *Antimicrob Agents Chemother* 1:148, 1972.
78. McOsker DE, Beck LW: Characteristics of accommodated (hardened) skin. *J Invest Dermatol* 48:372, 1967.

Chapter 6

Immunology
S. MADLI PUHVEL, PhD

Most studies on the immunology of acne have dealt with the response of patients with acne to specific microorganisms within acne lesions. There have been recent studies suggesting that patients with acne conglobata may be immunodeficient, but comprehensive investigations of the general immunologic status of patients with acne vulgaris are lacking. This Chapter reviews the immunologic findings which have related *Propionibacterium acnes* to acne vulgaris, and offers suggestions as to possible mechanisms whereby these findings may be of relevance in the pathogenesis of acne.

P. acnes is the predominant microorganism within the normal pilosebaceous follicles of human skin.[1] Thus, when these structures become the focus of pathogenic changes in acne vulgaris, it is not surprising that this anaerobic diphtheroid is almost invariably found in all stages of the acne process.[2,3] The role of *P. acnes* in the pathogenesis of acne is a question yet to be resolved. Acne is not a bacterial disease; yet the bacterial element appears to be essential, for why otherwise would antibiotic treatment with a variety of differently acting antibiotics be effective in alleviating the symptoms of acne in so many patients?

Other chapters in this book have dealt with the free fatty acid hypothesis of acne pathogenesis, which explains the role of *P. acnes* in acne as being primarily a source of intrafollicular lipases. However, in addition to being a source of lipases, there is evidence that *P. acnes* may be more directly involved in inducing the inflammatory stages of acne. Studies comparing the effects of

48 PATHOGENESIS

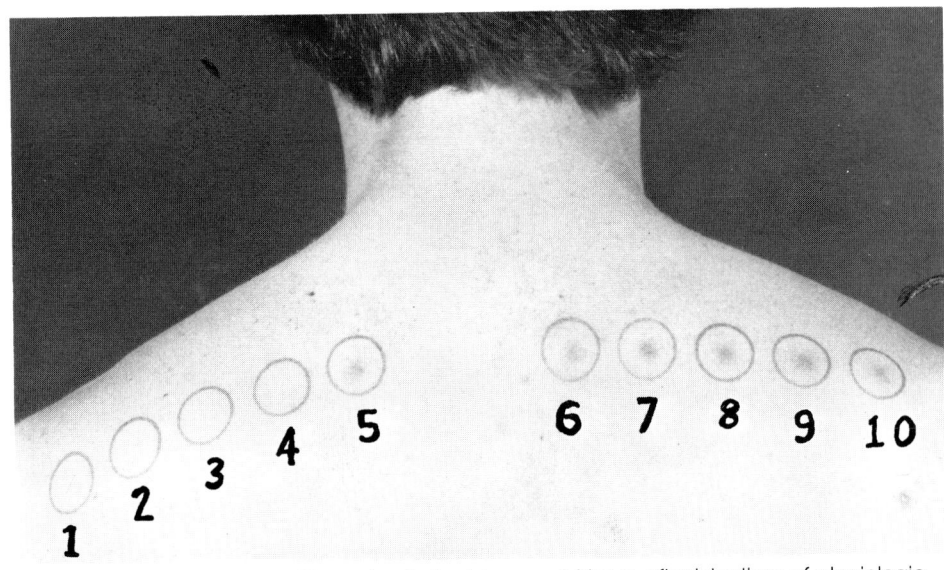

Figure 1. Back of patient with moderate facial acne, 24 hours after injections of physiologic concentrations of different comedonal components. 1) saline; 2) 500 μg purified sebaceous lipids; 3) 200 μg purified sebaceous fatty acids; 4) 50 μg squalene; 5) 2 x 10⁵ live P. acnes; 6) 2 x 10⁵ killed P. acnes; 7) 2 x 10⁵ live P. acnes plus 300 μg sebaceous lipids; 8) 2 x 10⁵ live P. acnes plus 200 μg fatty acids; 9) 30 μg insoluble keratinous material extracted from comedones; 10) 60 μg water-soluble material extracted from comedones. Note absence of visible inflammatory response to lipids. Reproduced with permission from Puhvel SM, Sakamoto M: An in vivo evaluation of the inflammatory effect of purified comedonal components in human skin. J Invest Dermatol 69:401, 1977. Copyright © 1977, Williams & Wilkins, Baltimore.

intradermal injections of physiologic amounts (ie, the amounts present in open comedones in acne) of skin surface lipids, free fatty acids, squalene, and *P. acnes* have demonstrated that physiologic amounts of *P. acnes* are more inflammatory in human skin than are the lipid components of comedones (Figure 1). Furthermore, patients with acne have a greater inflammatory response to *P. acnes* injections than do control individuals without acne.[4] Thus, there is evidence to suggest that the role of *P. acnes* in the pathogenesis of acne may be more complex than merely one as a source of intrafollicular lipases.

Adult patients generally have low, but titratable, levels of circulating serum antibodies to *P. acnes*.[5] This includes patients who have skin diseases other than acne, where the sebaceous follicles are not the prime target of the disease. In other words, the presence of *P. acnes* in normal pilosebaceous follicles stimulates significant antibody production in the host. However, in patients with inflammatory acne, the antibody titers are usually further elevated.[6] There is very good correlation between the severity of the inflammatory acne and the level of circulating antibodies to *P. acnes*. In patients with acne conglobata, bacterial agglutination titers of 1 : 40,000 have been found. These antibodies are most likely gamma G immunoglobulins. In a study conducted by Izumi and Kligman (unpublished observations, 1970) of 11 patients with acne conglobata, 5 had elevated gamma G levels and 2 had elevated gamma A levels. Gamma M levels were normal. The anti-*P. acnes* antibodies can be titrated by a variety of standard serologic techniques (SM Puhvel, unpublished observations, 1971): by direct bacterial agglutination; by agglutination of latex particles which have been coated with *P. acnes;* or, by complement-fixation, immunodiffusion, or antibody precipitation tests, using either soluble bacterial extracts or soluble extracellular bacterial products as antigen.

The antibody response in patients with inflammatory acne appears to be selective for *P. acnes,* and not a general response to all bacteria existing within the acne lesions. This is evinced by the finding[7] that antibodies to *Staphylococcus epidermidis* are not higher in patients with acne in comparison to control individuals without acne, even though *S. epidermidis* can be isolated in significant numbers from the acne lesions. A possible explanation of the antibody response of acne patients to *P. acnes* rather than to *S. epidermidis* may be related to the immunogenicity of the former organism.

P. acnes is a very potent stimulator of the reticuloendothelial system in animals.[8,9] This has been known since the advent of extensive research of the immunotherapy of cancer. Presently, two of the most widely used systems of nonspecific immunostimulators for the immunotherapy of certain types of malignancies are bacille Calmette Guérin (BCG) and killed *Corynebacterium parvum* vaccine. *C. parvum* is an anaerobic diphtheroid. It was demonstrated that strains known as *C. parvum* are often serologically and biochemically the same as *P. acnes.*[10] The latest edition of *Bergey's Manual*[11] no longer lists *C. parvum* as a separate entity; instead, the organisms formerly so labelled are now considered identical with *P. acnes*. It is interesting to note that one of the predominant organisms of the normal bacterial flora of human skin has such a potent effect as an immunostimulant and as an antitumor agent in other systems. The mechanism of action of *P. acnes* in immunotherapy of cancer is being investigated by numerous groups. Although not completely elucidated, it appears that the main function of *P. acnes* is in stimulating an increased production and activity of macrophages.[12] Resistance to tumors in laboratory animals was found to parallel an increase in reticuloendothelial phagocytic activity, through an increase in the production and function of tissue macrophages.[13] Further data[14] suggested that the antitumor effect of *P. acnes* is independent of the T-lymphocyte system, and treatment of animals with *C. parvum (P. acnes)* vaccine was shown to suppress production of T-lymphocytes in mice.[15]

It was suggested[16] that acne may play a biological role in stimulating the general immunologic competence of patients with this disease; *ie*, the frequent intrusions of masses of *P. acnes* into the dermis from inflamed sebaceous follicles in acne patients may have somewhat the same effect on the host's reticuloendothelial system as treatment with microinjections of *P. acnes* vaccine. Such a possibility could be tested by a study of the immunologic competence of cells from patients with acne, as compared to cells from age-matched, control individuals without acne, or alternatively by epidemiologic studies. One epidemiologic study[17] of the disease history of 605 men with leukemia demonstrated that significantly more leukemia patients had had acne, as compared to an age-matched, leukemia-free control group. This study does not support the concept that patients with acne are more immunocompetent than control individuals without acne, if, indeed, lack of immunologic competence is involved in the development of leukemia.

In acne patients, neither the potential stimulatory effect of exposure to *P. acnes* nor the development of high levels of circulating antibodies to *P. acnes* appears to have a beneficial effect in alleviating the acne. On the contrary, the highest antibody titers to *P. acnes* can be associated with the most severe forms of the disease. In the heydey of the use of vaccine therapies in the early 1900's, reports describing the use of acne bacillus appeared in the medical literature.[18,19] A vaccine consisting of a mixture of staphylococci and *P. acnes* became commercially available for the treatment of acne. To date, there is no evidence that bacterial vaccine treatments are beneficial in acne. In fact, Costello and Washburn[20] reported that, in some patients, vaccine therapy may have an adverse effect.

The hypersensitivity response of acne patients to *P. acnes* antigen was investigated,[21] using both cellular and extracellular bacterial antigens. In a study of 46 patients with varying degrees of acne and 46 control individuals without acne, it was found that 79% of the test group, as compared to 23% of the control group, had an immediate cutaneous hypersensitivity reaction to 10 μg intradermal injections of *P. acnes* antigen. Moreover, there was a strong correlation between the severity of the acne and the strength of the immediate hypersensitivity response. Patients with acne conglobata demonstrated immediate hypersensitivity to 1 μg injections of *P. acnes* antigen. However, significant delayed cutaneous hypersensitivity to *P. acnes* antigen could not be demonstrated in patients with acne, including patients with acne conglobata, according to the findings of Izumi and Kligman (unpublished observations, 1970).

The possibility that severe cystic acne may involve a delayed hypersensitivity reaction was suggested by the histologic picture of the acne lesions, which were characterized by a predominantly lymphocytic infiltrate.[22] Also, the successful use of intralesional corticosteroids in the treatment of cystic acne theoretically may be influenced by the immunosuppressive, as well as the anti-inflammatory, effect of corticosteroids. It was recently found[23] that the transformation response of peripheral lymphocytes to *P. acnes* antigen stimulation was significantly greater in patients with severe nodulocystic acne than in acne-free control individuals. This finding suggests that some form of cell-mediated response to *P. acnes* is present in a significant number of patients with severe acne. Therefore, despite negative skin tests, cell-mediated immunity to *P. acnes* in acne patients warrants further analysis, using more extensive *in vitro* techniques in the study of this problem.

In summary, no generalized abnormalities in immunologic responsiveness in patients with acne vulgaris have been demonstrated. There appears to be a response to *P. acnes* antigen which is manifested by elevated levels of serum antibodies and intensified immediate hypersensitivity reactions to *P. acnes*. This is sometimes accompanied by an intensified lymphocyte transformation response to *P. acnes* antigen *in vitro*, particularly in patients with the severe inflammatory forms of acne. However, the significance of these immunologic responses to *P. acnes* in relationship to the pathogenesis of acne vulgaris remains unclear.

The immunologic status of patients with acne conglobata appears to differ from that of patients with acne vulgaris. Izumi and Kligman (unpublished observations, 1970) were the first to suggest that patients with acne conglobata have a suppressed cellular immune response. Their studies for delayed cutaneous hypersensitivity to common recall antigens (*eg*, purified protein derivative [PPD], mumps, Varidase®) in 11 patients with acne conglobata produced only 2 positive reactions from a total of 33 tests.

More recently, studies[24,25] on cell-mediated immunity in patients with acne conglobata confirmed Izumi and Kligman's findings. In a study of 35 patients, Rajka[24] found that 25 individuals had a reduced or absent delayed reactivity to skin tests with tuberculin, streptococcal vaccine, staphylovaccine, mumps, and Schick toxin. Palatsi[25] reported negative reactions to tuberculin, Schick toxin, oidiomycin, trichophytin, and 25 common contact allergens in 5 patients with febrile acne conglobata (acne fulminans). Also, dinitrochlorobenzene (DNCB) sensitization was unsuccessful in the 4 patients in whom it was attempted. The lymphocyte transformation response to nonspecific mitogens such as phytohemagglutinin (PHA) was normal in patients with acne conglobata, and also in patients with the more common forms of nodulocystic acne.[23-25] Also of interest is the observation made by Palatsi[25] that patients with ordinary cystic and papulopustular acne, in contrast to those with febrile acne conglobata, did not demonstrate a suppression in response to cutaneous tests with both tuberculin (10 TU/ml) and oidiomycin. Thus, a definite suppression in the cell-mediated immune system in patients with acne conglobata has been demonstrated. Again, the question of whether the immune unresponsiveness is a result of the disease, or vice versa, remains unanswered.

REFERENCES

1. Puhvel SM, Amirian DA, Reisner RM: Quantification of bacteria in isolated pilosebaceous follicles in normal skin. *J Invest Dermatol* 64:208, 1975.

2. Shehadeh NH, Kligman AM: The bacteriology of acne. *Arch Dermatol* 88:829, 1963.
3. Marples RR, Izumi AK: Bacteriology of pustular acne. *J Invest Dermatol* 54:252, 1970.
4. Puhvel SM, Sakamoto M: An *in vivo* evaluation of the inflammatory effect of purified comedonal components in human skin. *J Invest Dermatol* 69:401, 1977.
5. Woodruff MFA, Clunie GJA, McBride WH, et al: "The Effect of Intravenous and Intramuscular Injection of *Corynebacterium parvum*," in Halpern H (Ed): *Corynebacterium parvum*, pp 383-388. New York: Plenum Press, 1975.
6. Puhvel SM, Barfatani M, Warnick MA, et al: Study of antibody levels to *Corynebacterium acnes*. *Arch Dermatol* 90:421, 1964.
7. Puhvel SM, Warnick MA, Sternberg TH: Levels of antibody to *Staphylococcus epidermidis* in patients with acne vulgaris. *Arch Dermatol* 92:88, 1965.
8. Adlam C, Scott MT: Lymphoreticular stimulatory properties of *Corynebacterium parvum* and related bacteria. *Med Microbiol* 6:261, 1973.
9. Halpern BN, Prevot AR, Biozzi G, et al: Stimulátion de l'activité phagocytaire du système réticuloendothelial provoquée par *Corynebacterium parvum*. *J Reticuloendothel Soc* 1:77, 1964.
10. Cummins CS, Johnson JL: *Corynebacterium parvum:* a synonym for *Propionibacterium acnes? J Gen Microbiol* 80:433, 1974.
11. Buchanan RE, Gibbons NE (Eds): *Bergey's Manual of Determinative Bacteriology*, ed 8, pp 602-639. Baltimore: Williams and Wilkins, 1974.
12. Smith LH, Woodruff MFA: Comparative effect of two strains of *Corynebacterium parvum* on phagocytic activity and tumor growth. *Nature* 219:197, 1968.
13. Klapschmidt RF, Pulliam LA: Changes in the opsonin and cellular influences on phagocytosis during the growth of transplantable tumors. *J Reticuloendothel Soc* 11:1, 1972.
14. Scott MT: Biological effects of the adjuvant *Corynebacterium parvum:* evidence for macrophage-T cell interaction. *Cell Immunol* 5:465, 1972.
15. Castro JE: The effect of *Corynebacterium parvum* on the structure and function of the lymphoid system in mice. *Eur J Cancer* 10:115, 1974.
16. Shuster S: Biological purpose of acne. *Lancet* 1:1328, 1976.
17. Gibson R, Graham S, Lilienfeld A, et al: Epidemiology of diseases in adult males with leukemia. *J Natl Cancer Inst* 56:891, 1976.
18. Fleming A: On the etiology of acne vulgaris and its treatment by vaccines. *Lancet*, p 1035, 1909.
19. Engman MF: Treatment of acne vulgaris with acne bacillus suspensions. *Interstate Med J* 17:943, 1910.
20. Costello MJ, Washburn JC: "Acne mixed" undenatured bacterial antigen in treatment of acne vulgaris. *Arch Dermatol Syphilol* 38:405, 1938.
21. Puhvel SM, Hoffman IK, Reisner RM, et al: Dermal hypersensitivity of patients with acne vulgaris to *Corynebacterium acnes*. *J Invest Dermatol* 49:154, 1967.
22. Lever WF: *Histopathology of the Skin*, ed 4, pp 188-189. Philadelphia: JB Lippincott, 1967.
23. Puhvel SM, Amirian DA, Weintraub J, et al: Lymphocyte transformation in subjects with nodulocystic acne. *Br J Dermatol* 97:205, 1977.
24. Rajka G: On cell-mediated immunity in acne conglobata. *Acta Derm Venereol (Stockh)* 57:141, 1977.
25. Palatsi R: Delayed hypersensitivity and febrile acne conglobata. *Acta Derm Venereol (Stockh)* 57:51, 1977.

Chapter 7

Hormones
F. J. G. EBLING, PhD, DSc

It is obvious that androgenic hormones play a role in the development of acne vulgaris. Although acne occasionally occurs in the neonatal stage, it is predominantly a condition of adolescence. Moreover, acne is associated with increased sebum production, and male hormones have been shown to stimulate sebaceous secretion in both man[1] and experimental animals.[2]

On the other hand, androgens cannot be implicated as the sole or prime cause of acne, since the disease is not an inevitable result of sexual development. Also, in males at least, neither plasma nor urinary testosterone levels are abnormally high in acne patients.[3-5] In addition, although testosterone will increase sebaceous secretion when given to prepuberal boys or eunuchs, it produces no such effect in normal adult men, in whom the sebaceous glands are already maximally stimulated by endogenous androgens.[6] Thus, high sebum production may, in some female acne patients, be a result of above average androgen levels, whereas in male patients, other factors (such as an increased response of the sebaceous glands, possibly due to the synergistic action of other hormones) must be sought. This Chapter examines in detail the evidence for the above propositions, and reviews some of the possible therapeutic consequences.

Sebaceous Secretion in Acne

Pochi and Strauss[7] first reported a relation between severity of acne vulgaris and the rate of sebum secretion as measured on the forehead, although there was too much overlap between acne sufferers and nonsufferers to characterize any single individual as having acne or not by his sebum production. Cunliffe and Shuster[8] obtained similar results, and made the further claim that, when their 221 patients were grouped according to severity of acne, there was no overlap between the ranges of sebum production. Their findings were amply confirmed in a further study.[9] Powell and Beveridge,[10] on the other hand, obtained so much overlap that they concluded there was no statistically significant relation between the rate of sebum secretion and the presence of acne. These authors also estimated the number of sebaceous glands by staining the small areas of lipid with osmium tetroxide on collecting papers. As expected, they found no difference in the number of sebaceous glands between acne sufferers and nonsufferers. However, they noted that sebum production showed an approximately linear relation to the sebaceous gland count in both groups. They were quite correct; an analysis of their data revealed a high degree of correlation, giving coefficients of 0.98 ($P < 0.001$) for 10 normal individuals and 0.93 ($P < 0.001$) for 20 patients with acne. This suggests that it would be useful and valid to correct the sebum production by the number of glands. On this basis, Powell and Beveridge's data[10] can be coaxed to reveal that their acne patients produced, on an average, nearly 50% more sebum per gland than did the controls ($P < 0.01$).

Androgen Levels in Acne

There is general agreement that testosterone levels are not abnormally high in males with acne. The finding of Pochi et al[3] that the concentration of testosterone in the plasma did not significantly differ between acne sufferers and nonsufferers was confirmed by Förström et al[4] (Table I) and by Lim and James,[5] who carefully measured the levels of total plasma 17-β-hydroxysteroids in a small group of males.

The situation may be different in women. Förström et al[4] found a highly significant elevation of plasma testosterone in women with acne.

Although figures published by Mauvais-Jarvis et al[11] were somewhat less dramatic (Table II), the findings were partially confirmed by Lim and James.[5] Comparing 26 female acne patients ranging in age from 14-35 years with 18 normal females of similar age, they found the mean level of free 17-β-hydroxysteroids to be significantly higher in the acne group, even though only 4 of those had basal plasma 17-β-hydroxysteroid levels outside the normal range.

Androgens and Sebaceous Secretion

Androgens have been shown to stimulate sebaceous activity in man[1,12,13] and in a range of experimental animals.[2,14] Jarrett[15] found a signifi-

Table I — Plasma Testosterone in Males in ng/100 ml*

Reference	Normal	# Patients	Acne	# Patients
Pochi et al[3]	720 ± 110	(16)	590 ± 33	(26)
Förström et al[4]	763 ± 92	(17)	641 ± 84	(23)

*Means ± Standard Error of the Mean

Table II — Plasma Testosterone in Females in ng/100 ml*

Reference	Normal	# Patients	Acne	# Patients
Mauvais-Jarvis et al[11]	45 ± 10	(10)	58 ± 5	(6)
Förström et al[4]	59 ± 3	(27)	119 ± 21	(31)

*Means ± Standard Error of the Mean

cant increase in sebum production within a week after administering injections of 25 mg of testosterone to adolescent boys. Strauss and Pochi[16] administered 100 mg a day of methyl testosterone to an 11-year-old boy, and observed that sebum secretion rose within 1-2 weeks, and reached 3-4 times the initial value in 6-8 weeks (Figure 1). The glands markedly enlarged. Similar effects could be produced in eunuchs, but not in normal adults.[6]

Figure 1. Sebum output of 11-year-old boy given 2 courses of oral methyl testosterone (100 mg/day). Reproduced with permission from Strauss JS, Pochi PE: The quantitative gravimetric determination of sebum production. J Invest Dermatol 36:293, 1961. Copyright © 1961, Williams & Wilkins, Baltimore.

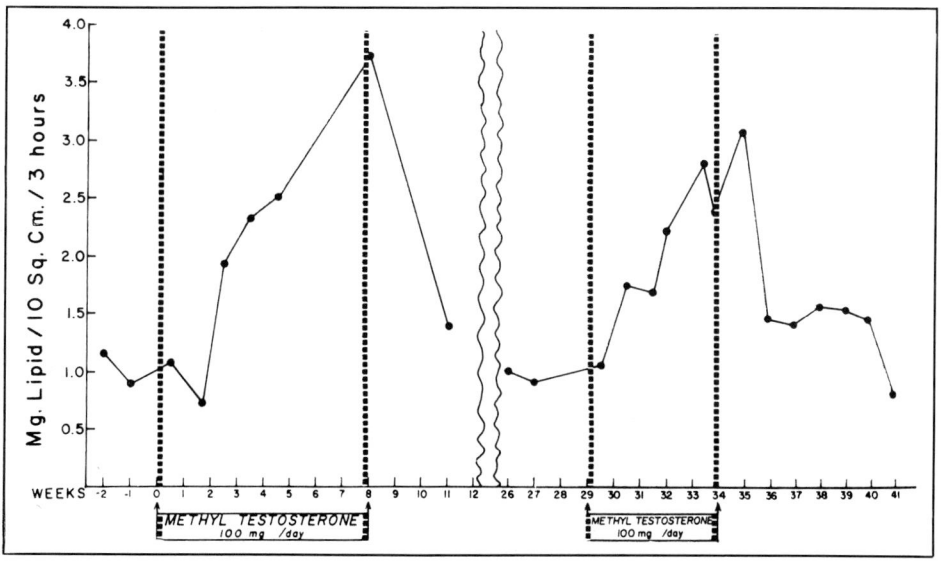

Testosterone increases sebum production in castrated male or spayed female rats.[2,17,18] The action involves an increase in mitotic rate, and the glands become enlarged.[19] A number of other androgens were also shown to be similarly effective: 5α-dihydrotestosterone was as potent as testosterone; androstenedione was less so. However, both these compounds appeared to be more potent than testosterone in hypophysectomized-castrated rats, as was 5α-androstane-3β,17β-diol.[2]

That progesterone might have an action similar to that of various androgens, and thus be a factor in female acne, has been debated. While some response to large doses cannot be ruled out, doses of progesterone within the range effective for androgens have no significant effect on the rate of sebum production.[17]

Possible Role of the Pituitary

Experiments with animals have produced strong evidence that pituitary hormones affect sebaceous secretion in various ways. If the role of the pituitary in human acne remains problematic, it is reasonable to suspect that animal findings may be relevant to the human condition, since hormonal responses of human sebaceous glands appear, from all evidence, to be no different from those of the rat.

It is important at the outset to recognize the various ways in which pituitary hormones might act on the skin. First, indirect actions by way of the endocrine organs, which are themselves pituitary-dependent, must be distinguished from direct actions, in which no intervening organ is concerned (Figure 2). It is obvious that if the sebaceous glands are affected by gonadal or adrenocortical steroids, then the gonadotropic or adrenocorticotropic hormones will indirectly produce similar effects. Similarly, if thyroid secretion also influences the sebaceous glands, as seems probable, so will thyrotropic hormone.

Second, the effect of a hormone on its target organ may or may not be dependent on the presence of another hormone. Thus, Houssay[20] stated that regulatory effects are comprised in no single hormone; pituitary or thyroid hormones act "in correct synergistic balance or antagonistic balance" together with corticosteroid hormones.

The idea that pituitary hormones have such a permissive or synergistic action in conjunction with androgenic steroids is now a clearly established fact, not only regarding the sebaceous glands, but also the preputial glands and the prostate. The first evidence for this function of the pituitary was the finding that, in the rat, hypophysectomy greatly reduces the response of the sebaceous glands to testosterone, whether measured by gland size[21-23] or by sebum output.[24] When the responses to testosterone of castrated and hypophysectomized-castrated rats were carefully compared in matched litter mates (Figure 3), testosterone substantially increased sebaceous secretion in

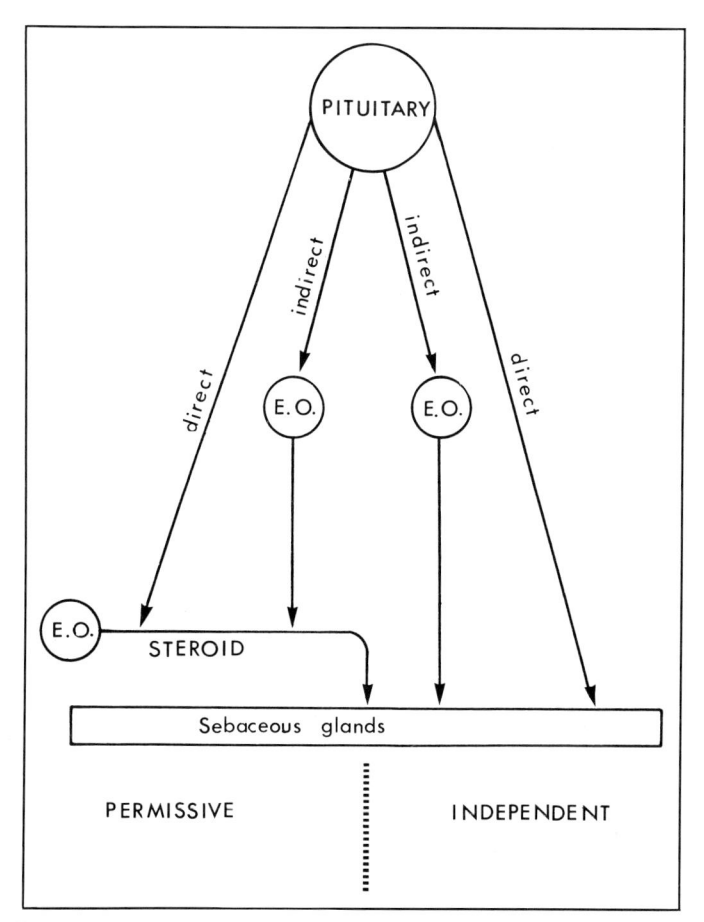

Figure 2. Possible ways in which pituitary hormones may affect sebaceous glands. Effect may be direct or indirect; it may also be independent or permissive, in the sense that the pituitary hormone facilitates the response to another hormone, eg, a steroid. E.O. = Endocrine Organ. Reproduced with permission from Ebling FJ, Ebling E, Randall V, et al: The sebotrophic action of bovine growth hormone (BGH) in the rat. *Br J Dermatol* 92:325, 1975.

the castrated rats, but had no significant effect in the hypophysectomized ones. However, a limited response to testosterone in hypophysectomized rats can be detected if sufficient data are analyzed. The comparison of 44 testosterone-treated rats with their untreated litter mate controls, using a two-way Student's T-test, revealed a statistically significant response—about 20% of that produced in rats with intact pituitaries.[2]

The response of the sebaceous gland to testosterone in hypophysectomized-castrated rats was completely restored by a porcine growth hormone[24] and a bovine growth hormone[25] of unimpeachable source (Figure 3). In this experiment, 27% of the total effect was accounted for by an independent action of the growth hormone, and the remainder as a synergistic action.[25] Similar effects have been shown with synthetic α-melanocyte-stimulating hormone (α-MSH). In the dose used, this peptide had a significant independent effect amounting to 47% of the total, leaving a synergistic component of over 50%.[26]

A synergistic partnership between pituitary hormone and androgens is not confined to the sebaceous glands. Although the preputial glands are less severely affected by hypophysectomy than are the sebaceous glands in their response to testosterone, the full response is restored by bovine growth hormone or by α-MSH. Similar synergistic effects can also be shown for the prostate.

Growth hormone and α-MSH are not the only peptides which can act as synergists. Prolactin will restore the response of the sebaceous glands,[24] and has also been implicated in the response of the prostate.[27] Thyrotropic hormone similarly increases the response of the sebaceous glands,[28] but the extent to which this is a synergistic effect in combination with testosterone, or an independent effect due to increased thyroid hormone, which is itself

Figure 3. Sebum production in castrated (C) and hypophysectomized-castrated (H) litter-mate rats with or without bovine growth hormone (G) or testosterone (T) treatment. Means ±S.E. for groups of 11 rats. Reproduced with permission from Ebling FJ, Ebling E, Randall V, et al: The sebotrophic action of bovine growth hormone (BGH) in the rat. Br J Dermatol 92:325, 1975.

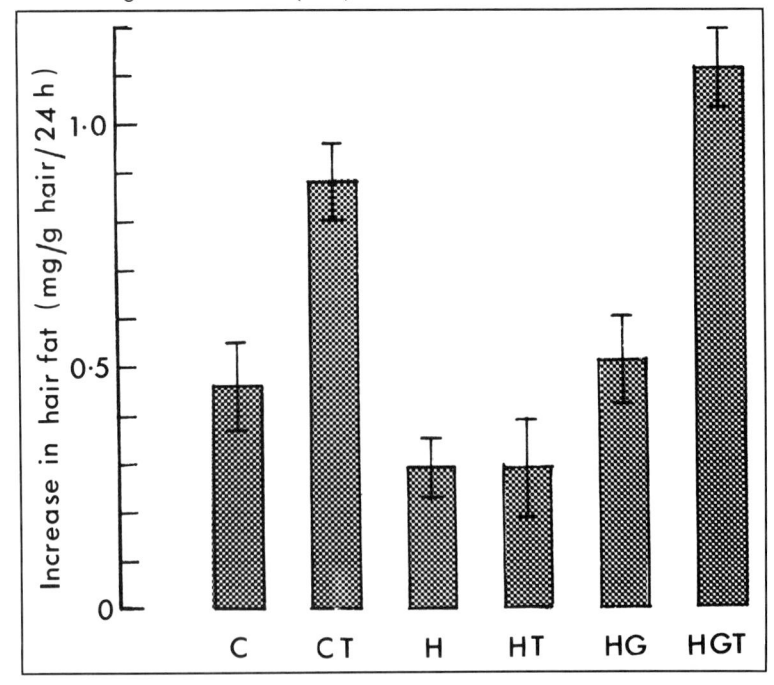

known to affect sebum production, is undetermined.

The evidence that the pituitary affects the responses to androgens of the sebaceous glands and, to a lesser extent, of other target organs, is thus considerable. The peptide sequences involved remain a problem, since, in experimental animals, the synergistic effect appears to be common to a range of pituitary hormones, rather than to a single identifiable "sebotropic hormone" as originally proposed.[29,30]

These facts suggest that the increased response of the sebaceous glands to androgens in acne patients might perhaps be the result of a synergistic action by pituitary hormones. Whether there is any clinical evidence that the pituitary affects sebaceous activity, or could be involved in acne, is thus an important question. Acromegalics are often noted to have oily skin, and there is some clear evidence that their sebum secretion rates are abnormally high. Burton et al[31] measured sebum production in 4 men and 7 women with untreated acromegaly; in each group, the mean rate was found to be significantly greater than that of normal controls of the same age range. It was possible to make measurements before and after pituitary irradiation by yttrium implants in 5 patients. In each of them, sebum secretion was diminished by the treatment. Data for a total of 20 treated and untreated acromegalics showed the rate of sebum production to be well-correlated with both log serum growth hormone concentration and plasma cortisol.

If growth hormone is an important factor, as indicated by a raised level of sebum secretion in acromegalics, one might also expect to find low sebum production in individuals with isolated growth hormone deficiency. Only a few such cases have been investigated. Two out of 3 individuals examined by Goolamali et al[32] had extremely low sebum secretion rates. Of 4 male and 3 female ateliotic dwarfs seen by Pochi and Strauss,[1] the mean rates were slightly, but not significantly, below normal. Some information is also available from patients with hypopituitarism of diverse etiology, but it is more difficult to interpret. Goolamali et al[32] found, in both men and women with pituitary hypofunction, mean rates which were substantially and significantly below those of normal control individuals. It seems unlikely that this was due to lowered output of adrenocortical, thyroid, or gonadal hormones, since all were receiving replacement therapy for these deficiencies. Pochi and Strauss[1] similarly obtained low figures for 6 women with hypopituitarism—3 had received both adrenocortical and thyroid hormones; one had received cortisone only; one, thyroxine only; and one, neither. There is thus reasonable, if not conclusive, evidence that acne is associated with abnormally high sebum secretion and that, at the same time, sebum secretion is correlated with growth hormone levels.

Could acne therefore be associated with raised growth hormone levels? Some light is shed on the problem by examining the clinical evidence from acromegalics. In the view of Faglia,[33] the incidence of acne is higher in acromegalics than in the normal population: of 28 acromegalic women, 12 had acne; in 4 of the 12, the acne was severe. Eight of 19 acromegalic men were similarly affected. It is more difficult to determine whether or not the occurrence of acne was correlated with serum growth hormone levels, since only limited single measurements were available, but there did appear to be some correlation.

Action of Hormones at the Target Site

The response of the target organ to testosterone involves two processes. First, the steroid immediately becomes attached to a binding protein in the cytoplasm of the cells and is transferred within 30 minutes to the nucleus.[34] The steroid is simultaneously reduced to 5α-dihydrotestosterone, which is generally believed to be the tissue-active androgen (Figure 4). The possible role of increased 5α-reduction of the androgen in acne is indicated both by the demonstration that sebaceous glands in acne-prone regions of patients show abnormally high 5α-reductase activity *in vitro*,[35] and by the finding of abnormally high amounts of 5α-androstanediols in the urine of female acne patients.[11]

The removal of the pituitary from rats greatly reduces the response of the sebaceous glands to testosterone, but has much less effect on their responses to 5α-dihydrotestosterone and 5α-androstane-3β,17β-diol, and also to androstenedione, another metabolite of testosterone.[36,37] That the response to testosterone can be restored by a range of peptide hormones as mentioned previously suggests that the pituitary hormones might act to promote synthesis of the steroid-metabolizing enzymes. However, extensive studies have failed to establish that hypophysectomy has any effect on the 5α-reductase activity of rat skin, either *in vivo* or *in vitro*.

An alternative explanation might be that the pituitary hormone affects synthesis of the receptor protein, for which testosterone has less affinity than its metabolites. The fact that the anti-androgenic steroid, cyproterone acetate, will selectively block binding of 5α-dihydrotestosterone without impairing 5α-reductase activity indicates, with other supporting evidence, that the androgen receptor and the enzyme are different proteins. Perhaps either explanation is too simple; perhaps the responses of the sebaceous gland are modified through a range of effects produced by a spectrum of hormones. That this may be the case is suggested by the findings that both bovine growth hormone and α-MSH have independent as well as permissive (or synergistic) effects with testosterone; moreover, when the pituitary hormones are given in consort, they appear to exhibit a mutual synergism.

Inhibition of Sebaceous Secretion

Several types of steroids inhibit sebaceous activity. Estrogens undoubtedly do so, as demonstrated in both human and animal experiments.

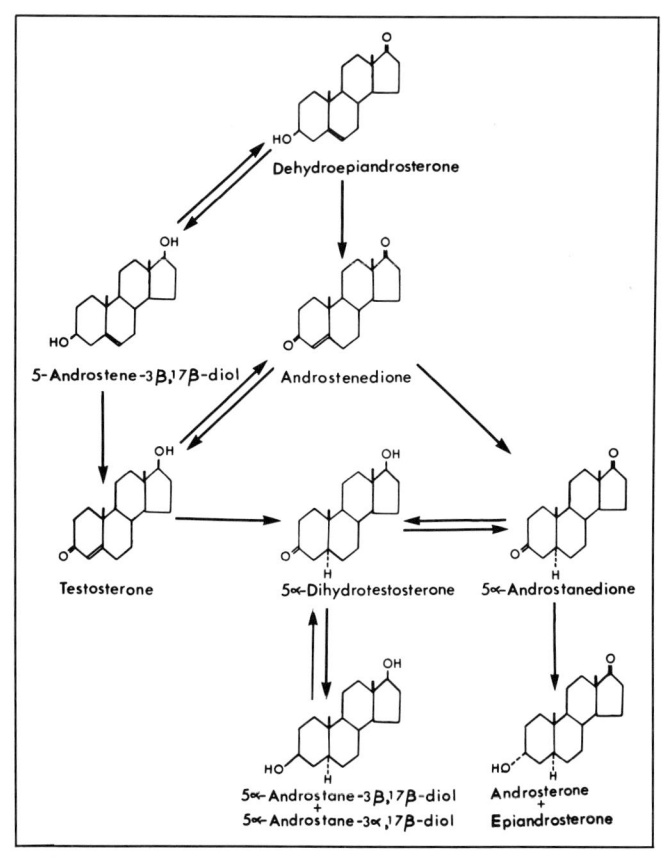

Figure 4. Major pathways of androgen metabolism in skin.

What has been debated is whether or not they are effective in physiological doses, and whether their action is peripheral and local, or by way of some systemic mechanism (*eg*, by suppression of endogenous androgen production). This problem has been fully discussed elsewhere,[17] and the conclusion was drawn that, although indirect effects cannot be ruled out, estrogens exert a major peripheral action on the sebaceous glands. Even so, topical application of estrogens has consistently proved somewhat less effective than systemic administration in reducing sebum production.

Jarrett[38] and Strauss and Pochi[12,13,16] showed clearly that systemically administered estrogens could reduce sebum production in human males and females. In rats, estrogens reduce the size and rate of secretion of the sebaceous glands, even when testosterone is given concurrently.[39,40] What is of particular interest is that, although androgens act, at least in part, by increasing cell division, estrogens appear to have little effect in this respect

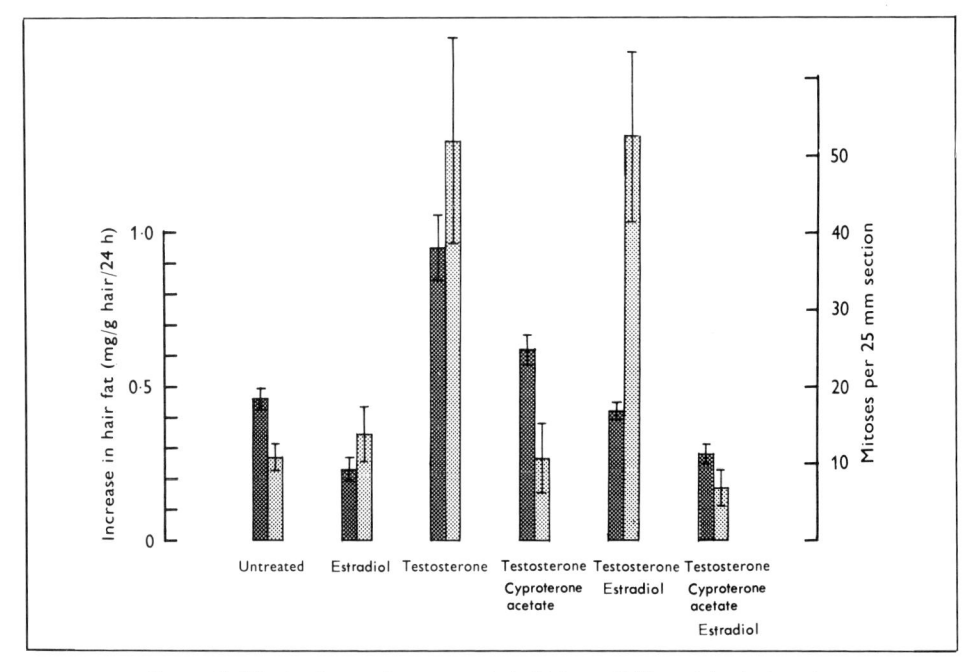

Figure 5. Effects of cyproterone acetate (2.0 mg/24 hour injected s.c. in 0.25 ml 1% carboxymethylcellulose solution) and estradiol (2-4 μg/24 hour from implant) on sebum secretion (left columns) and mitosis in sebaceous glands (right columns) in castrated male rats treated with testosterone (0.2 mg/24 hour from implant). Means ±S.E. for groups of 6 rats.

(Figure 5). Thus, it must be presumed that estrogens act principally by reducing intracellular lipid synthesis.

The discovery that certain nonestrogenic steroids (eg, A-norprogesterone, 17α-methyl-B-nortestosterone, or cyproterone acetate) will act as antiandrogens in the sense that they antagonize the action of androgens at their target sites has opened up further possibilities of reducing sebaceous secretion.[41] In theory, it might be expected that such compounds, in contrast to estrogens, would act at the same point as androgens and reduce sebaceous gland activity, at least in part, by inhibition of sebaceous mitosis. Experiments on rats with 17α-methyl-B-nortestosterone[42] and cyproterone acetate[40] (Figure 5) confirmed that this is so. It is also of particular interest that a dose of 2 μg a day of estradiol has a greater effect in reducing secretion than 5 mg of cyproterone acetate; furthermore, the two compounds in these doses have an additive effect when given simultaneously. Thus, their points of action must be quite distinct.

Anti-androgens have been used with some success in the treatment of both hirsutism and acne vulgaris in females. Hammerstein and Cupceancu[43]

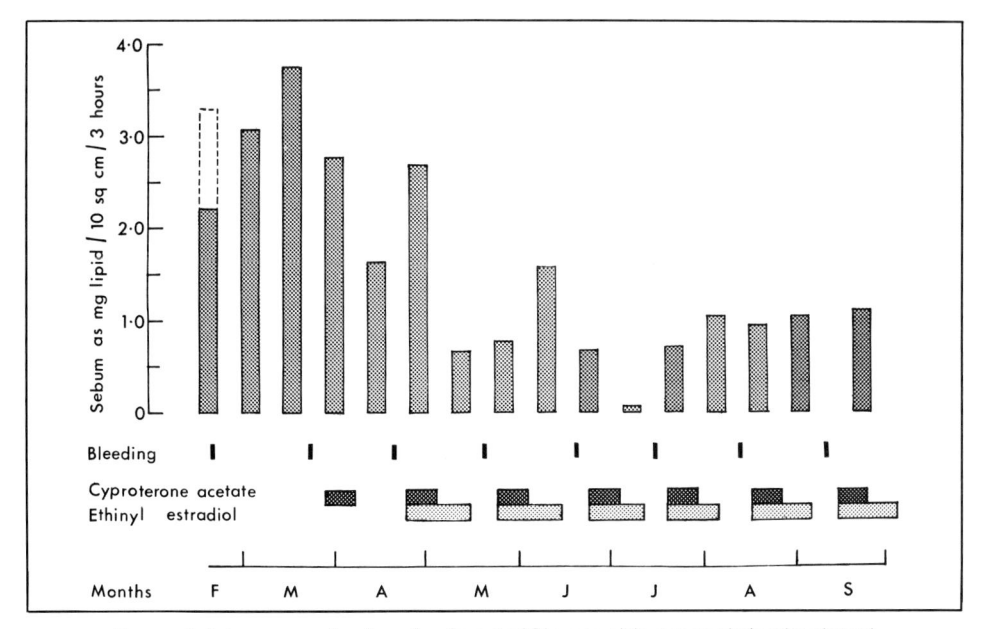

Figure 6. Sebum secretion from forehead of 21-year-old woman during treatment with cyproterone acetate and ethinyl estradiol. First measurement (shaded part of histogram) was for a 2-hour period only. Patient had history of increasing hirsutism from age 16, but no other symptoms of virilization or any evidence of endocrine abnormality. Reproduced with permission from Ebling FJ, Thomas AK, Cooke ID, et al: Effect of cyproterone acetate on hair growth, sebaceous secretion and endocrine parameters in a hirsute subject. *Br J Dermatol* 97:371, 1977.

devised a so-called "reversed two-phase therapy," in which 100 mg of cyproterone acetate is given orally each day from the 5th to the 14th days of the menstrual cycle, combined with 50 μg of ethinyl estradiol from the 5th to the 25th days. Braendle et al[44] treated 329 female patients in this way, and reported that 90% of those with acne showed improvement or disappearance of symptoms after 3 months. The treatment is anticonceptive, and no pregnancy was observed in more than 2000 treatment cycles; however, pregnancy was carefully excluded before treatment was started, since it was emphasized that cyproterone acetate could affect the development of a male fetus.

How does such treatment work? Barnes et al[45] carried out a careful study of 2 hirsute female patients treated in the manner described above. Before medication, both had urinary and plasma testosterone levels markedly above those in nonhirsute control individuals; after medication, these levels progressively fell. However, even after considerable improvement in the hirsutism, the plasma testosterone levels remained well above normal. The authors argued that the mechanism of action of the combined therapy was two-fold. There was, without doubt, a clear suppression of androgen production. But, since similar reductions could be produced by conventional contraceptive pills without greatly affecting hirsutism, the authors concluded that the more important action of cyproterone acetate in improving hirsutism must be a peripheral anti-androgenic effect.

The combined cyproterone acetate and estradiol therapy effectively reduces sebaceous secretion. Detailed study of a female patient (Figure 6) indicated a marked reduction in sebaceous secretion after 2 cycles of treatment, and a subsequent steady improvement of pustular acne.[46]

Anti-androgens and estrogens are not the only compounds which might reduce sebaceous secretion and thus have potential use in the treatment of acne. Steroids exist which inhibit 5α-reductase activity but are not anti-androgenic. Such a substance ought to inhibit the action of testosterone, but not that of 5α-dihydrotestosterone, in sebaceous secretion. There is some experimental proof of this proposition.

REFERENCES

1. Pochi PE, Strauss JS: Endocrinological control of the development and activity of the human sebaceous gland. *J Invest Dermatol* 62:191, 1974.
2. Ebling FJ: Hormonal control and methods of measuring sebaceous gland activity. *J Invest Dermatol* 62:161, 1974.
3. Pochi PE, Strauss JS, Rao GS, et al: Plasma testosterone and estrogen levels, urine testosterone excretion, and sebum production in males with acne vulgaris. *J Clin Endocrinol* 25:1660, 1965.
4. Förström L, Mustakallio KK, Dessypris A, et al: Plasma testosterone levels and acne. *Acta Derm Venereol (Stockh)* 54:369, 1974.
5. Lim LS, James VH: Plasma androgens in acne vulgaris. *Br J Dermatol* 91:135, 1974.
6. Strauss JS, Kligman AM, Pochi PE: The effect of androgens and estrogens on human sebaceous glands. *J Invest Dermatol* 39:139, 1962.
7. Pochi PE, Strauss JS: Sebum production, casual sebum levels, titratable acidity of sebum, and urinary fractional 17-ketosteroid excretion in males with acne. *J Invest Dermatol* 43:383, 1964.
8. Cunliffe WJ, Shuster S: Pathogenesis of acne. *Lancet* 1:685, 1969.
9. Burton JL, Shuster S: The relationship between seborrhea and acne vulgaris. *Br J Dermatol* 84:600, 1971.
10. Powell EW, Beveridge GW: Sebum excretion and sebum composition in adolescent men with and without acne vulgaris. *Br J Dermatol* 82:243, 1970.
11. Mauvais-Jarvis P, Charransol G, Bobas-Masson F: Simultaneous determination of urinary androstanediol and testosterone as an evaluation of human androgenicity. *J Clin Endocrinol Metab* 36:452, 1973.
12. Strauss JS, Pochi PE: "The Hormonal Control of Human Sebaceous Glands," in Montagna W, Ellis RA, Silver AF (Eds): *Advances in Biology of Skin*, vol 4, *The Sebaceous Glands*, pp 220-252. Oxford: Pergamon Press, 1963.
13. Strauss JS, Pochi PE: The human sebaceous gland: its regulation by steroidal hormones and its use as an end-organ for assaying androgenicity *in vivo*. *Recent Prog Horm Res* 19:385, 1963.
14. Ebling FJ: "Hormonal Control of Mammalian Skin Glands," in Muller-Schwarze

D, Mozell MM (Eds): *Chemical Signals in Vertebrates*, pp 17-33. New York: Plenum, 1977.
15. Jarrett A: The effects of progesterone and testosterone on surface sebum and acne vulgaris. *Br J Dermatol* 71:102, 1959.
16. Strauss JS, Pochi PE: The quantitative gravimetric determination of sebum production. *J Invest Dermatol* 36:293, 1961.
17. Ebling FJ: "Sebaceous Glands," in Marzulli FN, Maibach HI (Eds): *Dermatotoxicology and Pharmacology*, pp 55-92. Washington DC: Hemisphere, 1977.
18. Shuster S, Thody AJ: The control and measurement of sebum secretion. *J Invest Dermatol* 62:172, 1974.
19. Ebling FJ: "Hormonal Control of the Sebaceous Gland in Experimental Animals," in Montagna W, Ellis RA, Silver AF (Eds): *Advances in Biology of Skin*, vol 4, *The Sebaceous Glands*, pp 200-219. Oxford: Pergamon Press, 1963.
20. Houssay BA: Hormonal factors of growth. Proceedings of the Sixth Pan-American Congress of Endocrinology. *Excerpta Medica* 112:11, 1965.
21. Ebling FJ: The action of testosterone on the sebaceous glands and epidermis in castrated and hypophysectomized male rats. *J Endocrinol* 15:297, 1957.
22. Lasher N, Lorincz AL, Rothman S: Hormonal effects on sebaceous glands in the white rat. II. The effect of the pituitary-adrenal axis. *J Invest Dermatol* 22:25, 1954.
23. Lasher N, Lorincz AL, Rothman S: Hormonal effects on sebaceous glands in the white rat. III. Evidence for the presence of a pituitary sebaceous gland tropic factor. *J Invest Dermatol* 24:499, 1955.
24. Ebling FJ, Ebling E, Skinner J: The influence of pituitary hormones on the response of the sebaceous glands of the male rat to testosterone. *J Endocrinol* 45:245, 1969.
25. Ebling FJ, Ebling E, Randall V, et al: The sebotrophic action of bovine growth hormone (BGH) in the rat. *Br J Dermatol* 92:325, 1975.
26. Ebling FJ, Ebling E, Randall V, et al: The synergistic action of a α-melanocyte-stimulating hormone and testosterone on the sebaceous, prostate, preputial, Harderian and lachrymal glands, seminal vesicles and brown adipose tissue in the hypophysectomized-castrated rat. *J Endocrinol* 66:407, 1975.
27. Horrobin DF: *Prolactin: Physiology and Clinical Significance*. Lancaster: Medical and Technical Pub, 1972.
28. Ebling FJ, Ebling E, Skinner J: The effects of thyrotrophic hormone and of thyroxine on the response of the sebaceous glands of the rat to testosterone. *J Endocrinol* 48:83, 1970.
29. Lorincz AL, Lancaster G: Anterior pituitary preparation with tropic activity for sebaceous, preputial and Harderian glands. *Science* 126:124, 1957.
30. Woodbury LP, Lorincz AL, Ortega P: Studies on pituitary sebotropic activity. II. Further purification of a pituitary preparation with sebotropic activity. *J Invest Dermatol* 45:364, 1965.
31. Burton JL, Libman LJ, Cunliffe WJ, et al: Sebum excretion in acromegaly. *Br Med J* 1:406, 1972.
32. Goolamali SK, Burton JL, Shuster S: Sebum excretion in hypopituitarism. *Br J Dermatol* 89:21, 1973.
33. Ebling FJ: The role of the pituitary in acne. *Cutis* 17:469, 1976.
34. King RJB, Mainwaring WIP: *Steroid-Cell Interactions*. London: Butterworth, 1975.
35. Sansone G, Reisner RM: Differential rates of conversion of testosterone to dihydrotestosterone in acne and in normal human skin. *J Invest Dermatol* 56:366, 1971.
36. Ebling FJ, Ebling E, McCaffery V, et al: The response of the sebaceous glands of the hypophysectomized-castrated male rat to 5α-dihydrotestosterone, androstenedione, dehydroepiandrosterone and androsterone. *J Endocrinol* 51:181, 1971.
37. Ebling FJ, Ebling E, McCaffery V, et al: The responses of the sebaceous glands of

the hypophysectomized-castrated male rat to 5α-androstanedione and 5α-androstane-3β,17β-diol. *J Invest Dermatol* 60:183, 1973.
38. Jarrett A: The effects of stilboestrol on the surface sebum and upon acne vulgaris. *Br J Dermatol* 67:165, 1955.
39. Ebling FJ: "Steroid Hormones and Sebaceous Secretion," in Briggs MH (Ed): *Advances in Steroids,* vol 2. London: Academic Press, 1970.
40. Ebling FJ: The effects of cyproterone acetate and oestradiol upon testosterone-stimulated sebaceous activity in the rat. *Acta Endocrinol (Kbh)* 72:361, 1973.
41. Ebling FJ: "Antiandrogens in Dermatology," in Martini L, Motta M (Eds): *Androgens and Antiandrogens.* New York: Raven Press, 1977.
42. Ebling FJ: The action of an anti-androgenic steroid, 17α-methyl-B-nortestosterone, on sebum secretion in rats treated with testosterone. *J Endocrinol* 38:181, 1967.
43. Hammerstein J, Cupceancu B: Behandlung des Hirsutismus mit Cyproteronacetat. *Dtsch Med Wochenschr* 94:829, 1969.
44. Braendle W, Boess H, Breckwoldt M, et al: Wirkung und nebenwirkung der cyproteroneacetatbehandlung. *Arch Gynaekol* 216:335, 1974.
45. Barnes EW, Irvine WJ, Hunter WM, et al: Cyproterone acetate: a study involving two volunteers with idiopathic hirsutism. *Clin Endocrinol (Oxf)* 4:65, 1975.
46. Ebling FJ, Thomas AK, Cooke ID, et al: Effect of cyproterone acetate on hair growth, sebaceous secretion and endocrine parameters in a hirsute subject. *Br J Dermatol* 97:371, 1977.

Chapter 8

Free Fatty Acid Hypothesis: Summarized

ROBERT E. KELLUM, MD

The need to understand the pathogenic mechanisms of acne vulgaris has preoccupied clinicians and investigators for years. Prior to 1960, a loose consortium of hormones, dirt, dietary factors, psychological factors, and bacterial infections (presumably staphylococcal) was nebulously thought to be responsible for the pathogenesis of acne. Consequently, most patients were burdened with long, unworkable diets, reams of misinformation, and possibly even harmful treatments. Myths abounded regarding the cause of acne; traditional and foul-smelling complex pharmaceutical concoctions were dispensed, and acne pathogenesis remained entirely obscured behind an aura of mystery and trial-and-error. The fact that acne began and proliferated during the rising hormonal levels of pubertal years was unquestioned; that certain genetically-acquired skin types seemed predisposed to the more severe and scarring acne lesions was apparent; that skin oiliness was associated with disastrous acne sequelae in some, while others with similar greasy skin were spared was obvious, albeit perplexing. All these diverse facts and observations lacked any cohesive, integrated, or logical basis for evaluation or interpretation.

In 1960, Strauss and Kligman[1] reported that sebum, separated from its free fatty acids and injected intradermally, caused no inflammation, while total skin surface lipids or the isolated free fatty acid fraction caused severe inflammatory changes in the skin.[2] From these observations, an investigative hypothesis evolved to explore, in an orderly scientific pattern, the various interrelated pathogenic factors of acne. With minor modifications, this hypothesis for the pathogenesis of acne still stands as the major working model for many investigators. This Chapter examines the current evidence for that major hypothesis around which many investigators have focused their scientific efforts for almost 20 years.

The free fatty acid hypothesis proposes that five key factors interact to cause acne. (Each of these factors is reviewed in detail in other sections of this book, and the reader is referred to these sections for background information. Only the interactions will be discussed here.) These factors are: 1) androgenic hormones; 2) lipids arising in the sebaceous glands; 3) the follicular bacteria, predominantly *Propionibacterium acnes;* 4) abnormalities of pilosebaceous anatomy and keratinization; and 5) genetic factors.

The free fatty acid hypothesis proposes that: 1) under the driving stimulation of androgenic hormones, human sebaceous glands enlarge, with resulting increased production of sebaceous lipids; 2) the major sebaceous lipid component, triglyceride, is hydrolyzed (split) in the sebaceous follicle by the action of esterase-lipases from *P. acnes* to yield free fatty acids; 3) certain free fatty acids act as irritants and/or comedogenic agents to damage the wall of the sebaceous follicle, leading to subsequent follicular rupture and extrusion of keratinous debris, lipids, and bacteria into the surrounding dermis, producing the initial inflammatory events of acne.

Evidence in Support of the Free Fatty Acid Hypothesis

ANDROGENIC HORMONES

Ample evidence exists for a key role of androgenic hormones in the pathogenesis of acne.[3-6] Strauss, Kligman and Pochi[4] demonstrated that androgens stimulate sebaceous production and estrogenic substances suppress sebaceous activity. Without androgens, acne doesn't develop. Prepuberal castrates and eunuchs show no acne.[7] The tissue-active androgen is probably dihydrotestosterone (DHT), converted from testosterone by the enzyme, 5α-reductase.[8] Individuals lacking the 5α-reductase enzyme display no acne.[9] Furthermore, Sansone and Reisner[10] demonstrated that the skin from acne patients converts testosterone to dihydrotestosterone at a rate 2-20 times that of normal skin. This, of course, raises the question of an abnormal end-organ response in acne patients. The active testosterone metabolites in human scalp and back skin were found to be DHT and 3 β-androstanediol.

SEBACEOUS GLAND LIPIDS

Sebaceous lipids are an essential factor in acne. As noted earlier, clinical development of acne has always been associated with increased sebaceous activity at puberty, and patients with acne produce large amounts of sebum.[6] Sebum is an irritant, and free fatty acids are the most irritating components of sebum.[2,11] In an analysis of lipids from isolated human sebaceous glands, however, only triglycerides, squalene, and wax esters were found.[12] No free fatty acids were present in these lipids extracted from human sebaceous glands. Within the lumen of the sebaceous follicle, however, and extending into the surface lipids, free fatty acid levels rise dramatically, presumably as a result of lipolysis by follicular bacterial enzymes.[13-15] Free fatty acids with chain lengths of around C_{12} produce the greatest irritation on human skin,[16] and free fatty acids with chain lengths from C_{12} to C_{18} were most strongly comedogenic, as tested in the rabbit ear.[17] Great variations exist in the amount of free fatty acids present in skin surface lipids of different individuals.

Thus, free fatty acids are constantly being liberated in the depths of the pilosebaceous follicle. The free fatty acid hypothesis proposes that these free fatty acids lead to the clinical stages of acne.

FOLLICULAR BACTERIA

The dominant organism in the depths of the sebaceous follicle, and the organism with the greatest lipolytic activity, is the anaerobic diphtheroid, *P. acnes*. Many investigators have confirmed the role of *P. acnes* in the liberation of free fatty acids from sebaceous gland triglycerides.[14,15,18] Other sources of lipolytic enzymes (*eg, cocci, yeast, etc*) do not seem to play a significant role in the liberation of free fatty acids *in vivo*, and the conclusion was made that the anaerobic diphtheroids are the major source of such activity. The clinical improvement of acne with the use of tetracycline demonstrates good correlation between suppression of free fatty acid levels and reduction in population of *P. acnes*.[13,19]

ABNORMALITIES OF FOLLICULAR ANATOMY AND KERATINIZATION

The anatomical structure of the sebaceous follicle, defined as a dilated follicular channel containing a diminutive hair and surrounded by huge clusters of sebaceous glands, is probably essential to the development of acne.[17,20] Kligman[20] emphasized the probable significance of comedo formation as one of the early essential stages of acne. Comedones consist of follicular impactions of keratin, sebaceous lipids, and entrapped follicular bacteria. Thus, rather than the normal sloughing of the keratinizing cells within the follicle, "retention hyperkeratosis," with accumulation and impaction of unusually adherent keratinocytes, leads invariably to visible open and closed comedones (blackheads and whiteheads). Some of these comedones evolve into the inflammatory lesions of acne.

Kligman contended that these abnormalities of keratinization are genetically preordained, with the degree and extent of follicular response and subsequent damage of the follicular wall subject to great individual variation. The free fatty acid hypothesis, however, proposes that it is the free fatty acids which trigger the development of these abnormal and altered keratinization patterns. Knutson[21] studied these abnormalities of follicular wall keratinization by electron microscopy, and demonstrated the unusual compacting and adherence of countless numbers of follicular keratinocytes. However, critical testing of this specific alternative within the depths of individual pilosebaceous follicles has not yet been possible.

Evidence Challenging the Free Fatty Acid Hypothesis

At the time of this writing, no challenges have been made to the multifactorial concepts of acne pathogenesis—hormones, lipids, follicular bacteria, and abnormalities in follicular anatomy and keratinization. The questions center around how these factors interact at the molecular level, and whether other, yet unknown factors may play a role.

Several studies have produced information which challenges the free fatty acid hypothesis in other areas. Fulton[22] conducted clinical studies of the topical application in human patients of bacterial lipase inhibitors (halopyridyl phosphorus compounds) to suppress the formation of free fatty acids. The potent bacterial lipase inhibitor, fospirate, was applied 2 times a day to the faces of 13 acne patients. Although the free fatty acids measured on the skin decreased dramatically in all patients, the bacterial counts of *P. acnes* and the number of acne lesions (open and closed comedones, papules, pustules, and cysts) remained unchanged, and the severity of clinical acne did not improve.

The apparent dramatic decrease in free fatty acids on the skin of these acne patients with no evidence of clinical improvement thus raises the question of the significance of free fatty acids in the pathogenesis of acne. A possible defect in the study was that it was carried on for only 5 weeks, and other investigators have demonstrated that acne lesions (open and closed comedones and inflammatory lesions) may develop over periods as long as 4 months.[23] These studies by Fulton have not been confirmed by other investigators.

Voss[24] believed that the role of free fatty acids in acne pathogenesis is, at best, circumstantial. He suggested that other metabolic activities of *P. acnes*, such as the possible significance of other bacterial enzymes to produce tissue inflammatory changes, or host immunologic response to the bacterial antigens of *P. acnes* (see Chapter 5), should be investigated.

Puhvel et al[25,26] reported increased immunologic reactivity to *P. acnes* in acne patients. They found elevated levels of serum antibodies to *P. acnes* and associated intensified immediate hypersensitivity reactions in acne patients (see Chapter 6). Puhvel and Sakamoto[27] questioned the role of free fatty acids in acne. More recently, Puhvel et al[28] reported that lymphocyte transformation from stimulation of *P. acnes* antigen was significantly greater in patients with severe nodulocystic acne as compared to control individuals without acne. This information suggests that patients with severe acne may be manifesting some type of cell-mediated immunity to the bacterial antigens of *P. acnes*. Whether abnormal immunologic responses to antigens from *P. acnes* could initiate the abnormal patterns of keratinization (retention hyperkeratosis), or could initiate the initial microscopic inflammatory events of acne, remains unanswered.

Relationships of Pathogenesis to Acne Therapy

Within the framework of the free fatty acid hypothesis, logic dictates that any therapeutic measure that reduces free fatty acids should be beneficial to the acne patient, and should offer confirming evidence for the hypothesis. Whether by reduction of sebum with superficial x-ray, estrogens, or anti-androgens, or by inhibition of triglyceride hydrolysis with systemic or topical antibiotics, benzoyl peroxide, *etc*, or by alteration of the dynamics of abnormal follicular keratinization with retinoic acid, all these therapeutic measures might be considered as confirmatory to the free fatty acid hypothesis. Other mechanisms of therapeutic effect may be operating, however, and further investigation is needed.

Summary

The free fatty acid hypothesis attempts to correlate all the facets of acne pathogenesis. It proposes that androgenic hormones stimulate the enlargement of human sebaceous glands, resulting in increased production of sebaceous gland triglycerides. These triglycerides are hydrolyzed within the pilosebaceous follicle by esterase-lipases arising from the predominant anaerobic follicular bacteria, *P. acnes*, to yield irritating and/or comedogenic free fatty acids which induce abnormal patterns of keratinization in follicular wall epithelium. These impactions of abnormal keratin distend the sebaceous follicle, with subsequent rupture of the follicular epithelium and extrusion of keratinous debris, bacteria, and a complex mixture of sebaceous lipids into the surrounding dermis.

At the time of this writing, the free fatty acid hypothesis has not yet been disproved. This author deeply believes in the basic premise of inferential reasoning: science advances only by disproof; no scientific hypothesis has been, or can ever be, proven.[29] Experimental hypotheses are not the personal property of any individual, group, investigative team, or nationality. They are universal possessions, formulated to be tested, to be challenged with carefully conceived experiments and, if possible, to be disproved—not to be guarded, or elevated to supreme heights. The greater sin is not to disprove a leading (popular) hypothesis, but to fail to formulate and develop a more viable hypothesis, to fail to define all the possible alternatives that might explain the proposed hypothesis, and to fail to expose each alternative to critical testing with all available investigative techniques.

REFERENCES

1. Strauss JS, Kligman AM: The pathologic dynamics of acne vulgaris. *Arch Dermatol* 82:779, 1960.
2. Strauss JS, Pochi PE: Intracutaneous injection of sebum and comedones: histologic observations. *Arch Dermatol* 92:443, 1965.
3. Strauss JS, Pochi PE: "The Hormonal Control of Human Sebaceous Glands," in Montagna W, Ellis RA, Silver AF (Eds): *Advances in Biology of Skin*, vol 4, *The Sebaceous Glands*, pp 220-254. Oxford: Pergamon Press, 1963.
4. Strauss JS, Kligman AM, Pochi PE: The effect of androgens and estrogens on human sebaceous glands. *J Invest Dermatol* 39:139, 1962.
5. Strauss JS, Pochi PE: The human sebaceous gland: its regulation by steroidal hormones and its use as an end-organ for assaying androgenicity *in vivo*. *Recent Prog Horm Res* 19:385, 1963.
6. Pochi PE, Strauss JS: Sebum production, casual sebum levels, titratable acidity of sebum, and urinary fractional 17-ketosteroid excretion in males with acne. *J Invest Dermatol* 43:383, 1964.
7. Hamilton JB: Male hormone substance: a prime factor in acne. *J Clin Endocrinol* 1:570, 1941.
8. Gomez EC, Hsia SL: *In vivo* metabolism of testosterone-4-C^{14} and Δ^4-androstene-3,17 dione-4-C^{14} in human skin. *Biochem* 7:24, 1968.
9. Imperato-McGinley J, Guerrero L, Gautier T, et al: Steroid 5α-reductase deficiency in man: an inherited form of male pseudohermaphroditism. *Science* 186:1213, 1974.
10. Sansone G, Reisner RM: Differential rates of conversion of testosterone to dihydrotestosterone in acne and in normal human skin—a possible pathogenic factor in acne. *J Invest Dermatol* 56:366, 1971.
11. Ray T, Kellum RE: Acne vulgaris: studies in pathogenesis: free fatty acid irritancy in patients with and without acne. *J Invest Dermatol* 57:6, 1971.
12. Kellum RE: Human sebaceous gland lipids. *Arch Dermatol* 95:218, 1967.
13. Freinkel RK, Strauss JS, Yip SY, et al: Effect of tetracycline on the composition of sebum in acne vulgaris. *N Engl J Med* 273:850, 1965.
14. Reisner RM, Silver DZ, Puhvel M, et al: Lipolytic activity of *Corynebacterium acnes*. *J Invest Dermatol* 51:190, 1968.
15. Kellum RE, Strangfeld K: Triglyceride hydrolysis by *Corynebacterium acnes in vitro*. *J Invest Dermatol* 52:255, 1969.
16. Kellum RE: Acne vulgaris: studies in pathogenesis: relative irritancy of free fatty acids from C_2 to C_{18}. *Arch Dermatol* 97:722, 1968.
17. Kligman AM, Katz AG: Pathogenesis of acne vulgaris. I. Comedogenic properties of human sebum in the external ear canal of the rabbit. *Arch Dermatol* 98:53, 1968.
18. Smith RF, Willett NP: Lipolytic activity of human cutaneous bacteria. *J Gen Microbiol* 52:441, 1968.
19. Strauss JS, Pochi PE: Effect of orally administered antibacterial agents on the titratable acidity of human sebum. *J Invest Dermatol* 47:577, 1966.
20. Kligman AM: An overview of acne. *J Invest Dermatol* 62:268, 1974.
21. Knutson DD: Ultrastructural observations in acne vulgaris: the normal sebaceous follicle and acne lesions. *J Invest Dermatol* 62:288, 1974.
22. Fulton JE Jr: Lipases: their questionable role in acne vulgaris. *Int J Dermatol* 15:732, 1976.
23. Orentreich N, Durr NP: The natural evolution of comedones into inflammatory papules and pustules. *J Invest Dermatol* 62:316, 1974.
24. Voss JG: Acne vulgaris and free fatty acids: a review and criticism. *Arch Dermatol* 109:894, 1974.

25. Puhvel SM, Barfatani M, Warnick MA, et al: Study of antibody levels to *Corynebacterium acnes*. *Arch Dermatol* 90:421, 1964.
26. Puhvel SM, Hoffman K, Sternberg TH, et al: Dermal hypersensitivity of patients with acne vulgaris to *Corynebacterium acnes*. *J Invest Dermatol* 49:154, 1967.
27. Puhvel SM, Sakamoto M: A reevaluation of fatty acids as inflammatory agents in acne. *J Invest Dermatol* 68:93, 1977.
28. Puhvel SM, Amirian DA, Weintraub J, et al: Lymphocyte transformation in subjects with nodulocystic acne. *Br J Dermatol* 97:205, 1977.
29. Platt JR: Strong inference. *Science* 146:347, 1964.

Chapter 9

Other Pathogenic Factors
RONALD M. REISNER, MD

This Chapter reviews the miscellaneous factors commonly related to acne and acneform eruptions, and presents a current pragmatic assessment of each and its relationship to acne. Some concern areas about which patients often have questions; others may serve as useful clues to aid in the treatment of stubborn or unexplained cases of acne. Many are still not fully resolved. Thus, as is often the case in medicine, the physician who is confronted with a problem requiring an action decision must, after weighing all the available evidence, use his best judgment to select the most appropriate course of treatment for the individual patient.

Medicaments

Medications may act to exacerbate existing acne or, more commonly, to produce acneform eruptions (see Chapter 3, 4, and 26). As noted elsewhere in this text, acneform eruptions are follicular reactions in which the comedo occurs but seldom, and then only after the formation of papules or pustules; the comedo is not, as it is in true acne, the initial development in the disease.

Halides—While iodides and bromides in sufficient amounts may cause exacerbation of active or dormant acne, they are most commonly known to produce a pustular eruption of sudden onset which extends well beyond the usual acne areas. Comedones in these halide eruptions appear, if at all, late in the course of acne, and in small numbers. Sources of iodides likely to be implicated include drugs used for the treatment of colds and asthma, radioopaque contrast materials, and some vitamin-mineral preparations.[1] Dietary iodide, such as that present in iodized salt, seafood, and some water supplies, was well-demonstrated to have no influence on the incidence of acne, and only slight influence on its severity.[2] Fad diets with high iodide supplementation, such as large quantities of kelp pills, seem to be related to flares of preexisting acne. Bromide, once popular in sedatives, analgesics, and cold remedies, is much less often encountered today.

Anticonvulsants—Diphenylhydantoin, phenobarbital, and trimethadione are among the better known anticonvulsant drugs which can produce acneform eruptions in susceptible individuals.[3]

Isonicotinic Acid Hydrazide (Isoniazid)—This drug produces an inflammatory papular eruption of wide extent in some patients, usually after several months or more of therapy.[4]

Hormones—A common acneform eruption which may be associated either with the systemic administration of adrenocorticotropic hormone (ACTH) or corticosteroids,[5] or with the topical application of potent corticosteroids,[6] is known as corticosteroid acne. It is usually of abrupt onset, consisting initially of inflammatory papules, some of which develop into pustules or closed and then open comedones; this is essentially the reverse of the usual sequential evolution in acne vulgaris (comedo first, inflammatory lesion subsequently). Therapy, in addition to decreasing or discontinuing corticosteroids when possible, consists of topical retinoic acid and systemic tetracycline.[7]

Tetracycline—In addition to a superinfection manifesting as a gram-negative folliculitis,[8] a rare pustular acneform eruption due to long-term tetracycline therapy has been described in association with an increased number of *Pityrosporon ovale*.[9,10]

Androgens—Increased androgens, particularly in females, eunuchs, and prepubertal children, have the capacity to produce true acne in susceptible individuals. Androgens may be increased indirectly by the exogenous administration of gonadotropins, or directly by the administration of testosterone, anabolic steroids, or androgenic progestational agents in contraceptive pills (see Chapter 22).

In a woman, the sudden onset of acne, particularly relatively severe acne, should promptly lead the physician to consider the rare, but very real, possibility of an increase in endogenous androgen associated with a virilizing syndrome. The acne in such situations may precede the onset of hirsutism or clitoral enlargement, and may be a valuable early clinical clue.

Miscellaneous Drugs of Uncertain Etiologic Significance—There have been isolated reports[11-14] suggesting, but not proving, the occasional relationship of the use of a variety of drugs with the development of acneform eruptions. Drugs included have been vitamin B_{12}, disulfiram, chloral hydrate, thiourea, thiouracil, quinine, lithium, and halothane (see Chapter 26).

External Contactants (Including Cosmetics)

The acne patient may well ask whether cosmetics or other materials applied to the skin will aggravate or cause acne. Patient awareness of the role of external contactants may help in explaining the problem of resistant acne or acne in unusual locations. Comedones are the significant feature of this group of true acnes precipitated by external contactants.

Occupational Acne—Occupational acne is characterized primarily by comedones, with variable numbers of papules, pustules, and nodulocystic lesions. It involves areas of skin, often located well outside the usual acne-bearing areas, which are exposed to allow contact with the acnegenic substances (see Chapter 3). Substances involved include chlorinated hydrocarbons[15] (the most potent of the occupational contactants); insoluble cutting oils; and petroleum oil, coal tar, and their derivatives. Management consists primarily of prevention, including avoidance of exposure, frequent changes of clothing with appropriate laundering, and compulsory bathing. In addition to eliminating exposure, the use of a potent comedolytic (eg, retinoic acid) for the predominantly comedonal component, as well as additional therapy appropriate to the type of lesion present, are indicated. Systemic exposure to some of these compounds occasionally occurs (eg, the case of the Japanese "epidemic" affecting several hundred people who ingested cooking oil contaminated with a chlorbiphenyl). The route by which the substance reaches the intraductal area appears to be via sebaceous gland excretion.[15]

Cosmetics—Kligman and Mills[16] proposed the term "acne cosmetica" to describe a low-grade, chronic eruption consisting primarily of closed comedones with occasional papulopustular lesions, and chiefly involving the cheeks and chin of women between 20-50 years of age (see Chapter 3). They attributed the eruption to the chronic use of cosmetics, especially facial creams, night creams, moisturizers, and similar preparations which contain weak acnegens as demonstrated in the rabbit ear model. Because variations in concentrations of individual ingredients and the additive or synergistic effect of ingredient combinations may significantly affect the final comedogenicity of any given preparation, it is almost impossible to determine from the ingredient list alone the exact degree of comedogenicity, if any, of a given preparation. Fulton[17] published a list of cosmetics graded according to their comedogenic potential in the rabbit ear, which may serve as a rough guide to the selection of cosmetics. However, because of frequent changes both in available cosmetics and their ingredients, such lists require frequent review to be practically useful.

Since a great many women are significantly helped to live with their acne by the use of cosmetics, such use should not be routinely interdicted. If adequate lists of relatively noncomedogenic cosmetics are not readily available, patients should be advised to minimize the use of cream-base preparations and use water-base lotion makeup for coverup. Fortunately, lipstick, rouge, eyelash makeup, and various cleansers do not appear to be comedogenic. Some sunscreens were described by Mills and Kligman[18] as being fairly potent acnegens; they should thus be considered as possible culprits if a case of acne cosmetica is suspected. Pomades are another source of acneform eruptions which produce an almost exclusively comedonal response. Discontinuation of comedogenic cosmetics is said to be curative, but this may require 6-8 months. Active therapy directed toward the lesion types present should be carried out, whether or not the patient is willing to discontinue the use of cosmetics.

Hygiene

Despite popular mythology to the contrary, there is no significant evidence that rest or the lack of it, too much sex or not enough, masturbation, amount of water intake, or constipation have any influence on the prevalence or severity of acne. The same is true of the direct effects of exercise or the lack of it. Exercise may indirectly produce mechanical trauma to acne-bearing areas from the use of various sports accessories (*eg*, straps, helmets, headbands, pads, tape, *etc*), which may in turn exacerbate pre-existing acne, especially inflammatory acne.[19]

Heat and humidity sometimes play a role in aggravating acne vulgaris, whether due to climate or to local factors such as clothing. This effect is magnified by concomitant friction. This appears to be a lesser form of the extensive, severe, and disabling type of acne known as tropical acne, seen in some individuals who leave a temperate climate for a hot, humid climate (see Chapter 1 and 3). In cases of climate-related disease, treatment is ineffective unless the exposure to heat and humidity is eliminated. Flares due to local heat, humidity, and friction, however, are temporary conditions, and can be treated.

Emotional Stress

Some, but not all, acne patients are commonly observed to undergo exacerbation of their acne during periods of stress, although any given individual will not necessarily experience exacerbations with every episode of stress. The mechanism by which this occurs is unknown, although a range of explanations has been proposed. Exacerbation may be due to the simple increase of mechanical manipulation as a response to the stress, resulting in follicular wall damage and the incitement of new inflammatory lesions. Exacerbation may be due, on the other hand, to complex perturbations of the pituitary-adrenal axis (*eg*, ACTH produces greater increases in urinary glucocorticoids in those with acne than in those without acne[20]), resulting in increased sebum production and even in unexplained increases in the free fatty acids of sebum.[21]

The lack of a fully satisfactory explanation does not prevent the physician from being sensitive to the emotional state of the patient and providing a sympathetic ear, judicious support, and reassurance. Occasionally, the *limited*, not long-term, use of appropriate psychotropic drugs is indicated, while continuing an intensive regimen of dermatologic therapy.

Perhaps more often than not, the patient's emotional responses are the result, rather than the cause, of the acne vulgaris and its exacerbations. It has been suggested that one clear-cut exception to this is the explosive acne conglobata-like eruption, pyoderma faciale (see Chapter 3), occurring exclusively on the face of postadolescent females; severe emotional trauma is regularly responsible for precipitating this type of eruption.[5]

Diet

Probably no single facet of the management of acne has been characterized by so much discussion shedding so little light as the role of diet. In general, advice has consisted of the proscription of one, several, and often many foods (see Chapter 24). Lists of forbidden foods have featured such items as chocolate, cola drinks, fish and other seafoods, iodized salt, nuts, pork and other fatty meats, fried foods, milk, cheese, citrus fruits, spices, and on and on.

Although extreme changes in diet have been reported to alter both the sebum excretion rate and sebum composition in humans,[22-24] there is no convincing evidence that alterations in diet influence the clinical course of acne. Properly controlled clinical studies would obviously be very difficult to do, essentially involving prolonged residence in a completely controlled metabolic unit setting. However, the few studies that have been done do not support the role of diet as an aggravating factor in acne.

A well-constructed, double-blind study[24] on the effect of large amounts of chocolate on acne patients revealed no significant differences in total lesion counts. This study was criticized[25] on the grounds that pustular lesions should have been counted separately from comedones, and that the counting should have been done earlier to identify any possible diet-related changes, based on the expectation that diet-related flares of acne occur 1-3 days after ingestion of the suspected food. It might well be argued that this sounds more like the description of a papulopustular acneform follicular reaction than one of true acne in which the initial lesion is a comedo which leads, after weeks or months, to inflammatory lesions. However, even this type of acute reaction to foods ingested in ordinary amounts either does not exist or must be quite rare.

In another study,[26] acne patients who believed that specific foods (including chocolate, milk, nuts, and cola drinks) were responsible for flares of their acne were fed large quantities of the suspected food. During observation in the days immediately following ingestion, no significant change in the number or character of acne lesions was observed, thus denying even the concept that selected foods could produce acute papulopustular eruptions in acne patients (see Chapter 12 and 24).

An interesting pustular eruption involving acne-prone areas in young adults who received intravenous hyperalimentation[27] with solutions which proved to be deficient in L-cysteine, L-tyrosine, L-glutaminic acid and L-aspartic acid provides an intriguing observation. Effectively pursued, this observation might shed light on the pathogenesis of follicular pustular reactions.

A recent review of diet in relation to acne[25] concluded, in part, that, while there is evidence in animals and man suggesting that sebaceous gland function can be altered by gross dietary manipulation, it remains to be determined whether more moderate dietary alterations would have similar effects. Such gross or moderate dietary alterations are likely to remain difficult, if not impossible, to study in the acne patient. Since there is no reliable evidence that the removal of any food or foods from the diet, or any other reasonable achievable dietary alteration, affects the course of acne, there seems no reason to add dietary restrictions to the problems the acne patient must already face. If an individual is firmly convinced that a single given food is responsible for the flaring of his acne, it seems sensible to avoid a campaign to convince the patient to eat that food. Intervention would only seem worthwhile if the patient had developed a pattern of food restrictions which resulted in a nutritionally inadequate diet. Conversely, reassurance concerning the diet is often gratefully received.

At today's level of knowledge, the best advice to an acne patient would seem to be: "What you eat has no effect on your acne, but it is common sense to eat a well-balanced diet for your general health."

REFERENCES

1. Hitch JM: Acneiform eruption induced by drugs and chemicals. *JAMA* 200:879, 1967.
2. Hitch JM, Greenburg BG: Adolescent acne and dietary iodine. *Arch Dermatol* 84:898, 1961.
3. Jenkins RD, Ratner AC: Diphenylhydantoin and acne. *N Engl J Med* 287:148, 1972.
4. Cohen LK, George W, Smith R: Isoniazid-induced acne and pellagra: occurrence in slow inactivators of isoniazid (editorial). *Arch Dermatol* 109:377, 1974.
5. Plewig G, Kligman AM: *Acne: Morphogenesis and Treatment*. New York: Springer-Verlag, 1975.
6. Kaidbey KH, Kligman AM: The pathogenesis of topical steroid acne. *J Invest Dermatol* 62:31, 1974.
7. Mills OH Jr, Leyden JJ, Kligman AM: Tretinoin treatment of steroid acne. *Arch Dermatol* 108:381, 1973.
8. Leyden JJ, Marples RR, Mills OH Jr, et al: Gram-negative folliculitis—a complication of antibiotic therapy in acne vulgaris. *Br J Dermatol* 88:533, 1973.
9. Weary PE, Russell CM, Butler HK, et al: Acneiform eruption resulting from antibiotic administration. *Arch Dermatol* 100:179, 1969.

10. Bean SF: Acneiform eruption from tetracycline. *Br J Dermatol* 85:385, 1971.
11. Michel PJ: Un cas d'acne important du visage consecutif a l'administration de vitamine B$_{12}$. *Bull Soc Fr Dermatol Syphiligr* 76:131, 1968.
12. Soper LE, Vitez TS, Weinberg D: Metabolism of halogenated anesthetic agents as a possible cause of acneiform eruptions. *Anesth Analg (Cleve)* 52:125, 1973.
13. Ruiz-Maldonado R, Pérez de Francisco C, Tamayo L: Lithium dermatitis. *JAMA* 224:1534, 1973.
14. Frank S: Uncommon aspects of common acne. *Cutis* 14:817, 1974.
15. Crow KD: Chloracne: a critical review including a comparison of two series of cases of acne from chlornaphthalene and pitch fumes. *Trans St Johns Hosp Dermatol Soc* 56:79, 1970.
16. Kligman AM, Mills OH Jr: "Acne cosmetica." *Arch Dermatol* 106:843, 1972.
17. Fulton JE Jr, Bradley S, Agundez A, et al: Noncomedogenic cosmetics. *Cutis* 17:344, 1976.
18. Mills OH Jr, Kligman AM: Acne aestivalis. *Arch Dermatol* 111:891, 1975.
19. Mills OH Jr, Kligman AM: Acne mechanica. *Arch Dermatol* 111:481, 1975.
20. Pekkarinen A, Sonck CE: Adrenocortical reserves in acne vulgaris: the urinary excretion of 17-ketosteroids and total 17-hydroxycorticosteroids. *Acta Derm Venereol (Stockh)* 42:200, 1962.
21. Krauss SJ: Stress, acne and skin surface free fatty acids. *Psychosom Med* 32:503, 1970.
22. MacDonald I: Dietary carbohydrates and skin lipids. *Br J Dermatol* 79:119, 1967.
23. MacDonald I: Effects of a skimmed milk and chocolate diet on serum and skin lipids. *J Sci Food Agric* 19:270, 1968.
24. Fulton JE, Plewig G, Kligman AM: Effect of chocolate on acne vulgaris. *JAMA* 210:2071, 1969.
25. Rasmussen JE: Diet and acne. *Int J Dermatol* 16:488, 1977.
26. Anderson PC: Foods as the cause of acne. *Am Fam Physician* 3:102, 1971.
27. Schlappner OL, Shelley WB, Ruberg RL, et al: Acute papulopustular acne associated with prolonged intravenous hyperalimentation. *JAMA* 219:877, 1972.

Chapter 10

Comedo Formation: Ultrastructure

DENNIS D. KNUTSON, MD

Acne is a disease of specialized cutaneous structures known as sebaceous follicles. These follicles are found in large numbers on the face, and in lesser numbers on the neck, upper extremities and trunk. The initial pathologic lesion of acne is the comedo, an impaction of keratinized cells within the sebaceous follicle.[1]

The beginning of a comedo can be seen through the electron microscope as an alteration in the normal keratinization of the epithelial lining of the sebaceous follicle infundibulum.[2] The infundibulum is the segment of the follicle distal to the point where the sebaceous ducts join the pilary canal to form the pilosebaceous canal. On the basis of the type of keratinized cells which line the normal infundibulum, the pilosebaceous canal can be subdivided into a terminal acroinfundibulum continuous with the epidermis and a proximal infrainfundibulum in continuity with the sebaceous duct[3] (Figure 1).

The acroinfundibulum terminates at the follicular orifice. It has an epithelial lining which keratinizes in a fashion similar to epidermis. The granular layer of the acroinfundibulum contains large, prominent, keratohyalin granules, and it produces a thick, protective, horny layer (stratum corneum) of adherent, compact, dense stacks of cornified cells (Figure 2).

The epithelial lining of the infrainfundibulum also keratinizes, but in a quite different and unique manner. The thin granular layer contains a few small keratohyalin granules. The horny layer is attenuated, and consists of rather flimsy cornified cells which are filamentous and loosely attached, and

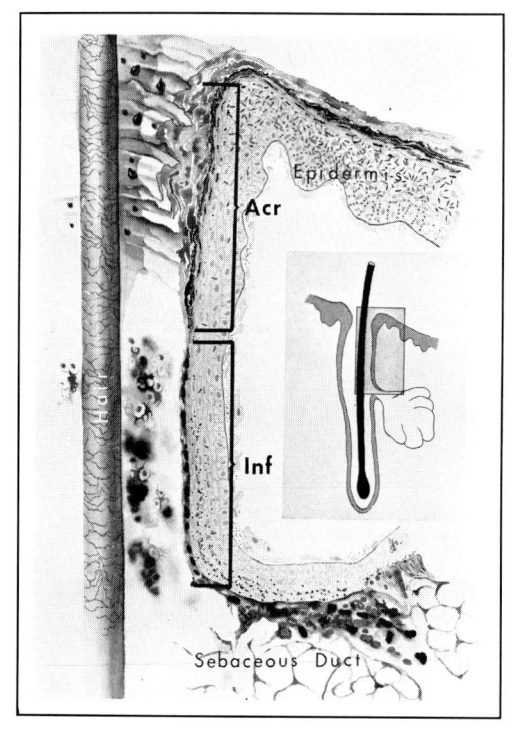

Figure 1. Schematic diagram of infundibulum of normal sebaceous follicle. Shaded box in inset diagram indicates area depicted in larger drawing. Keratinized layer of infrainfundibulum (Inf) is thin and disintegrates easily (see Figure 3 and 4). Thicker, more cohesive, keratinized layer of acroinfundibulum (Acr) is similar to horny layer of the epidermis (see Figure 2).

which disintegrate and slough as fine fragments into the stream of sebum flowing through the pilosebaceous canal. Between these rather indistinct keratinized cells are large clusters of lamellar granules (also called Odland bodies, keratinosomes, or membrane-coating granules), which are tiny lysosome-like structures extruded from cells of the granular layer (Figure 3 and 4). The function of the lamellar granules is unknown, although they contain hydrolytic enzymes which could be responsible for separation or disintegration of the keratinized cells.[4] While lamellar granules are present in the cornified layers of the epidermis and the acroinfundibulum, they appear more numerous in the disintegrating horny layer of the infrainfundibulum, a finding consistent with their possible enzymatic function.

The visible changes in keratinization which lead to comedo formation begin in the infrainfundibulum, where the follicular canal is filled with large

COMEDO FORMATION 83

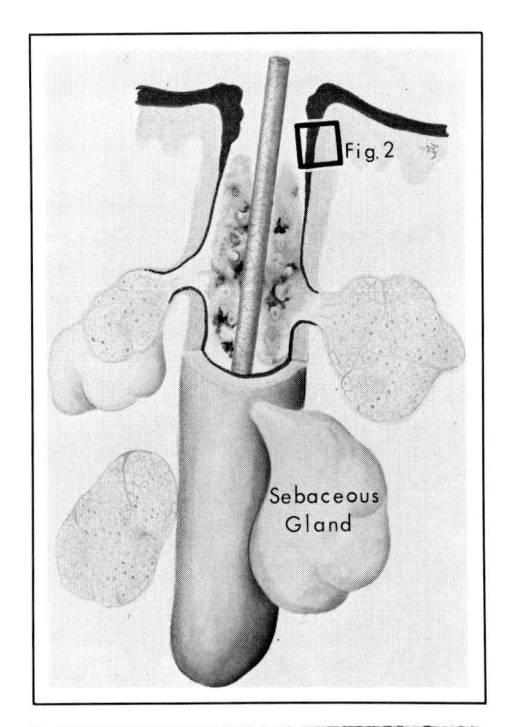

Figure 2. Acroinfundibulum. Keratohyalin granules are abundant. Distinct, compact, cornified cells comprise thick stratum corneum (reduced from ×4000).

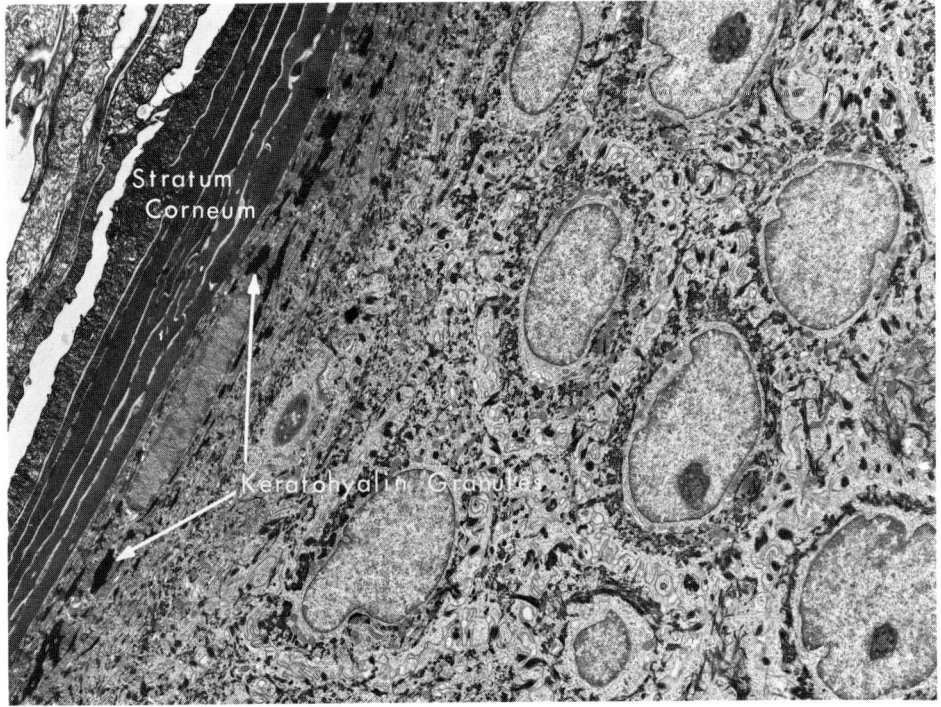

84 HISTOPATHOLOGY

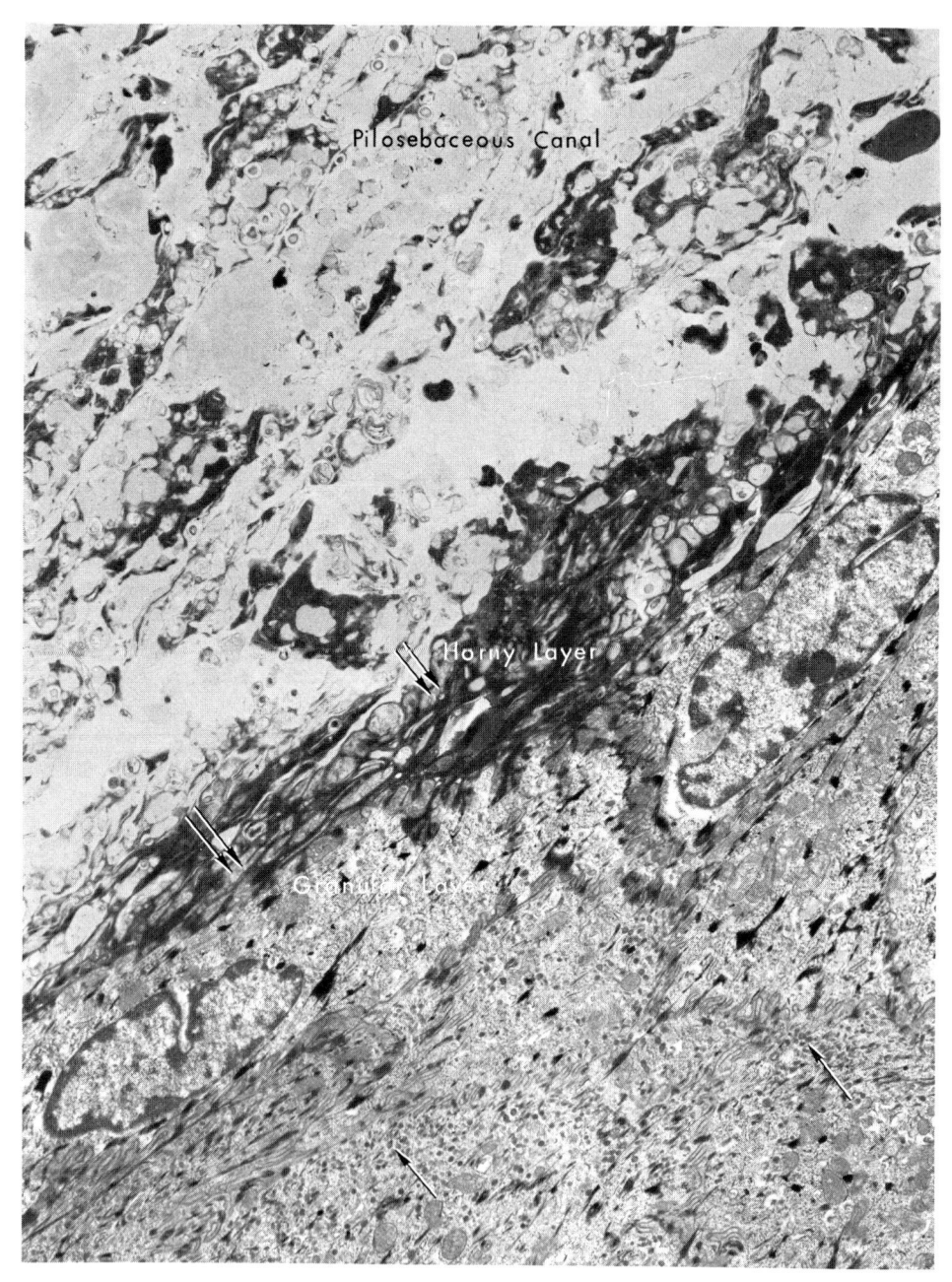

Figure 3. Infrainfundibulum. Numerous lamellar granules are formed within cells beneath granular layer (single arrows) and are discharged in clusters between cells of horny layer (double arrows). Adjacent to thin granular layer, horny layer consists of a few rows of poorly formed, keratinized cells which disintegrate and shed as fragments into the pilosebaceous canal (see Figure 4 for greater detail) (reduced from ×6000).

COMEDO FORMATION 85

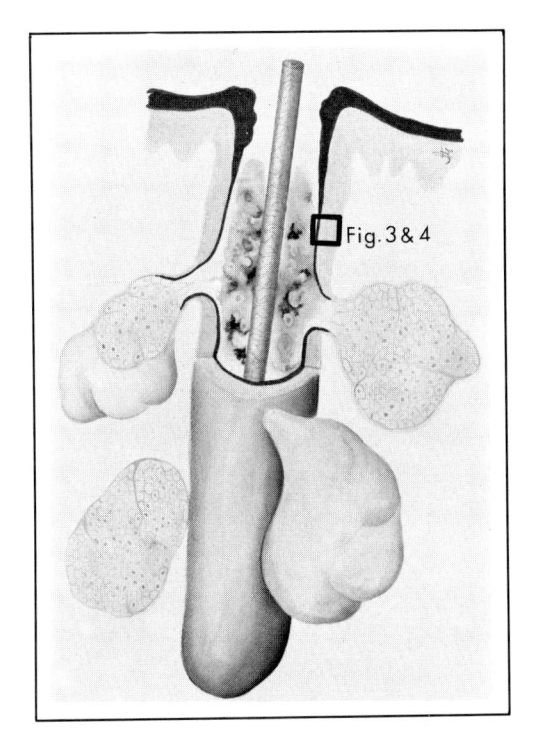

Figure 4. Higher magnification of the horny and granular layers of the infrainfundibulum. The keratohyalin granules are small and sparse. Large clusters of lamellar granules fill the spaces between the thin, filamentous, keratinized cells (reduced from ×20,500).

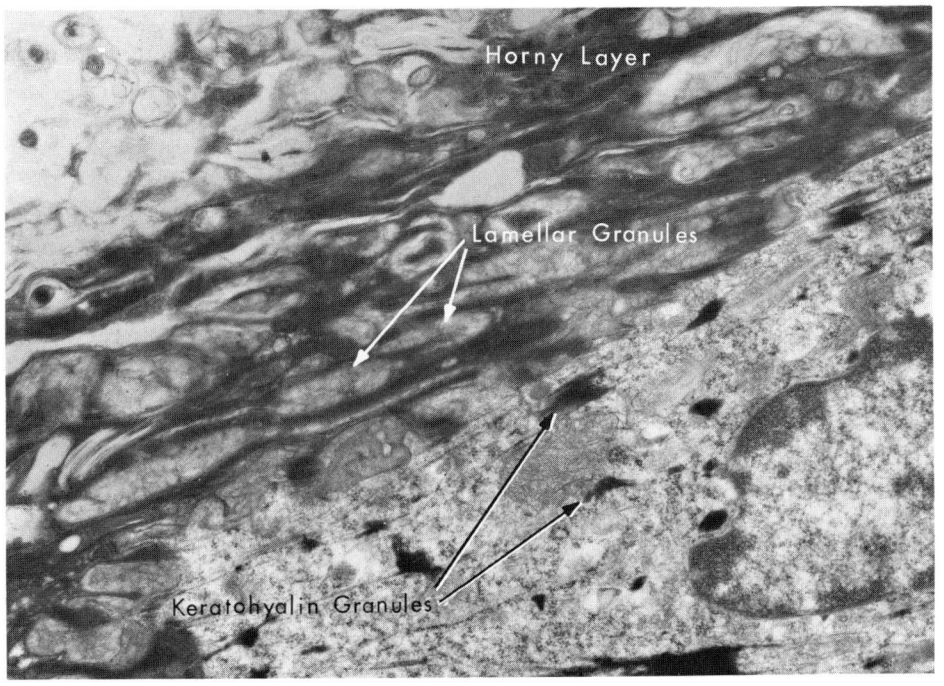

86 HISTOPATHOLOGY

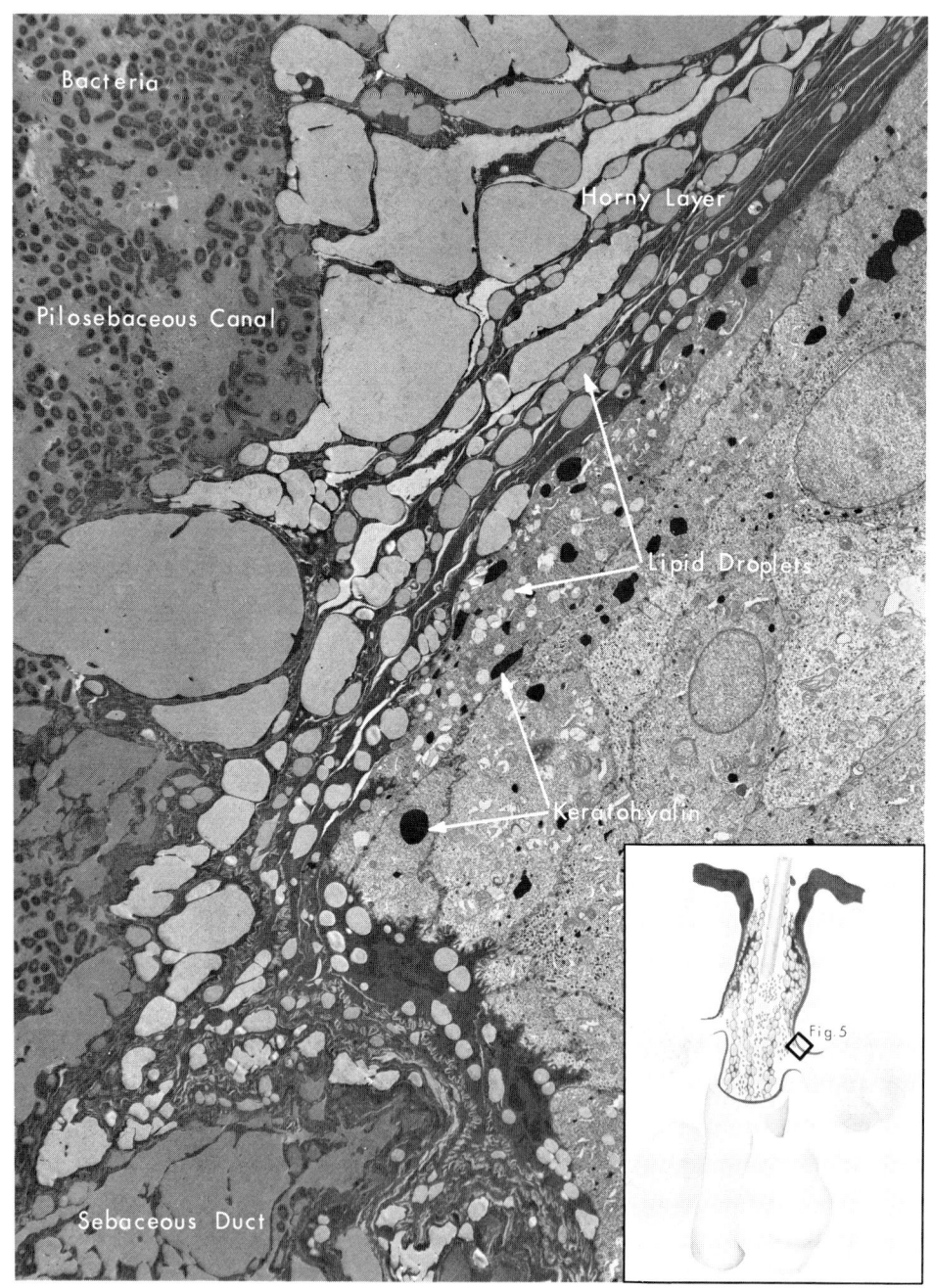

Figure 5. Electron photomicrograph of comedo formation beginning in infrainfundibulum. Large numbers of *P. acnes* present in pilosebaceous canal. Keratohyalin is prominent. Cells of horny layer remain intact and begin to adhere to each other. Many cells contain lipid droplets not seen in normal infundibulum (compare to Figure 3 and 4) (reduced from ×3100).

COMEDO FORMATION 87

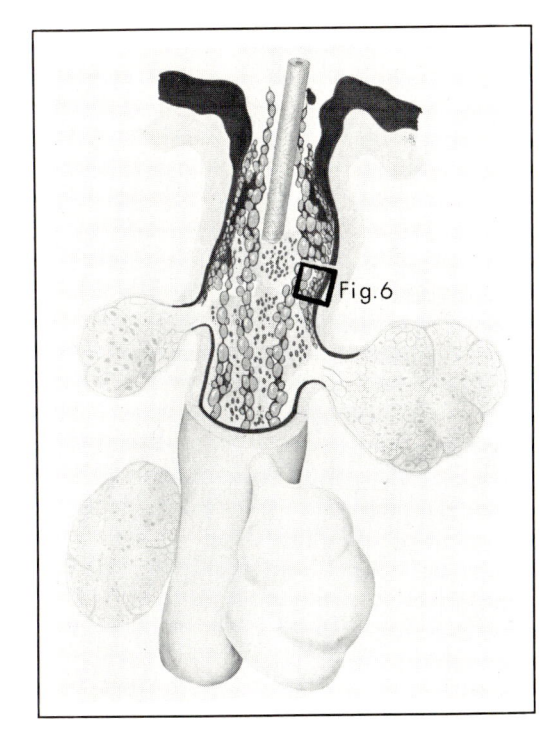

Figure 6. Higher magnification of granular and horny layers of early comedo. Clusters of lamellar granules are sparse (double arrows). Except for presence of lipid droplets, horny cells appear identical to those formed by the normal acroinfundibulum (reduced from ×11,400).

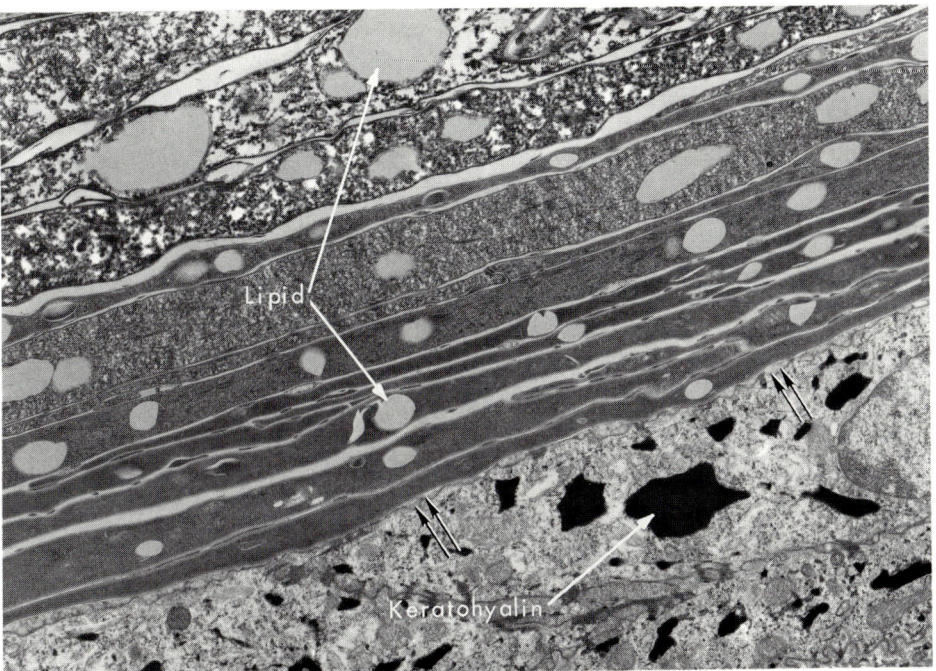

88 HISTOPATHOLOGY

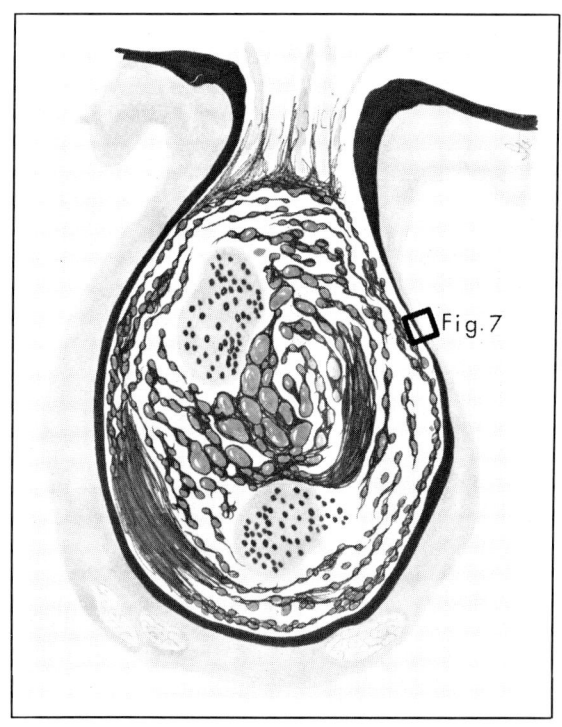

Figure 7. Portion of a mature closed comedo. Flattened, compact keratinized cells often containing lipid droplets (small arrows) make up hard outer shell of comedo contents. Keratohyalin is prominent; lamellar granules are sparse. Large arrow points to center of comedo (reduced from ×3300).

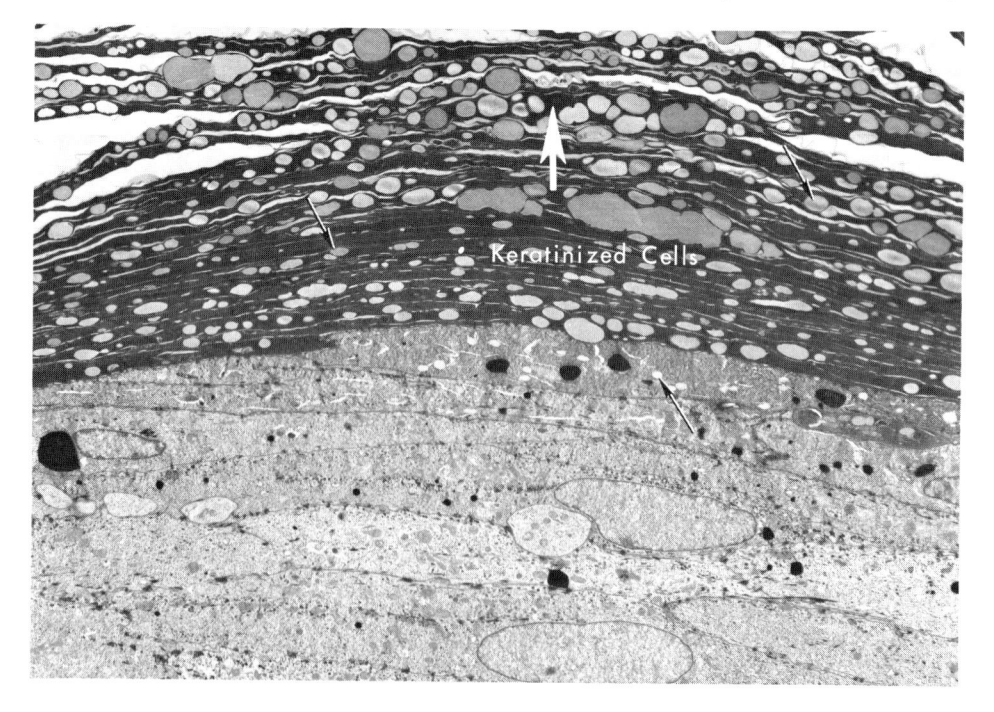

COMEDO FORMATION 89

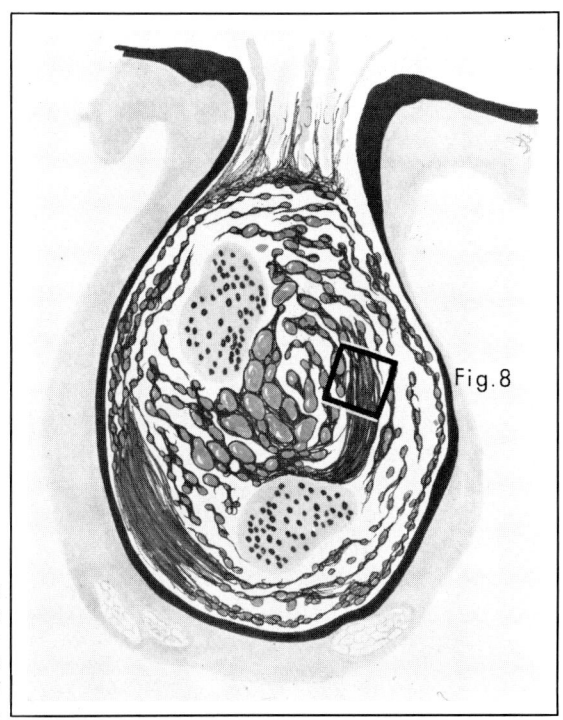

Figure 8. Horny cells deep within a closed comedo. Some cells (between arrows) appear less compact and contain fewer lipid droplets than others (darker areas in upper left and lower right corners) (reduced from ×3600).

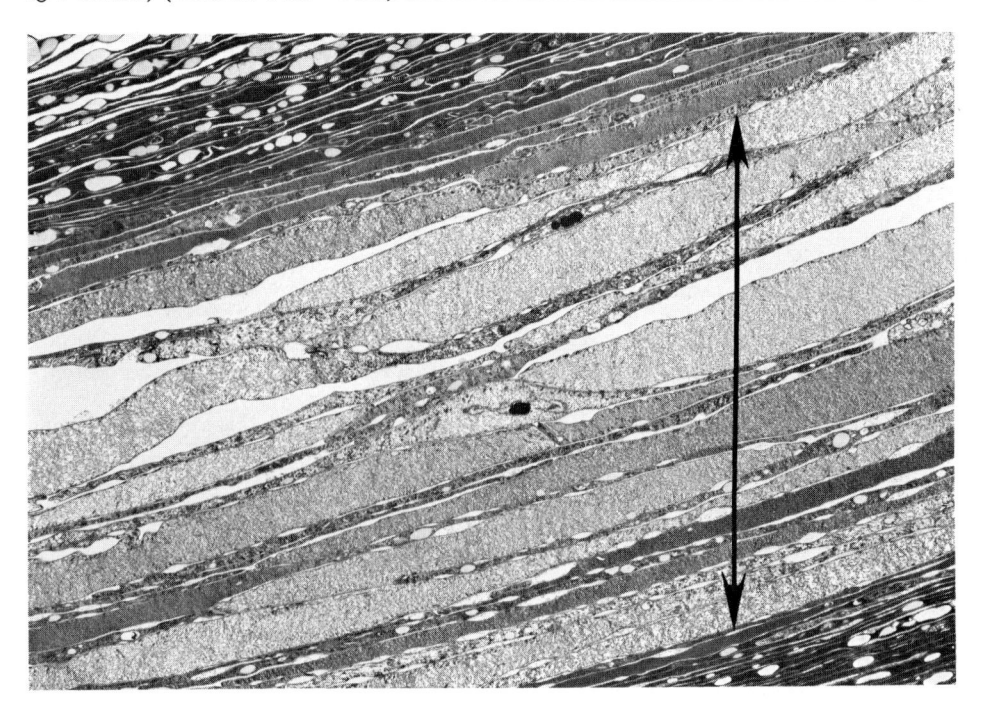

numbers of the bacteria, *Propionibacterium acnes*. The keratohyalin granules of the granular layer increase in size and number, and the cornified layer of the infrainfundibulum thickens (Figure 5). The keratinized cells in the early comedo then take on some of the characteristics of the typical keratinized cells of the acroinfundibulum and the epidermis. They form as compact, discrete, horny cells which adhere to each other and do not fragment easily. Unlike the cornified cells of the acroinfundibulum or epidermis, however, the horny cells of the early comedo contain large lipid deposits. The lamellar granules, which are numerous in the normal infrainfundibulum, are greatly decreased in number in the developing comedo (Figure 6).

As the abnormally keratinized cells aggregate and the infrainfundibulum distends, a mature comedo develops. The keratinized cells filling the chamber of the mature closed comedo appear, for the most part, similar to those lining the early comedo (Figure 7). In some areas of the comedo chamber, however, the horny cells appear swollen, and they are more loosely attached. Some of these cornified cells lack the lipid deposits which are so prominent in the early comedo and in the cells forming the outer keratin shell of the mature comedo (Figure 8).

As the comedo evolves, it has two possible fates. The horny impaction may continue to accumulate until it ultimately dilates the follicular orifice to form an open comedo; or, the epithelial lining surrounding the impaction may become disrupted, and it may then incite an inflammatory reaction accompanied by the various inflammatory lesions of acne.[5]

Acknowledgments: Figure 1 and all electron photomicrographs reproduced with permission from Knutson DD: Ultrastructural observations in acne vulgaris: the normal sebaceous follicle and acne lesions. *J Invest Dermatol* 62:288, 1974.

REFERENCES

1. Strauss JS, Kligman AM: The pathologic dynamics of acne vulgaris. *Arch Dermatol* 82:779, 1960.
2. Knutson DD: Ultrastructural observations in acne vulgaris: the normal sebaceous follicle and acne lesions. *J Invest Dermatol* 62:288, 1974.
3. Wolff HH, Plewig G, Braun-Falco O: Ultrastructure of human sebaceous follicles and comedones following treatment with vitamin A acid. *Acta Derm Venereol [Suppl] (Stockh)* 74:99, 1975.
4. Gonzalez LF, Krawczyk WS, Wilgram GF: Ultrastructural observations on the enzymatic activity of keratinosomes. *J Ultrastruct Res* 55:203, 1976.
5. Kligman AM: An overview of acne. *J Invest Dermatol* 62:268, 1974.

Chapter 11

Noninflammatory and Inflammatory Acne

GERD PLEWIG, MD
ALBERT M. KLIGMAN, MD, PhD

Acne is a strictly follicular disease. Of the three kinds of follicles which occur on the face, namely, vellus follicles, terminal follicles, and sebaceous follicles, only the sebaceous follicles are of interest in acne, as the disease is entirely limited to them.

Sebaceous follicles, peculiar to man, are most numerous on the face and, to a lesser extent, on the back. They have special characteristics[1-3] (Figure 1). The canal, or infundibulum, is deep and cavernous. The terminal portion of the infundibulum, the acroinfundibulum, is similar to the contiguous epidermis, and keratinizes almost in the same fashion, thus forming a horny cell layer barrier. Below this is the epithelium, or infrainfundibulum. It comprises the major portion of the infundibulum, and extends down to the sebaceous ducts. Although the infrainfundibulum keratinizes also, only thin, fragile, loosely attached horny cells are produced; these horny cells do not form a functioning cornified layer.[4,5] Instead, horny detritus, which is mostly lost during histological sectioning, occupies the canal. The sebaceous ducts are short canals, which connect the sebaceous lobules, or acini, to the infrainfundibulum. The epithelium of the sebaceous ducts keratinizes in much the same way as the infrainfundibulum. In this way, separate streams of keratinized cells are created which flow into the infundibulum (or later, the comedo), where they can be identified in horizontal sections. These sections correspond

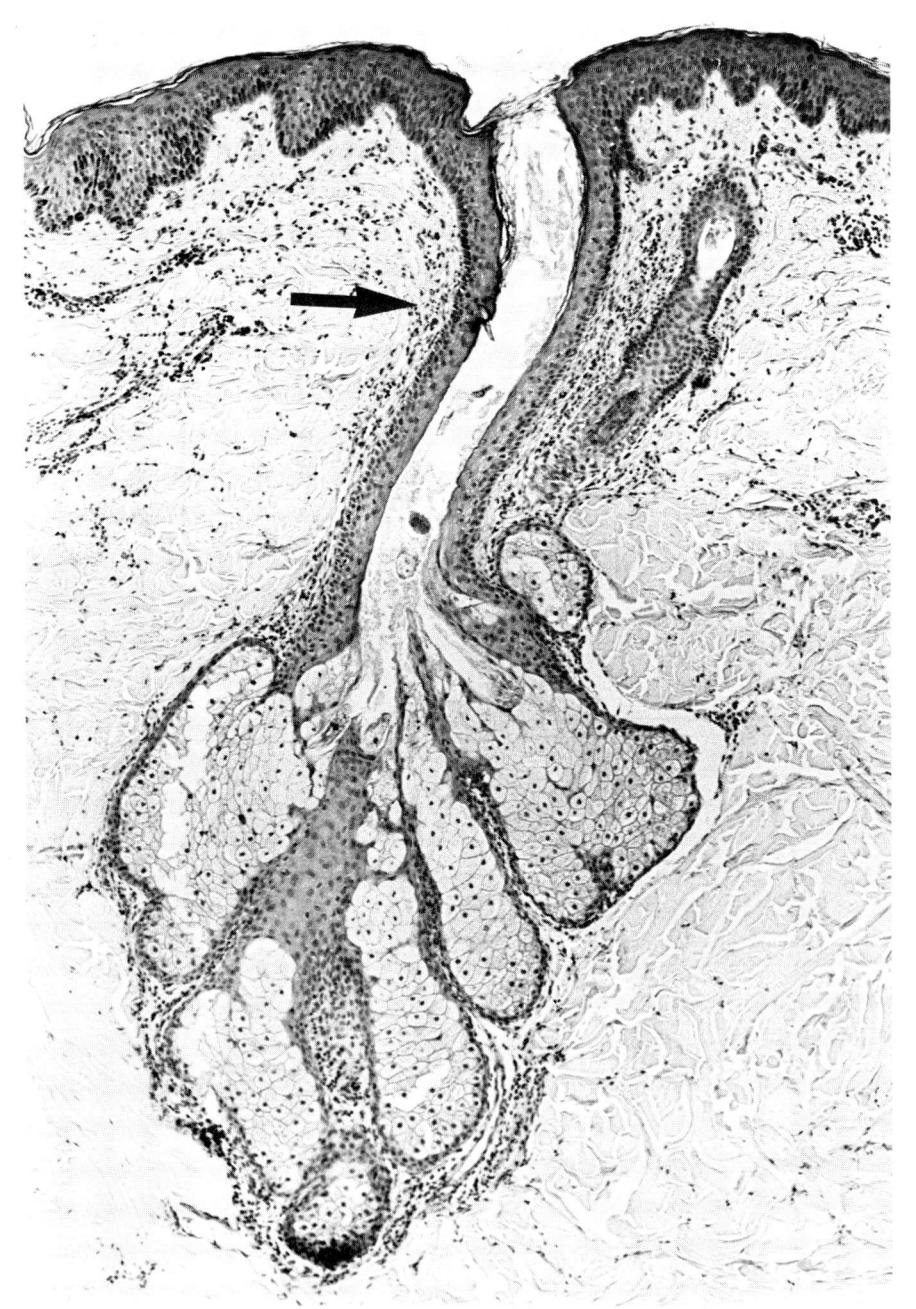

Figure 1. Sebaceous Follicle. The sebaceous lobules of this facial lesion are large. Their contents drain through sebaceous ducts into the infundibular canal. Below arrow is the infrainfundibulum; above and contiguous to epidermis is the acroinfundibulum. Pilary portion (center) is cut tangentially (H & E ×120).

to the number of sebaceous ducts in one follicle; usually there are 3-4.

Contiguous to the sebaceous ducts are the sebaceous glands. They are exceptionally large and multilobulated. Lipid-laden cells, or sebocytes, fill up the acini, and deliver their product, the sebum, into the sebaceous ducts. The sebum streams steadily through the long infundibular canal to the skin surface. Likewise, there is a steady stream of sebum from the sebaceous glands to the skin surface, once comedones have built up. Sebum is never retained in comedones; the "cork" concept, *ie*, plugging of the acroinfundibulum with horny cells and retention of sebum, is a myth.

Each sebaceous follicle contains one pilary unit. The hair root is hidden between the large acini, and is only found in serial sections. The pilary unit enters a short hair root-sheath canal into the lower portion of the infrainfundibulum. The pilary unit undergoes complete hair cycles with anagen, catagen, and telogen phases. In normal sebaceous follicles, only one hair is trapped in the huge canal. During the transformation of a sebaceous follicle into a comedo, hairs are trapped.[6] Old comedones contain numerous hairs, up to 15. The age of the comedo can be fairly well estimated by the number of hairs it contains.

Melanocytes are distributed regularly along both the basal layer of the epidermis and the upper portion of the follicular epithelium (*ie*, the acroinfundibulum).[2,7] Melanocytes are not usually present below this level. The restriction of active melanocytes to the upper portion of the follicle also holds true for comedones. Hence, only the tip of the comedo becomes pigmented. The pigment of the comedones is not the result of oxidation of fatty acids, nor is it the result of dirt and dust particles, as commonly believed.[8]

The normal infundibular canal contains a mixture of sloughed horny cells, sebum, dense masses of bacteria, and a hair. Within the acroinfundibulum, *Pityrosporon* sp. reside, often in beautiful bead-like patterns. These are considered to be innocuous in the overall picture of acne. Also found in the distal part of the canal are high numbers of aerobic bacteria, or cocci. The anaerobic diphtheroid, *Propionibacterium acnes*, almost exclusively occupies the deeper portions of the follicles (and comedones). Follicular mites, commonly called *Demodex*, do not appear in the skin of adolescents, but flourish in the sebaceous follicles of middle-aged and older persons.[1,9] *Demodex* do not play a role in acne.

Sebaceous or seborrheic filaments are the waxy "worms" that can be forced out of the sebaceous follicles of the alae nasae. The filament is a cylindrical tube of keratinized tissue, a dense stratum corneum enclosing a mass of sebaceous lipids and myriads of *P. acnes*[1,2,10] (Figure 2). Sebaceous filaments may precede comedo formation, but this is not always the case. For instance, on the nose, the sebaceous filaments do not progress into microcomedones, but remain at this stage. Using the cyanoacrylate technique, acne-prone persons can be identified by the finding of an abundance of seborrheic filaments.[2]

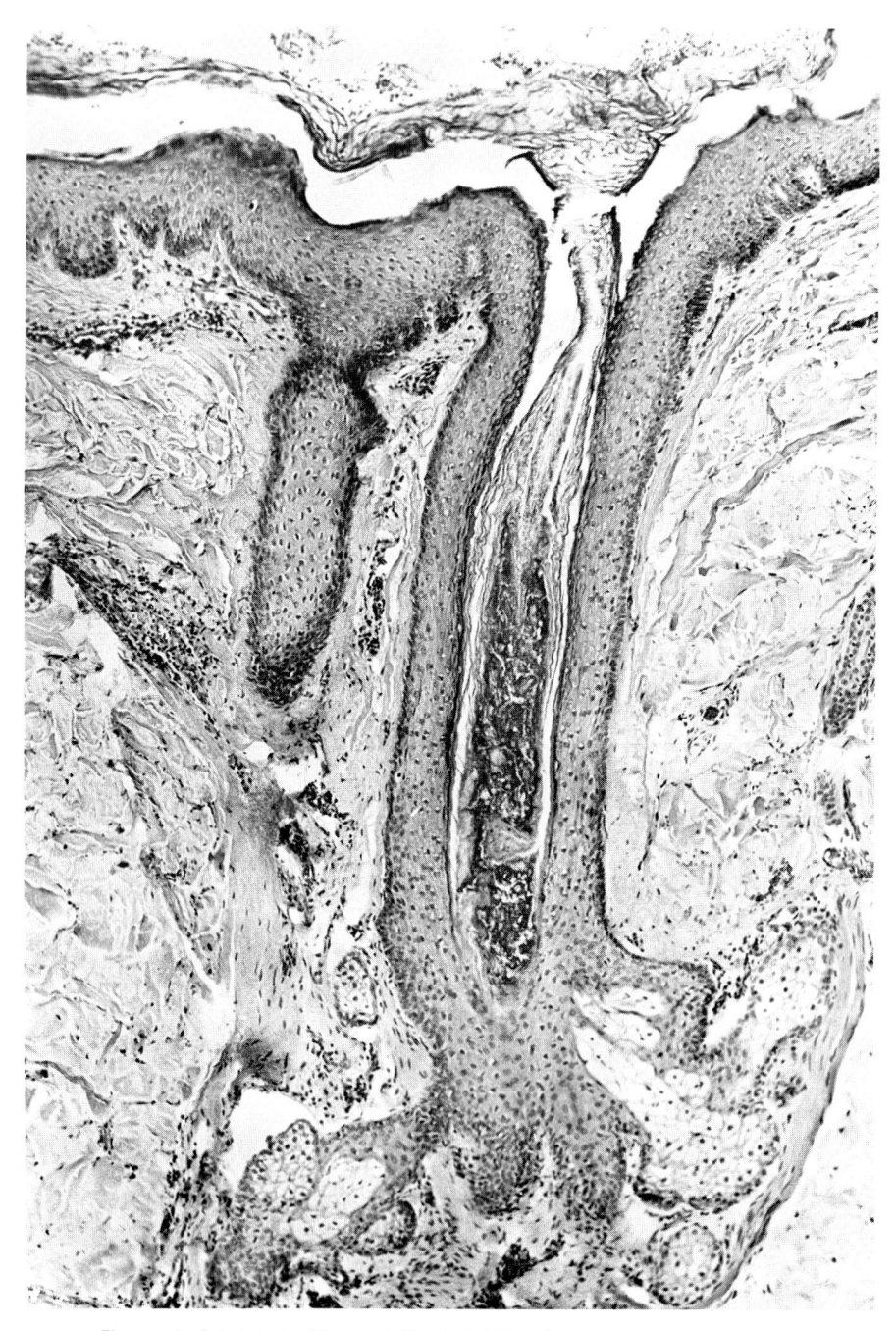

Figure 2. Seborrheic Filament. The infrainfundibulum now has a stratum granulosum and forms a horny, cylindrical framework. This cylindrical tube encloses a mass of *P. acnes*. Sebaceous glands are still intact (H & E ×120).

Evolution of the Comedo

PRIMARY COMEDONES

The comedo is the initial, primary lesion of acne. There are 3 types of comedones: the microcomedo; the closed comedo, or whitehead; and the open comedo, or blackhead. Microcomedones are an early distension of the follicle by horny cells; their existence can only be verified by histological techniques (Figure 3). Closed comedones are the first visible lesions, and resemble milia. The pore, the original acroinfundibulum, of the closed comedo is tiny, and can barely be seen with the naked eye. Open comedones are characterized by the dilatation of the comedonal orifice, and by their large size; these comedones occasionally measure up to 5 mm.

A specialized change in the pattern of keratinization of the infrainfundibulum marks the onset of comedo formation.[2,4,5] A granular layer appears; sturdier horny cells are produced; and, most importantly, these horny cells begin to adhere to each other to form a coherent, horny cell tissue made up of well-defined lamellae. The ultimate secret in comedo formation is bound up in the intercellular cement substance. We presently know very little about this other than that mucopolysaccharides are probably an important constitutent.

Microcomedones—These probably originate in follicles harboring sebaceous filaments. The transformation of a sebaceous filament into a microcomedo is a continuous process. The key change is the decreased dehiscence of the horny cells. The horny cells stick together tightly to form a solid mass which steadily expands. In addition to this hyperkeratosis of the retention type, there is an accelerated turnover of the comedonal epithelium. Measurements with radiolabeled substances such as 3H-thymidine or 3H-histidine showed a definite increase of horny cell production within the infrainfundibulum,[11] or, as it is now called at this anatomical stage, the comedo wall. Both processes—increased production and increased retention of horny cells—contribute to the formation of comedones. It should be emphasized that the acroinfundibulum, or pore region, does not participate in this proliferation-retention hyperkeratosis.

In microcomedones, the epithelial wall becomes acanthotic. The sebaceous glands are initially well-proportioned, but significantly regress in size with ongoing duration of the lesion. Bacteria, notably *P. acnes*, are abundant, and densely colonize the tortuous channels or lacunae. Two to 3 hairs indicate the age, still young, of the lesion.

Closed Comedones—Closed comedones are sequelae of microcomedones. Horny squamae are densely packed into concentric lamellae, often whorled into odd patterns. The channels become large and more irregular, and contain a solid growth of *P. acnes*. The comedonal epithelium now stretches out and becomes thinner; the sebaceous acini regress in size and dedifferentiate (Figure 4). The sebaceous ducts are fully keratinized and

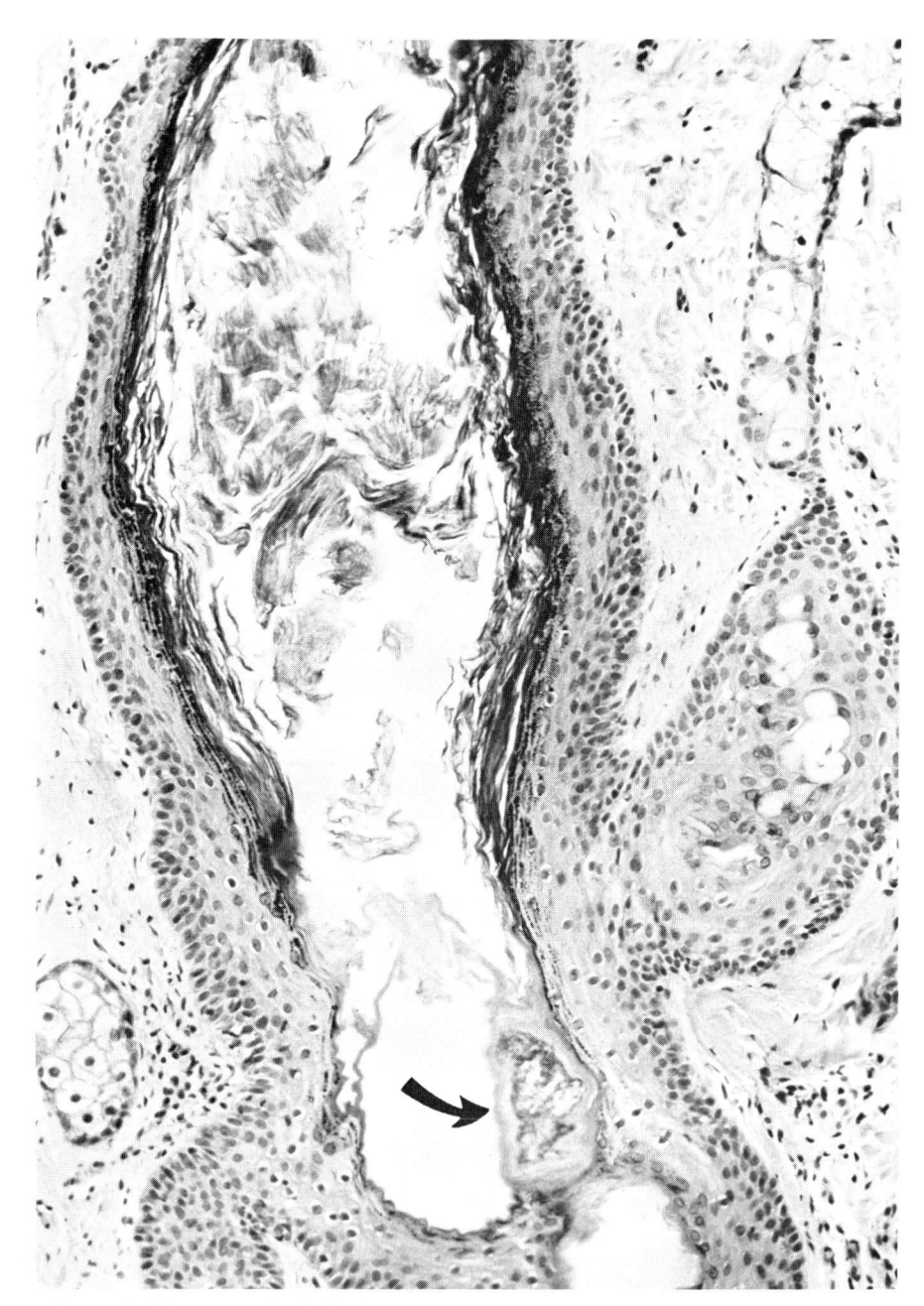

Figure 3. Microcomedo. Follicular canal is extended by accumulation of horny cells. Acanthotic epithelium and pronounced stratum granulosum indicate increased proliferation of corneocytes. Most of lacunae harboring *P. acnes* have been lost during sectioning except for a nidus at lower right (arrow). This embryonic stage of the comedo is not visible clinically, but is easily demonstrated with cyanoacrylate technique (H & E ×120).

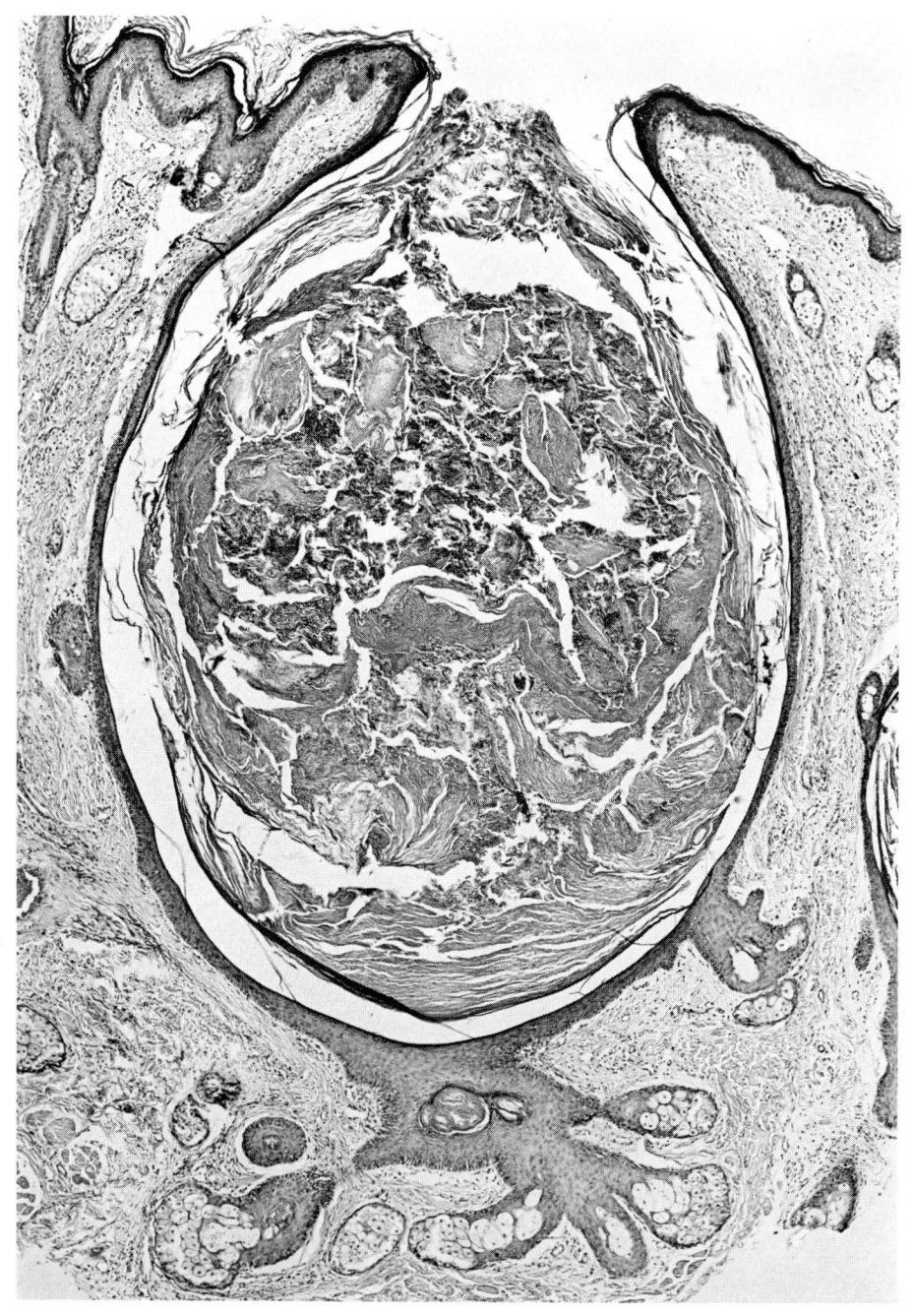

Figure 4. Closed Comedo. The ovoid-shaped kernel has extended the epithelium, now thinned out but still hyperproliferative. Pore is tiny and tight like a tobacco pouch. *P. acnes* colonizes in lacunae (not seen in this section). Sebaceous glands are atrophic (H & E ×80).

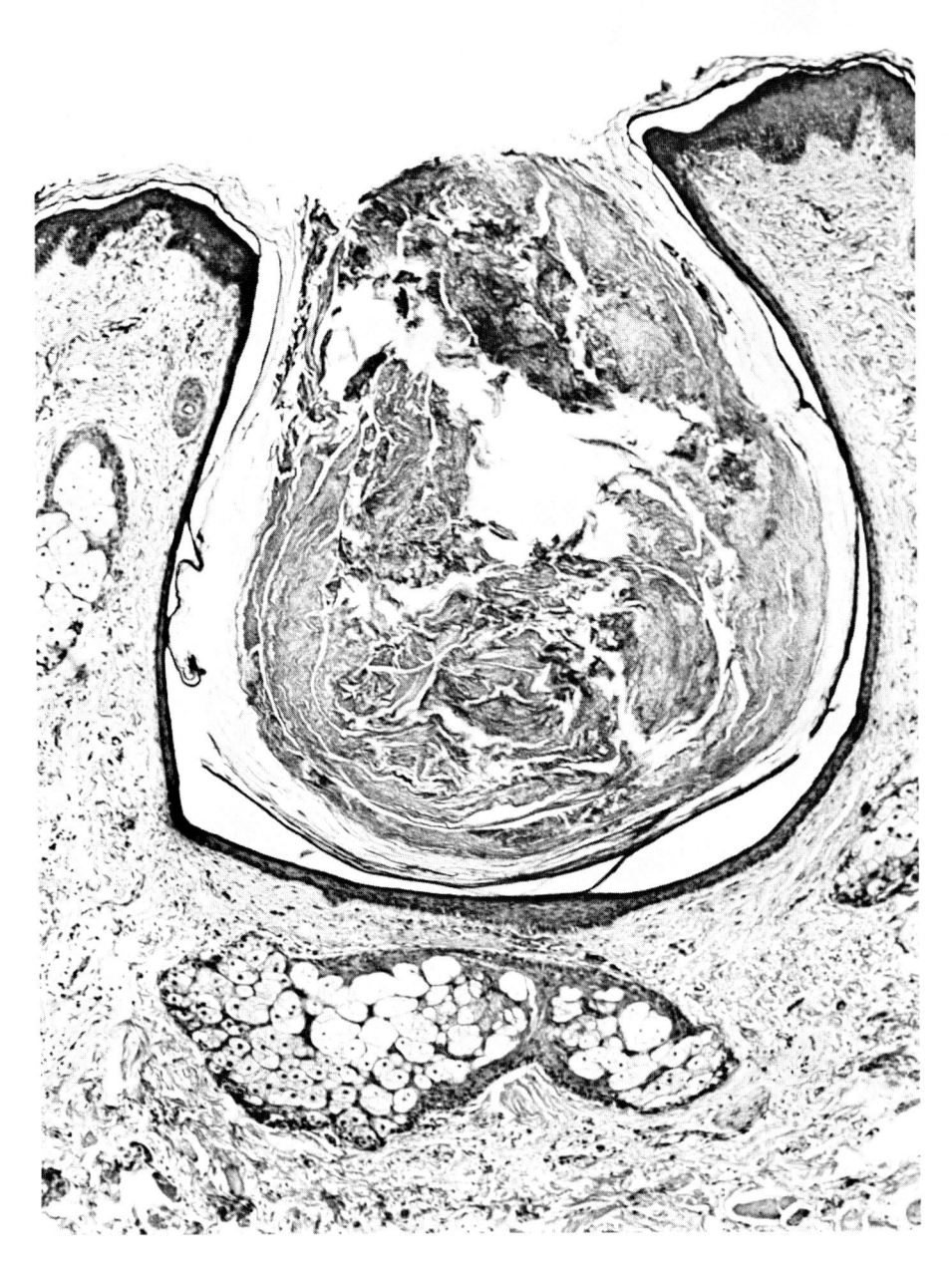

Figure 5. Open Comedo. Pore is wide open: contents are protruding. Epithelial lining is thinned out. One relatively large sebaceous lobule still present. Normally, sebaceous glands are reduced to small, hardly differentiating buds. Pilary unit not visible in this section (H & E ×80).

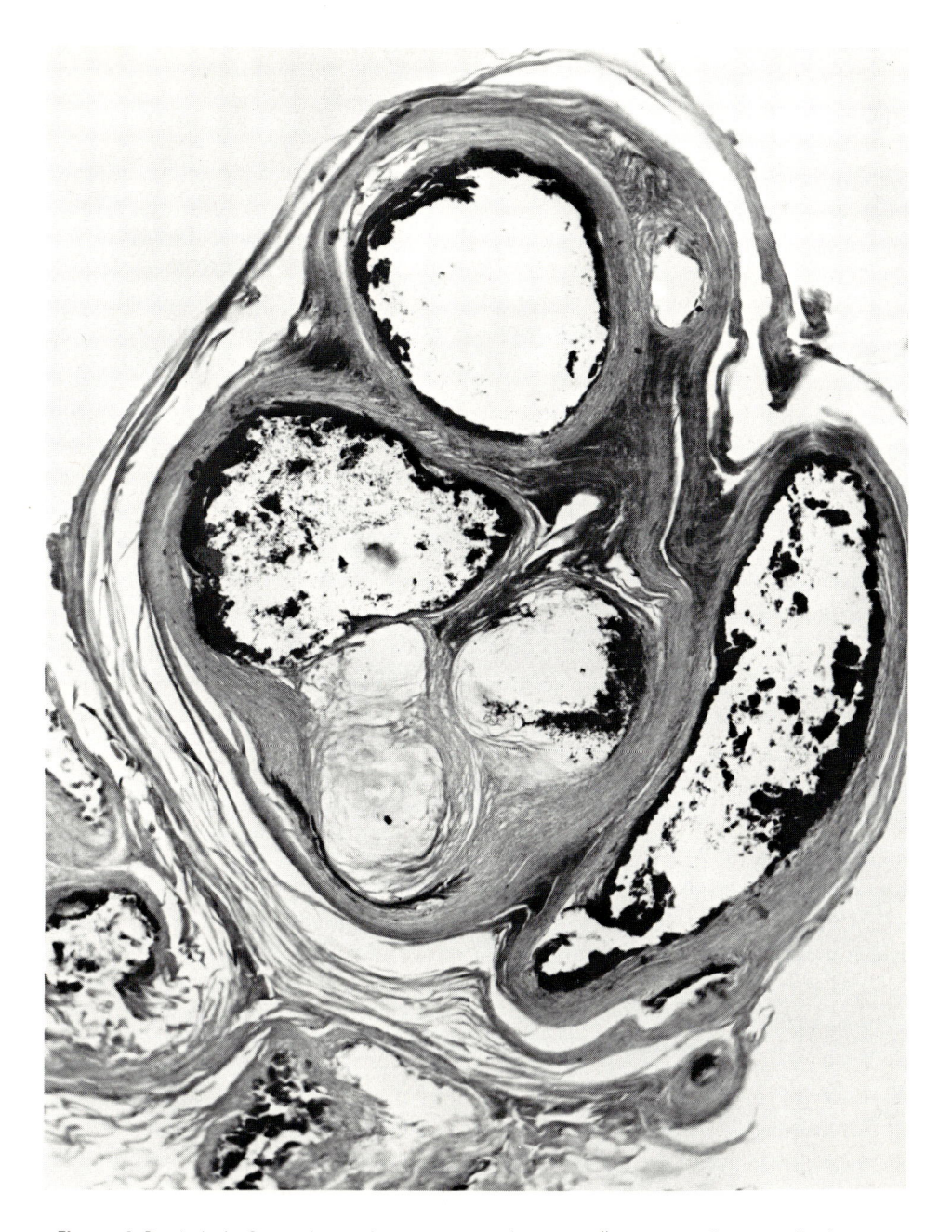

Figure 6. Bacteria in Comedones. An open comedo, manually expressed, was routinely processed and Gram-stained. It contains several large chambers which are filled with masses of P. acnes (partly lost during sectioning). Each chamber connects with a sebaceous duct below and the tip of the comedo above, and drains sebum out to skin surface (Gram's stain ×170).

become part of the comedonal wall. The pilary unit continues to produce hairs, many of which are trapped inside the comedo.

Open Comedones—Radioautographic studies have shown that the production of horny cells does not abate as the comedo enlarges. The pore region of the closed comedo extends and widens, thus giving birth to an open comedo. Unlike the activity in the closed comedo, horny material continually moves through the orifice of the open comedo in a glacier-like fashion, and is thus eroded. Soluble substances and liquid material such as sebum can escape more easily. In closed comedones, drainage is almost completely obstructed; therefore, the contents of these comedones are soft and of a paste-like consistency, as compared to the hard, dry, open comedones.

The comedo wall thins out with time (Figure 5). Richly filled with bacteria, the central channels fuse and become large cavities containing dense communities of *P. acnes* (Figure 6). The sebaceous glands disappear almost completely. The pilary unit is intact, and many hairs are caught within the kernel of the comedo; some manage to escape through the orifice (Figure 7). Old open comedones may be as hollow as an old tree. In such comedones, hardly any sebum is produced, as compared to that produced in the normal, uninvolved sebaceous follicle.

SECONDARY COMEDONES

The rupture and re-encapsulation of comedones create secondary comedones. A single comedo may repeatedly experience focal blow-ups (Figure 8). Rupture may occur early in the microcomedonal stage, or even earlier in the sebaceous filament stage, in individuals subject to early inflammation; or, rupture may occur somewhat later, at the closed comedo stage. These ruptures are therefore called "time bombs" of acne,[1,3] because they may explode at any time. Open comedones rupture less frequently. Secondary comedones can be distinguished from open comedones by the irregular shape and generally larger size of the former. Also, secondary comedones show histologic signs of a prior inflammatory episode.[12] Two types of lesions warrant further discussion: cysts, and polyporous comedones.

Cysts—These lesions are large, skin-colored, protruding, rubbery nodules, and resemble keratinous cysts. Their size often exceeds 20 mm in diameter (Figure 9). Cysts occur mainly on the back and, less frequently, on the face, and are typical of acne conglobata. When punctured, cysts release a cheesy, crumbly material.

Polyporous comedones—These lesions look like a cluster comprised of 2-20 blackheads, and occur mainly on the back in patients with acne conglobata. However, polyporous comedones are interconnected, and share common openings. These undermining tunnel systems are also called fistulated comedones. Histologically, the epithelial wall varies considerably between atrophy and acanthosis, with irregular sprouts of epithelium migrating through the dermis (Figure 10).

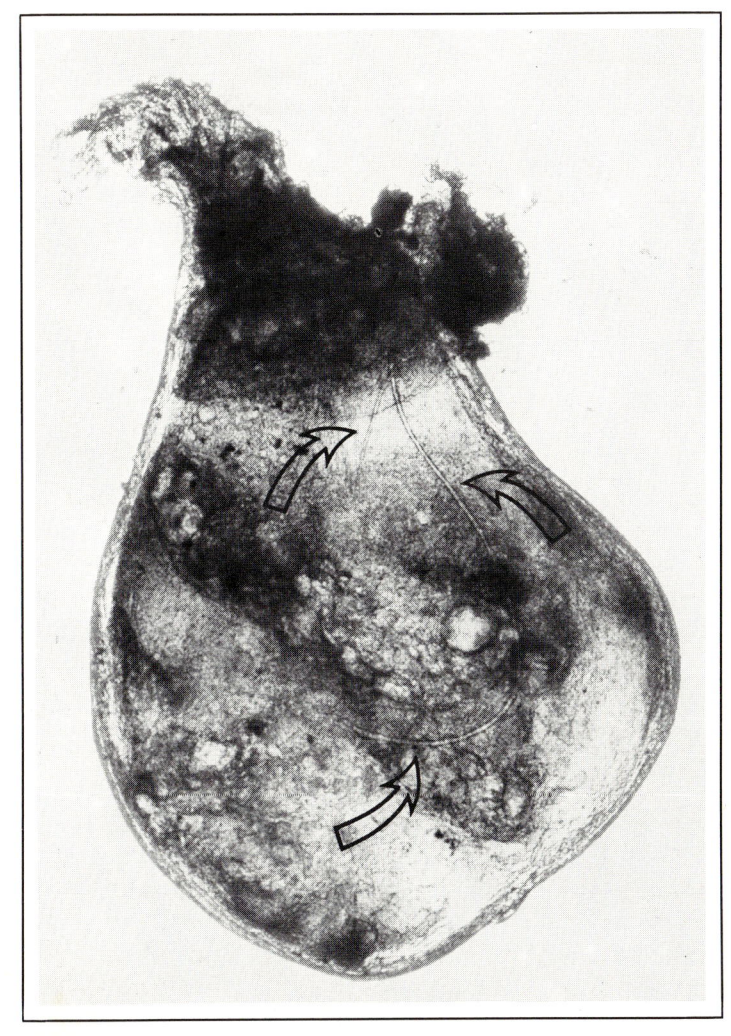

Figure 7. Hairs in Comedones. This open comedo was expressed with a comedo extractor, placed on a slide, immersed in oil, and covered with a cover glass. This makes entire comedo translucent. Several hairs are tangled in comedo (arrows); the few hairs indicate that comedo is only a few months old (Unstained ×50).

There are always, in secondary comedones, histologic signs of previous inflammation with streaked collagen bundles. Concentric layers of connective tissue surround the cysts and polyporous comedones. The sebaceous glands and hairs in both these lesions are virtually destroyed. Both types of lesions contain fewer bacteria and almost no channels within the horny masses.

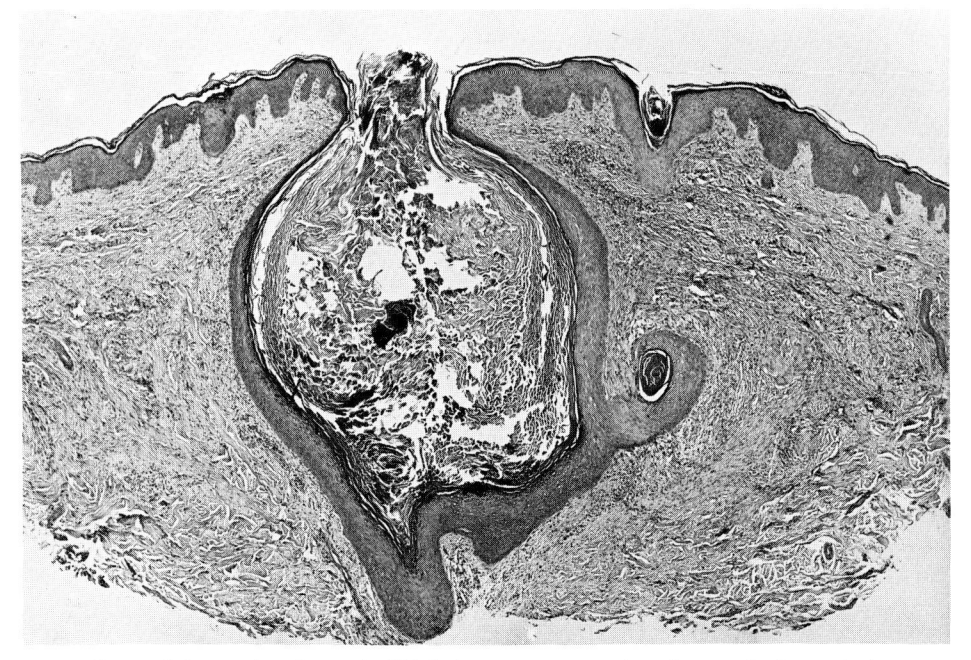

Figure 8. Secondary Comedo. This lesion was once a closed comedo. Repeated rupture and re-encapsulation led to bizarre shape. Epithelial wall is acanthotic with hypergranulosis. Pilary unit and all sebaceous glands have been destroyed. Comedo is embedded in a scarred dermal tissue (H & E reduced from ×50).

Inflammatory Acne Lesions

Inflammatory lesions always spring from comedones or from pre-comedonal lesions; their quality will depend on the extent and place of rupture. Comedones are generally not evident when observing the inflammatory lesions in acne. The reason for this is that the comedones frequently burst before attaining a size large enough to be seen. The inflammatory reaction itself tends to mask the underlying comedo. Expression of the contents of a papule or pustule allows for the extraction of the horny kernel.

There are several well-distinguished inflammatory acne lesions: the pustule; the papule; the nodule; the hemorrhagic nodule; and the draining sinus. Other types of lesions, such as the gelatinous ulcerations seen in acne fulminans, are extremely rare.[2,13]

PUSTULES

The dissolution of the epithelial lining which is close to the skin surface creates an intrafollicular abscess with some perifollicular involvement. The lower portion of the comedo usually stays intact (Figure 11). Healing will occur without scarring by re-encapsulation.

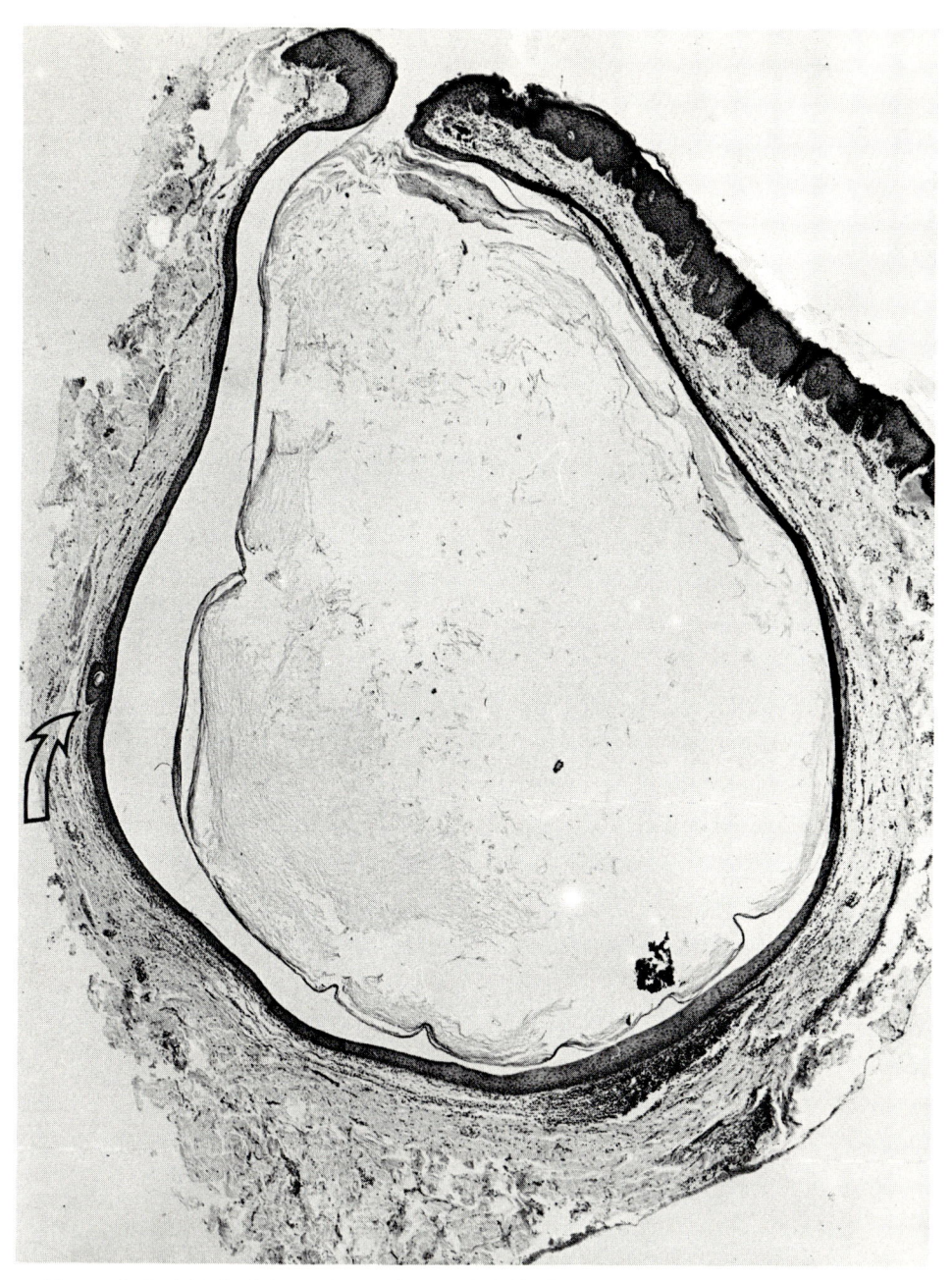

Figure 9. Cyst. Typical shape is round or oval. Epithelium is thinned out, producing noncoherent, loose, horny material. Pilary unit and sebaceous acini were destroyed during the many inflammatory breaks which occurred in this former comedo. A bud of undifferentiated cells (arrow), probably remnant of an acinus, is at left. A pocket of inflammatory cells is at bottom. Concentric rings of scarred dermis surround this gigantic lesion (H & E ×15).

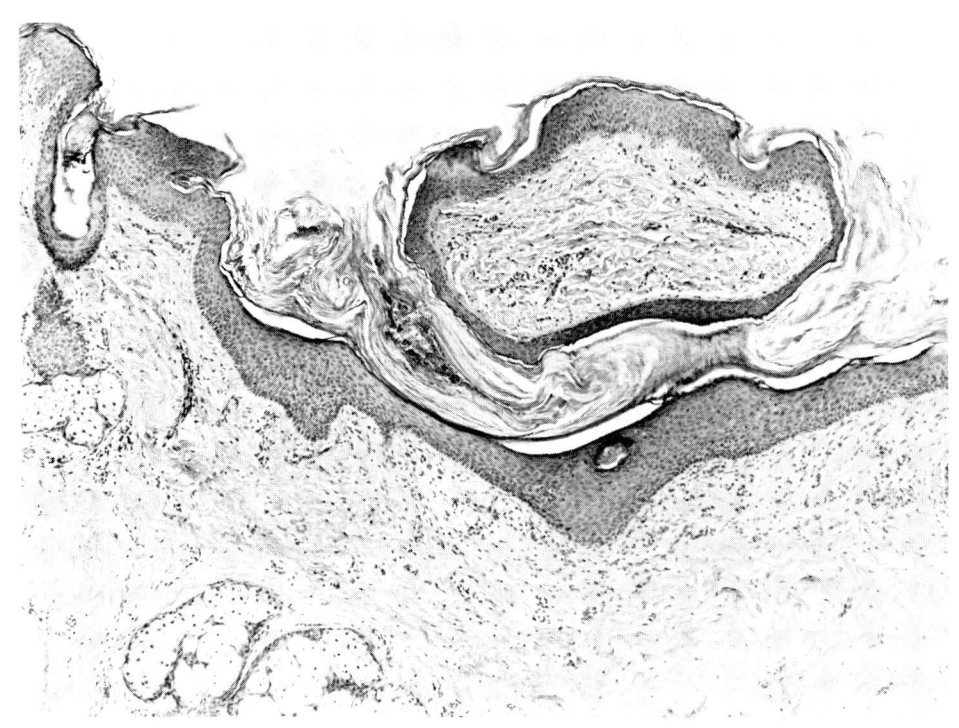

Figure 10. Polyporous Comedo. This secondary comedo is actually a scar. Groups of 2 or more follicles become linked by repeated localized ruptures. Tunnel system is lined by a bizarre epithelium with pigmented, horny tips protruding through wide openings. Sebaceous glands and pilary units have been destroyed. Bacteria are scarce, but *Pityrosporon* sp. commonly colonize between loose, horny lamellae. Dermal bed is scarred (H & E reduced from ×120).

PAPULES

This is a lesion similar to the acute pustule, but with more and deeper collapse of the comedo structure. Major portions of the comedonal epithelium are disrupted, and fragments of the horny kernel are displaced into the adjacent dermis. Neutrophils are numerous, and spread far into the tissue. The fragmented ends of the comedo will finally reunite. Scarring is inevitable.

Some papules persist for a long while; their clinical healing may take many weeks. This is not surprising, as the foreign material such as hairs, horny cell lamellae, lipids, bacteria, and epithelial cells have to be removed from the site of the lesion. Foreign-body giant cells and actual granulomas persist for long periods, well beyond the clinical healing of the lesion.

NODULES

This is the hallmark of serious acne. The nodule is a tender, firm, hot lesion, which often becomes fluctuant and sometimes crusted. Histologically, a nodule is the total explosion and collapse of a comedo (Figure 12). Frag-

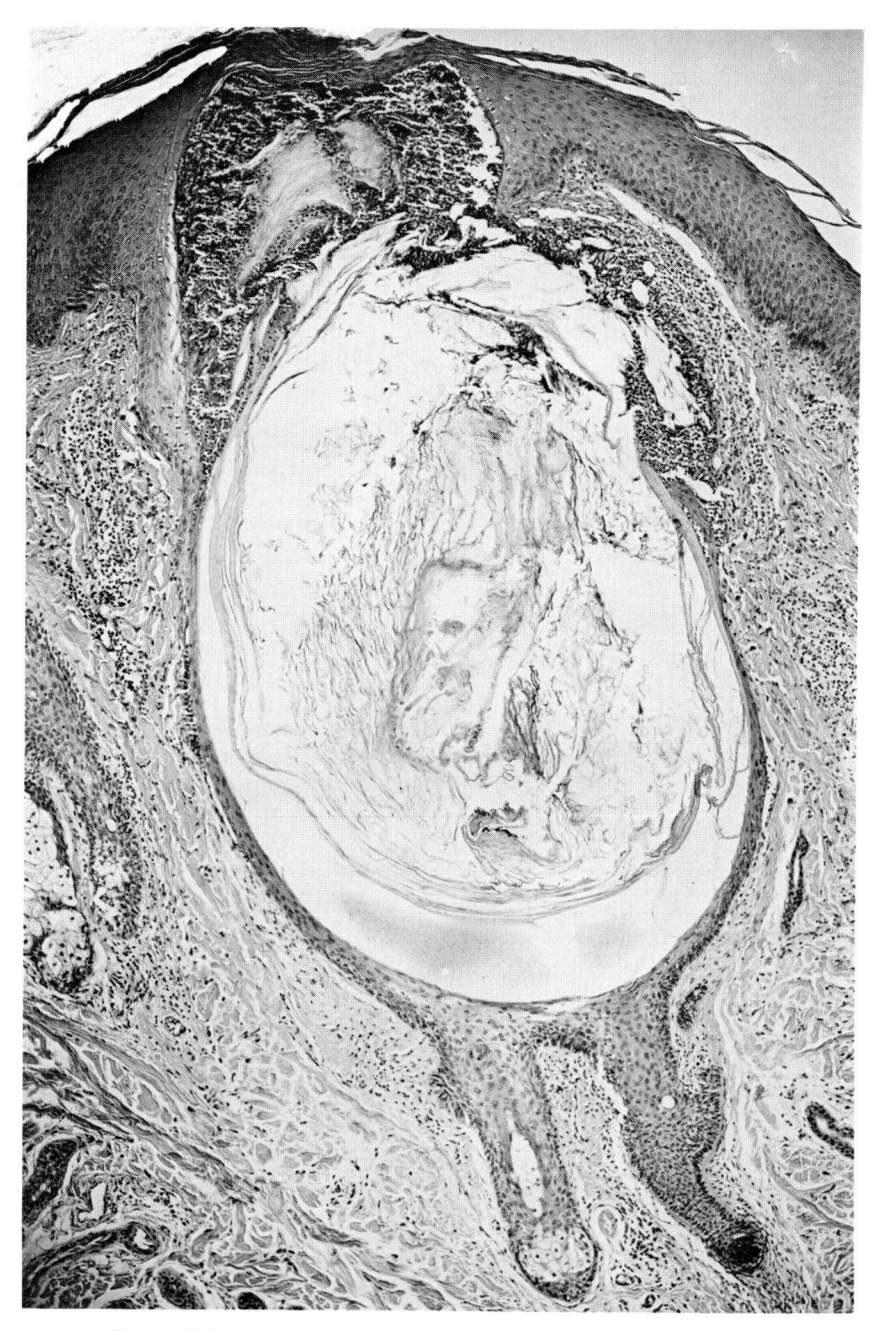

Figure 11. Pustule. This is a superficial lesion. A local blow-up occurred at upper part of comedonal epithelium. An apical abscess, limited to comedonal structure, has formed, and will soon be resolved. Comedo remains intact above pilary portion at bottom (H & E ×80).

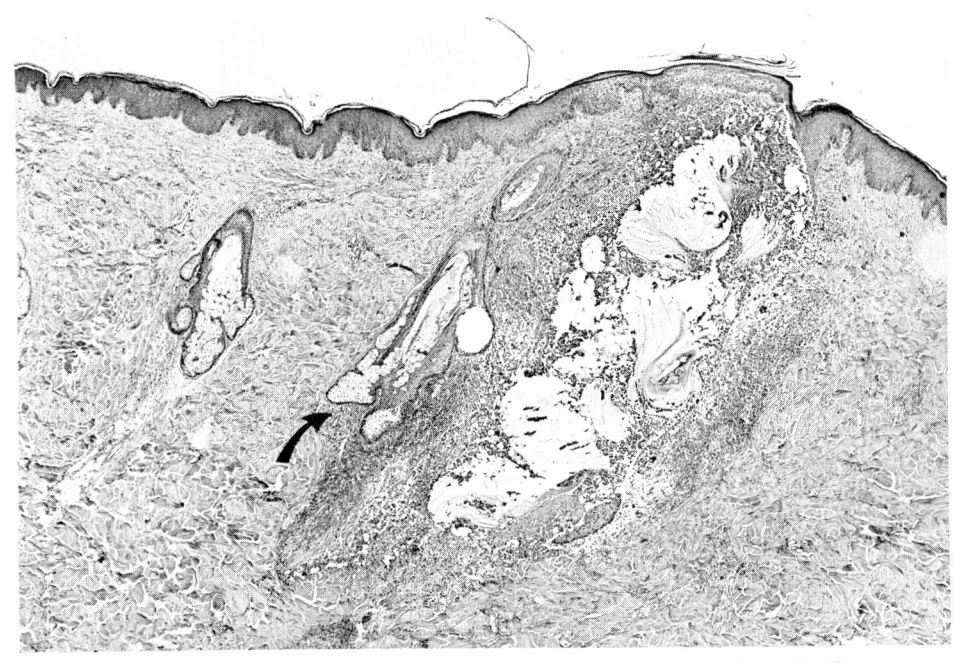

Figure 12. Nodule. This nodule developed from a closed comedo. Kernel is still in place, but entire epithelium has been destroyed. Deep-reaching, dense infiltrate consists of neutrophils. Normal sebaceous follicle at left (arrow) is almost engulfed by the inflammatory reaction. It will take weeks until this lesion is completely resolved; a scar is inevitable (H & E reduced from ×50).

ments of the horny nidus are dispersed into the tissue, which is densely infiltrated with neutrophils. The epithelium is ultimately completely destroyed. The abscess often reaches down to the adipose tissue. From the far-flung inflammatory reaction, a terrible scar is inevitable.

HEMORRHAGIC NODULES

Hemorrhagic nodules are the tell-tale signs of acne conglobata. They are ferocious lesions. These nodules clinically have a dull red hue; the necrotic abscess erodes blood vessels, resulting in bleeding into the central necrosis (Figure 13). The patients afflicted with these lesions seemingly lack means to confine the inflammation. In some instances, every living thing within a radius of a few centimeters of the hemorrhagic nodule is killed outright—sweat glands, vellus and sebaceous follicles, nerves, and blood vessels. Acute inflammation slowly gives way to chronic reaction. Histologic activity lasts for many months.

DRAINING SINUSES

This is a variant of the nodule, and a truly malevolent lesion. It is most

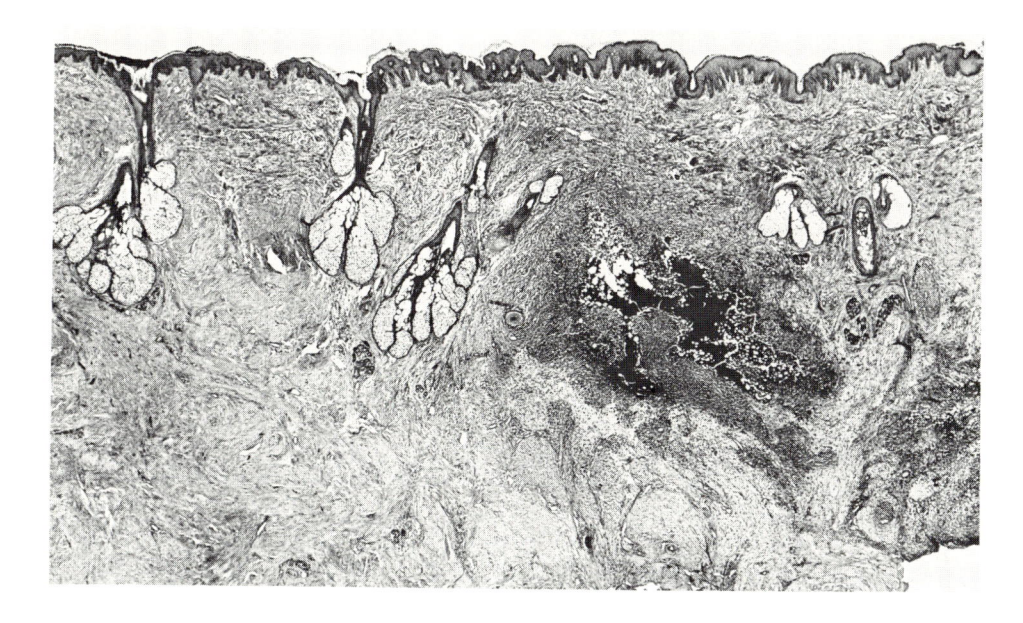

Figure 13. Hemorrhagic Nodule of Acne Conglobata. *above:* This nodule is characterized by an abscess that erodes blood vessels and destroys everything in its path (H & E reduced from ×60). *below:* A foreign-body reaction, manifested by ectatic blood vessels, giant cells, mononuclear cells, and histiocytes, follows the acute inflammation (H & E reduced from ×400).

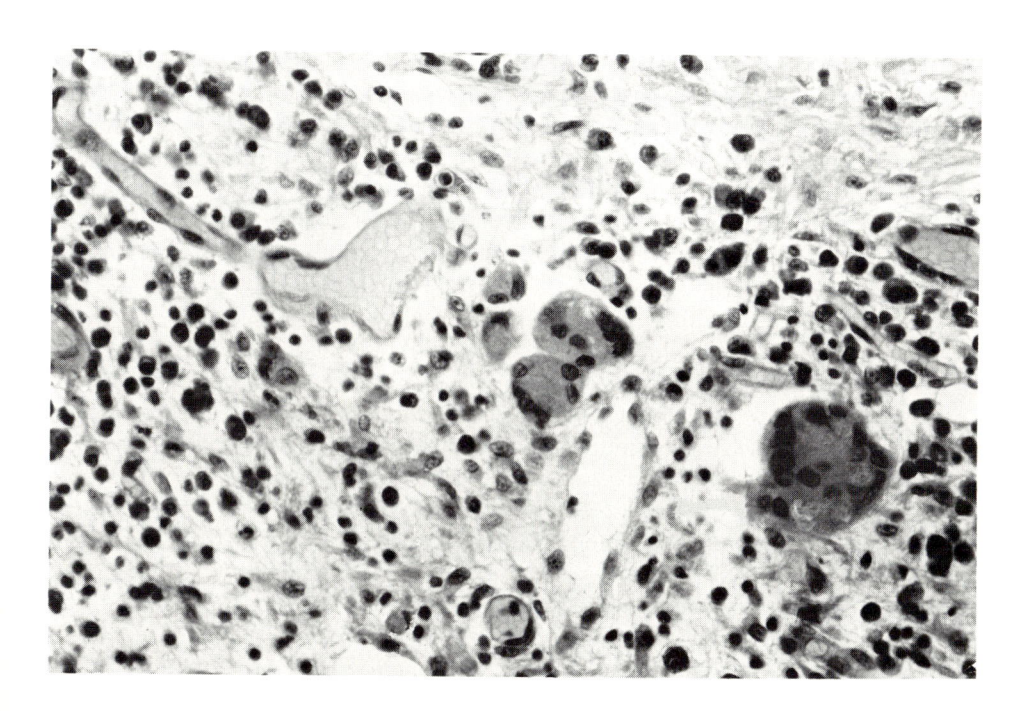

108 HISTOPATHOLOGY

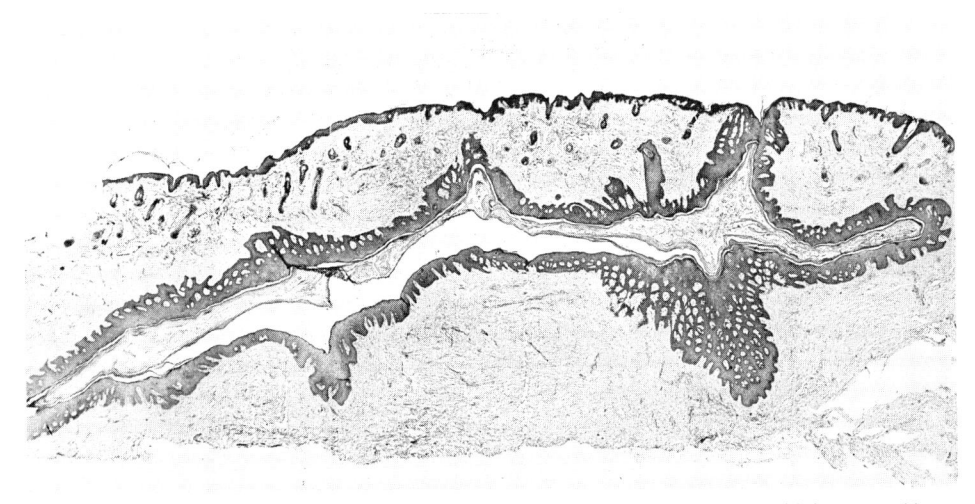

Figure 14. Draining Sinus. This long, linear lesion consists of elaborate galleries which connect to skin surface at multiple points. Acanthosis, papillomatosis, sprouts and tongues of epithelial cells are typical histological features. Sebaceous glands are usually absent. Lumen contains loose, horny material; bacteria are scarce. Dermis is scarred (H & E reduced from ×10).

common on the face, in the nasolabial folds, and on the neck beneath the mandibular line. Clinically, the draining sinus is an elongated, elevated, periodically inflamed lesion which sporadically discharges pus. The lesion smolders and rages for years. Histologically, a draining sinus is an elaborate gallery which opens to the skin surface at multiple points (Figure 14). It is an epithelialized, undermining system of tunnels with a bizarre epithelial wall; every cut reveals a different aspect. The lumen contains loose horny cell material, hairs, pockets of inflammatory cells, and a few bacteria. The surrounding connective tissue is grossly distorted. Granulation tissue (or, in later stages, scarring) is found everywhere. The inflammatory reaction engulfs other, hitherto uninvolved sebaceous follicles or comedones. The draining sinus is analogous to the pilonidal cyst.

HIDRADENITIS SUPPURATIVA-LIKE LESIONS

Hidradenitis suppurativa-like lesions in the axillae and groin, often extending over both the perineum and the entire intergluteal cleft including the buttocks, are indicative of the acne tetrad[2] (*ie*, hidradenitis suppurativa, dissecting folliculitis of the scalp, acne conglobata, and the pilonidal cyst). Hidradenitis is a misnomer. The lesion does not originate from infected or inflamed sweat glands—eccrine or apocrine. It is a true follicular lesion, starting either in the sebaceous follicles, which are rare in these intertriginous regions, or, more commonly, in the terminal hair follicles. A follicular abscess, which soon spreads and engulfs other neighboring follicles, develops. Heat

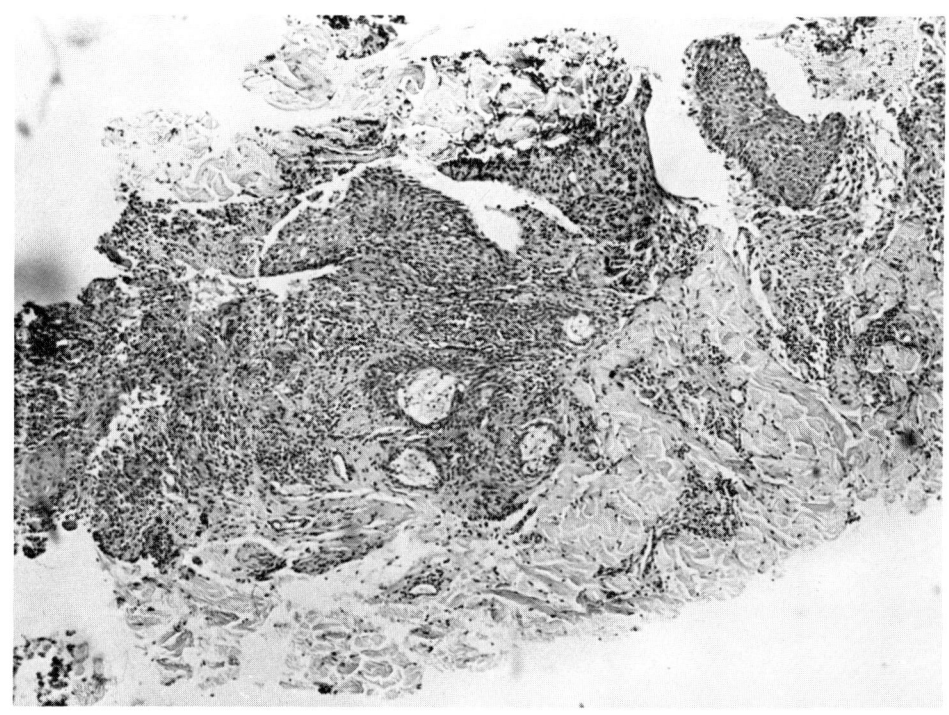

Figure 15. Acne Fulminans. This acne is a devastating one. Surface epidermis is destroyed. Only remnants of sebaceous glands and other structures remain.

and moisture promote the spreading of the lesions, which reach deep down into the sweat glands. In early lesions of so-called "hidradenitis suppurativa" in the acne tetrad, no primary involvement of sweat glands is seen in serial histological sections. Uncontrolled, dissecting inflammation bringing severe destruction to all surrounding tissues is found in similar lesions (eg, in dissecting folliculitis of the nape of the neck or of the hairy scalp).

ACNE FULMINANS

Ulcerative lesions are characteristic of acne fulminans. The epidermis is denuded. An abundant infiltrate of polymorphonuclear neutrophils is seen, with remnants of epithelium and sebaceous glands present[13] (Figure 15).

Acne Scars

The histological picture of acne scars is as variable as that of the polymorphic clinical lesions. Only a few types of scars will be discussed here; they are all late sequelae of ruptured comedones.

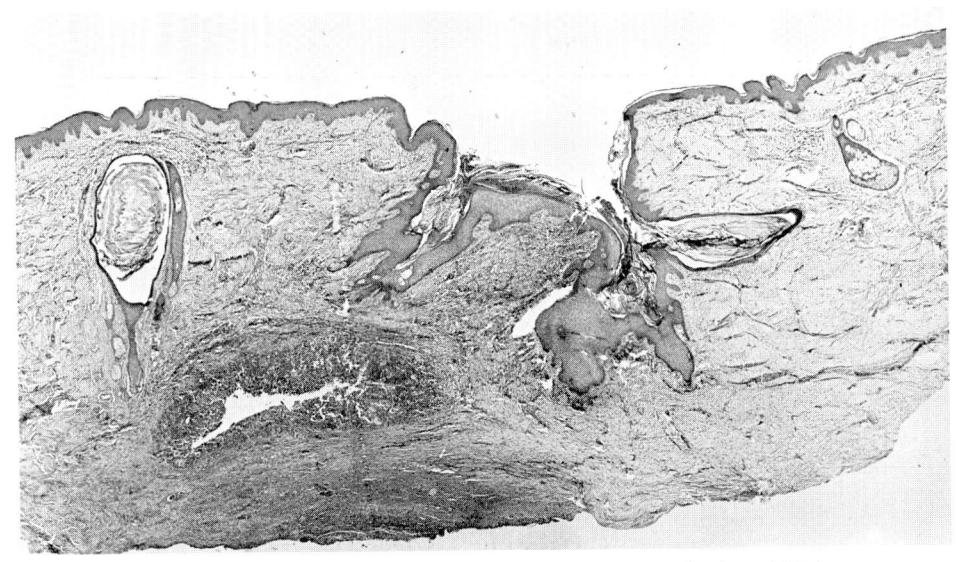

Figure 16. Crateriform Scar. Irregular scars are usually seen on the face. Histologically, they are more elaborate than clinically appears. Finger-like extensions of epithelium burrow deeply into dermis. Crater is filled with horny lamellae. Smoldering inflammation is underneath scar (H & E reduced from ×50).

"ICE PICK" OR CRATERIFORM SCARS

The follicular offspring of this type of scar is often discernible. The remnants of the original sebaceous follicle, or what is now the comedonal epithelium, burrow deep into the dermis in bizarre patterns (Figure 16). The epithelium is acanthotic. Small buds of the sebaceous glands are often the remnants of the once-huge sebaceous acini; or, the sebaceous glands may form anew. The surrounding tissue is always scarred with zones of fibrosis often containing mononuclear and giant cells. The disease dies clinically long before it reaches its histologic demise. Bevelling of the steep crater walls (*eg*, with dermabrasion) will more or less improve this scar.

COMPLEX SCARS

These scars are most often found on the face. Serial sectioning frequently reveals geographic features which are otherwise not immediately evident (Figure 17). Fistulae may connect 2 or more follicles. Some of the complex scars may earlier have been draining sinuses or conglobate nodules.

KELOIDAL SCARS

Keloidal scars do not appear spontaneously, but are derived always from previous inflammatory acne lesions. These elevated, lumpy growths are exophytic or endophytic (Figure 18). Dense, mostly horizontally compacted

NONINFLAMMATORY AND INFLAMMATORY ACNE **111**

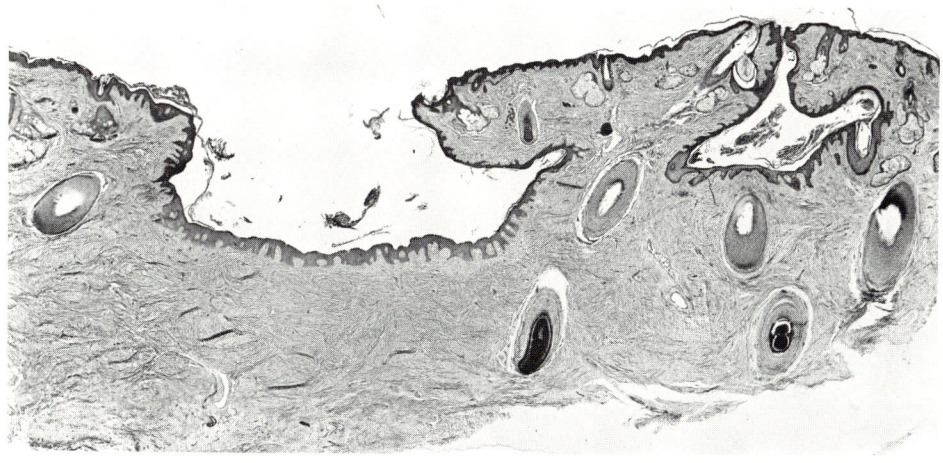

Figure 17. Complex Scar. Scars of this type, seen on the face, often have unexpected ramifications. Deep depressions, defects, fistulae, and troughs compose this lesion. Irregular, hyperplastic epithelium lines this horrendous defect. At least half a dozen follicles are linked. Serial sections reveal that the 2 pits are actually part of a single tunnel system. Dermis is also scarred (H & E reduced from ×20).

Figure 18. Keloidal Scar. Hypertrophic scars are lumpy growths, and are usually found on the back. Normal epidermis with intact sebaceous follicles is at far right and left (arrows). Whorling patterns of collagen bundles with some dilated vessels comprise this gigantic scar. All skin adnexa have been destroyed (H & E reduced from ×10).

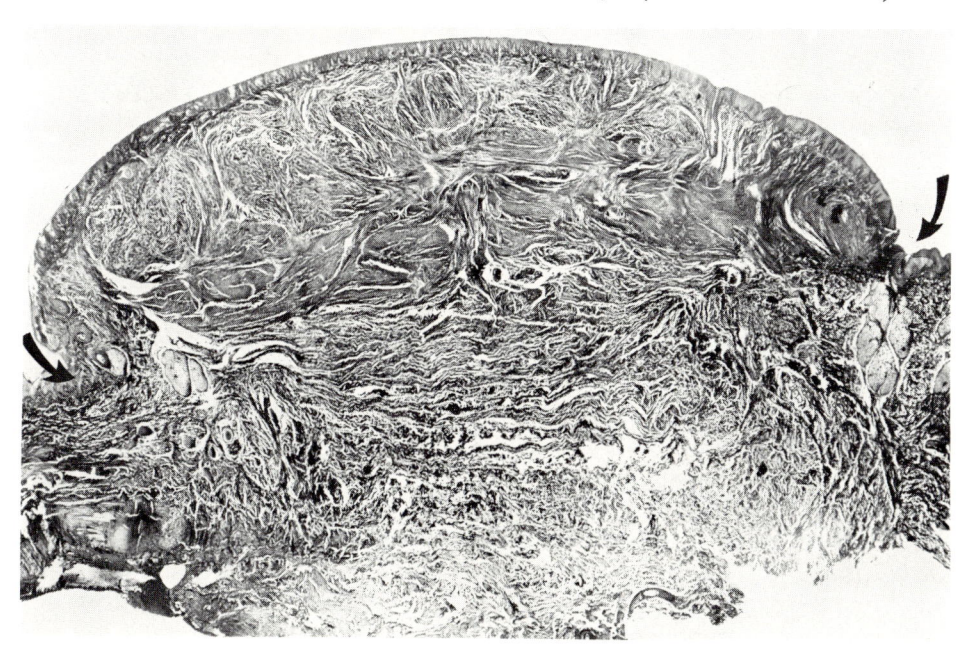

HISTOPATHOLOGY

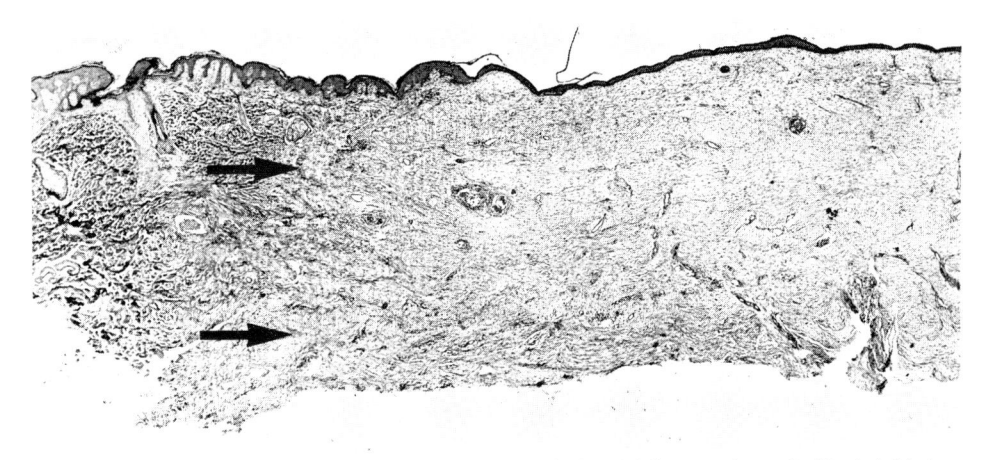

Figure 19. Atrophic Scar. This flat, depressed scar on the back is the counterpart of the keloidal scar. Normal tissue and epidermis is at left. Arrows mark one border of this lesion. Nidi of inflammatory pockets reside within fine collagen bundles. Ectatic vessels and numerous fibroblasts also present. All skin adnexa have been destroyed (H & E reduced from ×10).

collagen bundles of variable size, having lost much of their elastic tissue, are sharply demarcated from the surrounding normal skin. Almost all skin appendages at the site of this scar have been destroyed. Thin-walled, ectatic blood vessels are numerous, and characteristic of keloidal scars.

ATROPHIC SCARS

Atrophic scars are usually seen on the back in patients with acne conglobata. Some of these scars are cigarette paper-like thin (Figure 19). The epidermis is slightly depressed, atrophic, and void of rete ridges; there are no skin appendages.

CLOSED COMEDO-LIKE SCARS

Small, closed comedo-like, elevated, follicular-bound, whitish scars, sometimes with the original central hair still intact and protruding, are commonly seen on the back in acne conglobata patients. Clinically, these scars are often mistaken for comedones. Nothing can be pressed out by puncturing this fibrous mass. Histologically, these lesions are larger than clinically appears. The elastic stain is a diagnostic sign. Elastic fibers have generally been destroyed. The collagen bundles are coarse, densely packed, whorled, and eosinophilic.

CYSTS AND POLYPOROUS COMEDONES

These two lesions, described previously as secondary comedones, may also be considered specialized forms of acne scars, at least in their final stage, when they are completely quiescent and "burned out." This is especially true of the polyporous comedones.

Some scars, mostly on the face, contain foci of calcification and, possibly, bone formation. X-ray films taken with a soft technique may show either dozens or hundreds of little nodules in the skin.[14,15]

Acknowledgments: Figure 2, 3, 6, 12-14, 17, and 18 reproduced with permission from Plewig G, Kligman AM: *Acne: Morphogenesis and Treatment.* New York: Springer-Verlag, 1975. Copyright © 1975, Springer-Verlag, New York. Figure 15 reproduced with permission from Goldschmidt H, Leyden JJ, Stein KH: Acne fulminans: investigation of acute febrile ulcerative acne. *Arch Dermatol* 113:444, 1977. Copyright © 1977, American Medical Association, Chicago.

REFERENCES

1. Kligman AM: An overview of acne. *J Invest Dermatol* 62:268, 1974.
2. Plewig G, Kligman AM: *Acne: Morphogenesis and Treatment.* New York: Springer-Verlag, 1975.
3. Strauss JS, Kligman AM: The pathologic dynamics of acne vulgaris. *Arch Dermatol* 82:779, 1960.
4. Knutson DD: Ultrastructural observations in acne vulgaris: the normal sebaceous follicle and acne lesions. *J Invest Dermatol* 62:288, 1974.
5. Wolff HH, Plewig G, Braun-Falco O: Ultrastructure of human sebaceous follicles and comedones following treatment with vitamin A acid. *Acta Derm Venereol* [*Suppl*] (*Stockh*) 74:99, 1975.
6. Leyden JJ, Kligman AM: Hairs in acne comedones. *Arch Dermatol* 106:851, 1972.
7. Kaidbey KH, Kligman AM: Pigmentation in comedones. *Arch Dermatol* 109:60, 1974.
8. Blair C, Lewis CA: The pigment of comedones. *Br J Dermatol* 82:572, 1970.
9. Nutting WB, Green AC: Pathogenesis associated with hair follicle mites *Demodex* sp.) in Australian Aborigines. *Br J Dermatol* 94:307, 1976.
10. Plewig G, Wolff HH: Follikel-Filamente. *Arch Dermatol Res* 255:9, 1976.
11. Plewig G, Fulton JE, Kligman AM: Cellular dynamics of comedo formation in acne vulgaris. *Arch Dermatol Forsch* 242:12, 1971.
12. Plewig G: Follicular keratinization. *J Invest Dermatol* 62:308, 1974.
13. Goldschmidt H, Leyden JJ, Stein KH: Acne fulminans: investigation of acute febrile ulcerative acne. *Arch Dermatol* 113:444, 1977.
14. Ennis LM: Roentgenographic appearances of calcified acne lesions. *J Am Dent Assoc* 68:351, 1964.
15. Basler RS, Taylor WB, Peacor DR. Postacne osteoma cutis: x-ray diffraction analysis. *Arch Dermatol* 110:113, 1974.

Chapter 12

An Overview of Acne Treatment
RONALD M. REISNER, MD

The various therapeutic methods available for the management of acne, described here and throughout this book, are usually effective. In addition to presenting an introductory overview of current acne therapy, this Chapter emphasizes a vital aspect of the successful management of this chronic disease—one so obvious that it may easily be overlooked as the physician moves through a busy day's practice. Properly used, this aspect enhances therapeutic success and encourages patient cooperation. Improperly used, it may undermine the most medically sound treatment regimens, and may provoke both patient resistance to and dissatisfaction over the often prolonged course of therapy. It validates the sometimes maligned art of medicine, and gives real meaning to the doctor-patient relationship.

This vital aspect is quite simply the content of the first visit. It is during this critical, formative interchange that the bonds of mutual trust and understanding are formed. When treating adolescents, this relationship often involves the patient's family and friends as well.

Adequate time should be allotted during this first visit to sit quietly and discuss, in simple terms, and with the help of a drawing, the basic anatomy of the obstructive and inflammatory lesions of acne. This interview then serves as a basis for the greater acceptance of and cooperation with required therapy, especially in areas such as acne surgery, long-term antibiotic therapy, intralesional injection of corticosteroids, and the use of topical agents (alone or in combination with the above), which all require patient cooperation over many months or years.

Explanations of the chronicity of acne, its waxing and waning course, and, most importantly, the fact that amelioration and control rather than cure are the only realistic goals with presently available therapy, will avoid later disappointment over tacit expectations of cure. This author has seen patients whose dissatisfaction and even anger with their previous physician turned out to be based solely on the grounds that the acne was not cured. Such patients accept the reality of the present limited state of knowledge, once it is explained to them. It is also helpful to debunk the often destructive mythology that has arisen around acne. Although a specific youngster may not harbor any misconceptions, a sufficient number do wonder about one or more of them. Reassurance does much to relieve unspoken fears and guilt, and the patient's emotional health obviously benefits from an improved self-image.

It helps to explain to the patient that, while some people may hold such mistaken beliefs, there is no relationship of acne to dirt or being dirty; to sexual intercourse or the lack of it; to masturbation; to constipation; to venereal disease; to angry feelings (the normal turbulence of the adolescent seeking an independent identity); or, to contagion. Unless one is committed to the unproven concept that diet affects acne, the removal of dietary restrictions produces a healthy sense of normality and freedom. This is most gratifying to the adolescent already under stress because of his acne.

Adolescents especially may suffer severe loss of self-esteem in our appearance-conscious society as a result of their acne. Some may be more emotionally affected than others and may even withdraw from normal social interactions. While not trying to hide the fact that the acne really is present, and while communicating interest and concern for doing everything possible to keep the acne under maximum control, it is at the same time very important that the physician help the adolescent to keep his perspective.

Explicit reassurance should be given that most people, while not oblivious of the fact that the patient has acne, will not judge him on the basis of the acne, but rather on personality and accomplishments. This point can often be brought home successfully by asking the young patient if he judges friends on the basis of whether or not they have acne.

Adolescents and others with acne often spend inordinate amounts of time examining themselves closely in the mirror under bright lights, focusing attention on every lesion. The description of this practice will often elicit a smile of recognition and will further an appreciation of the physician's understanding, which then reminds the patient that this can lead to his developing distorted feelings that other people perceive him as "acne with a person attached," rather than as "a person who happens to have acne."

From this solid foundation of mutual trust and understanding, the physician can approach a rational therapy of acne with good expectations. The choice of therapy can be significantly aided by considering acne as falling into two major groups: noninflammatory acne and inflammatory acne. The following is a brief commentary on the agents used in treatment which are discussed in detail elsewhere in this text.

Treatment of Noninflammatory Acne

This is essentially an obstructive disease, characterized by compacted keratin, sebum, and bacteria which dilate the pilosebaceous duct, resulting in the development of open and closed comedones. Therapy consists basically of removal and then prevention or reduction of the formation of new comedones.

Comedo Removal—Current evidence now implicates not only closed comedones, but, at times, open comedones, as a source of inflammation and scarring.[1] Therefore, regular, atraumatic removal of comedones reduces the risk of possible future inflammatory lesions and scarring, and produces the immediately gratifying benefit of a prompt improvement in the patient's appearance (see Chapter 25).

If the physician performs the comedo removal, time is then afforded for discussion with the patient to reinforce and expand upon the content of the initial visit. Adjustment of the current therapeutic regimen as needed can also be seen to at this time. However, a well-trained assistant will often serve equally as well in performing comedo removal.

Peeling Agents—Many agents appear to function by producing desquamation, often accompanied by erythema. The effect of some may be due in part to an increased rate of turnover of the stratum corneum of the follicular duct, thus presumably preventing the opportunity for the compaction necessary to produce the comedo.[2] This may be helpful in reducing the development of new comedones, as well in easing the mechanical removal of existing ones. Peeling materials include: cleansing agents; astringents; topical preparations containing sulfur and/or salicylic acid and/or resorcinol; benzoyl peroxide (usually in 5% or 10% concentration); topical retinoic acid (usually in 0.025-0.1% concentration); cryotherapy, including the slush and spray techniques; and ultraviolet light (see Chapter 24).

With the exceptions of retinoic acid and benzoyl peroxide, there is no clear-cut evidence that the agents listed above have unquestioned comedolytic activity. However, the erythema and desquamation produced by these agents do seem to hasten the involution of minor inflammatory lesions such as small papules and pustules.

Recently, the combination of benzoyl peroxide and retinoic acid (see Chapter 16) has proven to be more effective than the use of either alone, both in the management of obstructive acne and in selected patients with inflammatory acne. While it has not been this author's experience that this combination therapy has successfully eliminated the need for systemic and/or topical antibiotics in the more severe types of inflammatory acne discussed below, it has proved a useful addition to our therapeutic armamentarium.

Cleansing agents such as soap and water or astringents are cosmetically useful in improving appearance by removing accumulated surface oil. Used one or more times a day as needed, cleansing agents can temporarily eliminate undesirable oiliness.

The topically applied agents are available in a number of forms, including lotions, creams, and, more recently, gels. The total effect of the agents in each of these groups is additive; depending on the nature of the individual's response, it is generally wise to proceed gradually and build up the intensity of therapy, striving ordinarily for very slight, virtually subclinical erythema and desquamation.

Treatment of Inflammatory Acne

Characterized by papules, pustules, and nodulocystic lesions, inflammatory acne carries the double burden of producing greater disfigurement during its active phases, therefore having a greater propensity to produce permanent scarring. In general, with the exception of mild forms of inflammatory acne, the measures described for the management of noninflammatory acne are not of great value here.

Acne Surgery—Pustular lesions which are not superficial enough to unroof with topical peeling agents and produce spontaneous drainage may be incised and drained. Cystic lesions are actually nodules which have undergone suppurative changes, and today it is seldom necessary to incise and drain any but the most fluctuant of such lesions. They are better treated in most cases with intralesional corticosteroids or cryotherapy, or prevented with systemic or topical antibiotic therapy (see Chapter 24 and 25).

Chemotherapeutic Agents—The most significant advance in the management of the more severe types of inflammatory acne has been the long-term administration of broad-spectrum antibiotics. A promising new development is the use of topical antibiotics. Both subjects are discussed in detail elsewhere in this book (see Chapter 17-19).

Intralesional Corticosteroid Therapy—One of the most useful methods in the day-to-day management of the more severe nodular and cystic forms of acne is the intralesional injection of dilute solutions of corticosteroids. It has been the experience of this author that saline dilution of the corticosteroid is preferable to its dilution in lidocaine or other local anesthetics, both because there is less stinging at the moment of injection and because, by the time the local anesthetic can act, the discomfort of the entire procedure is over. The use of disposable #30 needles further reduces the discomfort of the procedure; most patients tolerate it well and are grateful for its rapid effect. However, the hazards of corticosteroid-induced pseudoatrophy should be made clear to the patient (see Chapter 24 and 25).

Systemic Corticosteroid Therapy—Although systemic corticosteroids in sufficient dosage may themselves produce a papulopustular follicular acneform eruption, they are effective in reducing the inflammatory component of severe nodulocystic acne. They should be reserved for use in carefully selected patients with extensive severe nodulocystic acne which is unresponsive to other modes of therapy, because of the hazardous side effects associated with their use, particularly over long periods. Starting dosages of 30 mg a day of prednisone or its equivalent should be followed by tapering and discontinuation as soon as possible, preferably within a month or so. In rare situations, long-term therapy may have to be considered with the concomitant greatly increased risk of significant side effects. In this author's view, the primary value of these agents is for control of acute exacerbations of nodulocystic acne not otherwise responsive to currently available therapy (see Chapter 24).

Cyclic Estrogen-Progestogen Therapy—This form of therapy is based on the capacity of the estrogenic substances employed, usually ethinyl estradiol or mestranol, to suppress sebum production.[3] This capability is, at least, their most easily measured effect. Much more difficult to evaluate are other effects, such as the inhibition of ductal retention hyperkeratosis, which may well be of greater importance. Women so treated should be warned that they may experience a flare of their acne in the first few months of treatment. Ordinarily, if a good response is to be obtained, it will have occurred by the end of the fifth month of treatment (see Chapter 22).

In general, dosages in the range of 100 μg of ethinyl estradiol or its equivalent are necessary to produce both significant sebum suppression and noticeable improvement in acne in most patients. This dose level appears to carry a risk three times greater of producing thromboembolic phenomena, resulting at times in pulmonary embolism and death, than that of the 50 μg doses often used for contraception.[4] Statistically small as it may be, this one risk, when considered in relation to the acne which in itself carries no threat to life, and even without reference to the vast number of other side effects which have been described with such therapy, combined with the fact that it is by no means uniformly effective, raises very serious questions in this author's mind as to its role in the management of acne. Such therapy, in this author's view, should rarely be considered in the management of acne except when the need to control the acne justifies the risk, as in the case of those women who have extremely severe, recalcitrant nodulocystic acne, which has been clearly demonstrated to be unresponsive to an intensive regimen of other, potentially less hazardous modes of therapy. Therapy should then be undertaken only with complete awareness of all the appropriate history, and after the necessary physical examination and laboratory evaluations have been completed. Full recognition of the real risks involved in the use of these agents is essential.

Diuretics—The use of diuretics during the 7-10 days prior to the onset of menses has been proposed as being useful in the control of premenstrual exacerbations of acne. However, a recent double-blind study[5] suggested that diuretics are not more useful than placebo (see Chapter 24).

X-ray Therapy—This form of therapy is being used less and less, since newer and more effective measures for the control of the more severe forms of acne have been developed. If, in the physician's judgment, this method of treatment seems indicated, it should be undertaken only with full understanding of proper technique and associated risks (see Chapter 23).

Diet—To date, no genuinely convincing evidence exists to incriminate any single dietary item, or combination of items, in the production of acne exacerbations. For example, neither chocolate[6] nor dietary iodine[7] has been shown to be able to produce exacerbations of acne. Should a rare patient reliably demonstrate flaring of acne following ingestion of a given food, there is obviously no harm in eliminating this single item from the diet, at least for a significant period, in order to evaluate its influence (see Chapter 9 and 24).

Vitamin A—At present, no conclusive evidence has been presented for the value of systemic administration of vitamin A in the treatment of any form of acne. A well-designed, double-blind study[8] comparing the results of 150,000 units a day of oral vitamin A administered for 12 weeks to those of a lactose placebo revealed no difference in effectiveness. There does not seem to be a firm role at this time for oral vitamin A, in non-toxic dose levels, in the treatment of acne.

Vaccines—There does not appear to be any convincing evidence to date for the value of staphylococcal toxoids or other similar vaccines in the management of acne.

Cosmetics—The appropriate use of cosmetics may be of considerable help in reducing the immediate emotional impact of the disfigurement produced by acne. However, there is some evidence[9] that selected cosmetic agents may be responsible for the development of exacerbations of acne (see Chapter 3 and 24).

Sulfones—The use of diaminodiphenylsulfone in the dosage range of 100 mg, 3 times a week, for about 3 months, with subsequent gradual reduction, has been suggested[10] for the management of very severe, resistant nodulocystic and conglobate acne. While this author is unaware of any large, double-blind control studies to support this view, it is a therapeutic measure worthy of consideration in selected patients with acne as noted above, but full awareness of the risks of hemolytic anemia, methemoglobinemia, central nervous system toxicity (*eg*, headaches and nervousness), blurred vision, hematuria, *etc*, is necessary.

Miscellaneous—Patients with inflammatory acne may experience significant increased activity with exposure to excessive heat and humidity. While this may sometimes make it necessary to discontinue active sports such as football and wrestling, it is often possible to continue such activity by intensifying the treatment program. Local increases in heat and humidity, produced by occlusive clothing and/or mechanical irritation from wool or other rough textured clothing, may also exacerbate acne. Picking, squeezing, *etc*, may contribute to the rupture of follicular contents into the surrounding dermis, converting a noninflammatory or slightly inflammatory lesion into a destructive, scarring lesion.[11] As part of the explanation of the anatomy of the development of acne, a description of this phenomenon at the initial visit is, in this author's experience, much more effective in obtaining patient cooperation than the simple repetition of the injunction, "don't pick."

Summary

Although no cure for acne can presently be offered, the well-informed clinician who has established a good working relationship with the acne patient can employ a rationally selected, intensive regimen of therapy to provide maximum control of the disease. Through treatment and understanding, the physician can help the patient through this difficult period of life with a minimum of physical, as well as psychological, scarring.

REFERENCES

1. Orentreich N, Durr N: The natural evolution of comedones into inflammatory papules and pustules. *J Invest Dermatol* 62:316, 1974.
2. Kligman AM, Fulton JE Jr, Plewig G: Topical vitamin A acid in acne vulgaris. *Arch Dermatol* 99:469, 1969.
3. Strauss JS, Pochi PE: Effect of cyclic progestin-estrogen therapy on sebum and acne in women. *JAMA* 190:815, 1964.
4. *Estrogens and thromboembolism* (editorial). *Br Med J* 2:189, 1970.
5. Jelinek JE: Hydrochlorothiazide and the control of premenstrual exacerbation of acne. *Arch Dermatol* 105:79, 1972.
6. Fulton JE Jr, Plewig G, Kligman AM: Effect of chocolate on acne vulgaris. *JAMA* 210:2071, 1969.
7. Hitch JM, Greenburg EG: Adolescent acne and dietary iodine. *Arch Dermatol* 84:898, 1961.
8. Anderson JAD, Stokoe IH: Vitamin A in acne vulgaris. *Br Med J* 2:294, 1963.
9. Kligman AM, Mills OH Jr: "Acne cosmetica." *Arch Dermatol* 106:843, 1972.
10. Kaminsky CA, de Kaminsky AR, Schicci C, et al: Acne: treatment with diaminodiphenylsulfone. *Cutis* 13:869, 1974.
11. Baer RL, Witten VH (Eds): "Acne Vulgaris: Remarks on Recent Advances in Knowledge and Management," in *The Year Book of Dermatology, 1959-60*, pp 7-32. Chicago: Year Book Medical Pub, 1960.

Chapter 13

Vitamin A Acid Topical Therapy

CHRISTOPHER M. PAPA, MD

Tretinoin (vitamin A acid, trans-retinoic acid) is believed to be the tissue-active form of vitamin A (Figure 1). Applied topically, it is a potent pharmacologic agent, capable of altering epithelial growth and differentiation.[1,2] Since faulty follicular keratinization is thought to be the primary defect in acne (see Chapter 10, 14, and 16), the use of tretinoin makes good sense—the drug is targeted where it is most needed. Extensive clinical experience has shown tretinoin to be valuable in both the treatment and the prevention of acne. At this time, tretinoin and topical tetracycline are the only drugs approved by the FDA for the local treatment of acne.

During the past 10 years, many of the original misconceptions concerning the use of topical tretinoin have been re-evaluated. The drug was introduced when "peeling agents" were being sought in acne therapy. As the ultimate "keratolytic," tretinoin allegedly possessed a unique irritant activity. The skin would supposedly peel forever, because it could not accommodate to the effect of tretinoin.[3] This required a stringent regimen, as treatment was designed to keep the patient's skin in a high state of irritation. An unswerving commitment was expected of both patients and physicians.

Time and experience have proven these initial impressions erroneous. There is no relationship between the therapeutic benefits of topical tretinoin and any irritant or peeling effect.[4-7] Furthermore, the skin accommodates to the drug in a matter of days or weeks. Heroics are not required; the successful physician and the patient need only understand how to use tretinoin.

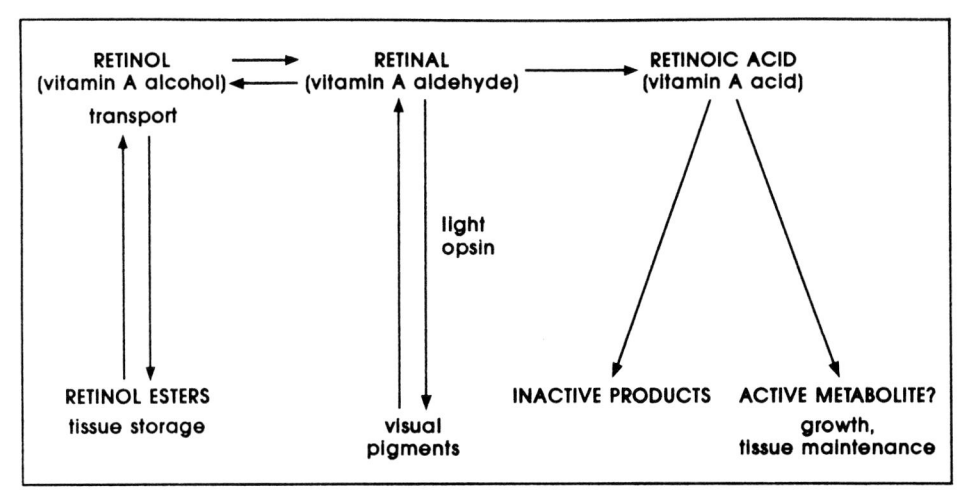

Figure 1. Physiological relationships of tretinoin to vitamin A.

The truism that patient instruction is an integral part of successful therapy is particularly meaningful in regard to tretinoin acne treatment. As the patient encounters anticipated events, he accepts them as encouraging signs of the predicted successful results. As evidence of the physician's prognostic prowess is demonstrated, patient confidence in the prescriber, as well as in the prescription, increases. Active patient participation minimizes impatience, minor discomforts, and the often petty annoyances which threaten to disrupt the long-term, harmonious relationships required in the management of a chronic disease such as acne.

Early Clinical Course of Tretinoin Therapy

EXPULSION OF COMEDONES

The comedo is the clinical expression of the primary obstructive defect in the sebaceous follicle. While it was long recognized that the removal of comedones was most desirable, the goal was elusive. The lesions are actually very deep compactions of adherent horny cells with admixed sebum, bacteria, and yeasts. Superficial peeling can do little to unseat such obstructions from the follicle (Figure 2 and 3). Until the advent of tretinoin therapy, only persuasive manual efforts with the comedo extractor could laboriously and painfully expel these masses.

The earliest evidence of the drug's activity is what can best be termed a "follicular flush." Within the first 2 weeks of treatment, the open comedones (or blackheads) literally catapult out of their recesses. It is a clearly visible event (Figure 4). During this stage, impressive alterations are taking place which explain the expulsion of the comedones. The epidermis and its down-

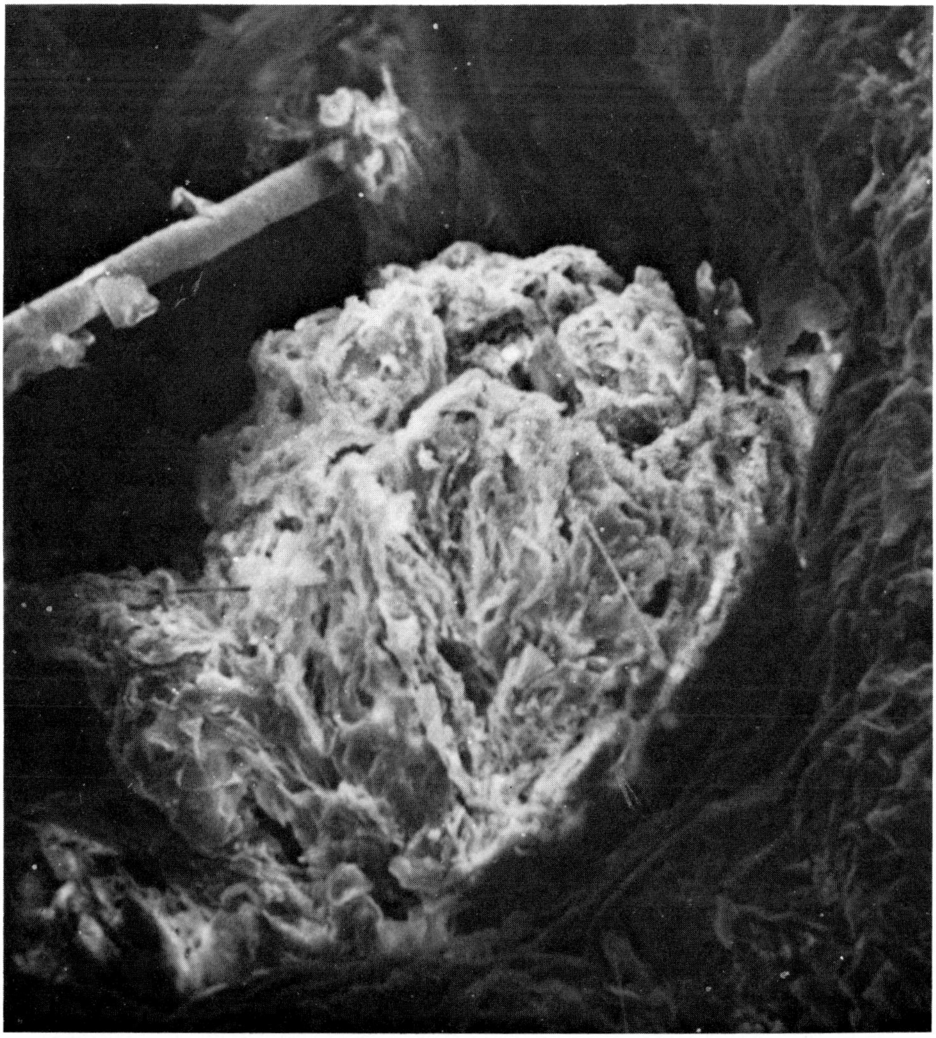

Figure 2. Scanning electron microscopic surface view of open comedo. Mass is a compaction of sloughed cells, lipids, and microorganisms. Tiny trapped hairs seen as linear streaks; compare with larger, normal hair (above comedo) from a nearby follicle (reduced from ×100).

growths that line the follicular canal are stimulated to grow at a more rapid rate, and the desmosomal attachments of the keratinocytes are diminished.[1-3] The loosened comedo is dislodged from within the follicle and is carried out onto the skin's surface. The ultrastructural changes in the follicular infundibulum which characterize the retention hyperkeratosis and basic obstruction are reversed with the application of tretinoin.[8]

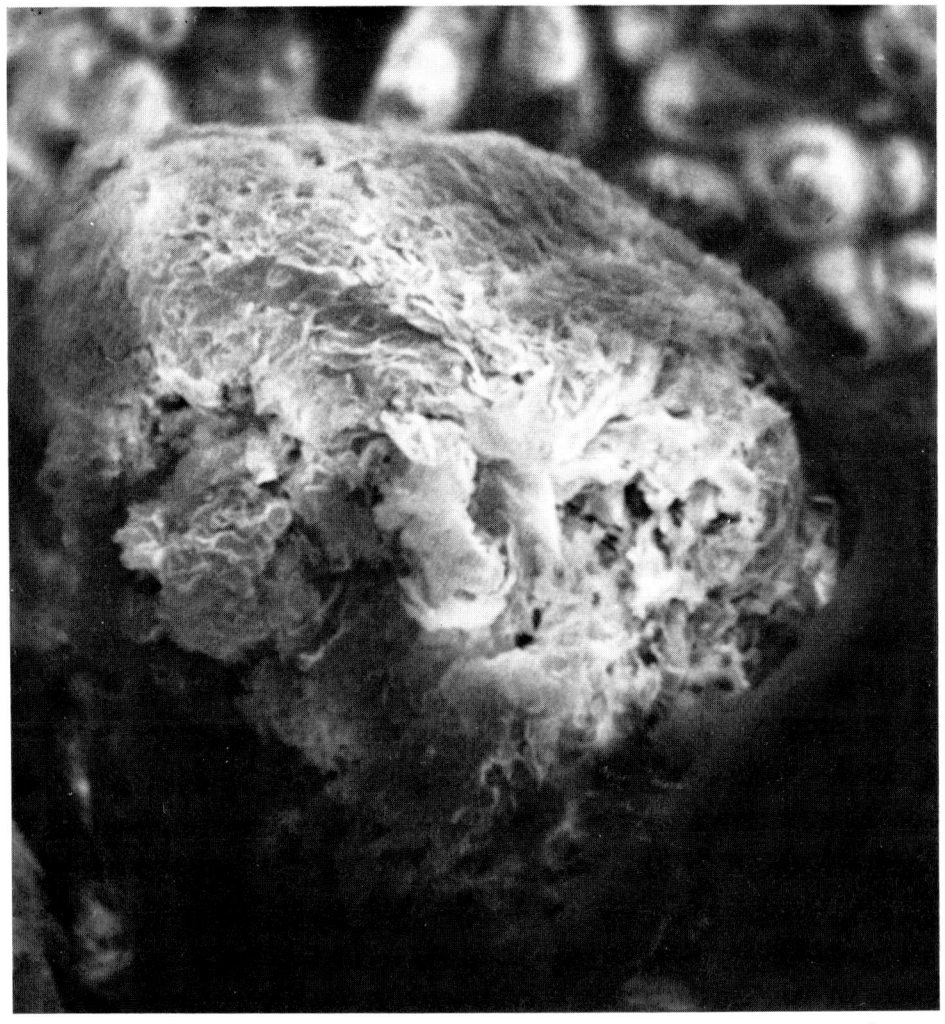

Figure 3. Deep follicular portion of comedo, separated chemically from surrounding dermis. Portion of lining capsule is removed, exposing compacted material. This emphasizes the futility of trying to remove plugs by washing or surface peeling (reduced from ×100).

RESOLUTION OF PAPULES AND PUSTULES

During the initial 2 weeks, there is also considerable resolution of the pre-existing papules and pustules. Early clinical observers were so impressed with the comedo expulsion that this additional effect was not stressed. Data obtained from the clinical studies required for drug registration and approval included objective counts of each lesion type. It was established that these pre-existing lesions respond to tretinoin as well.[9]

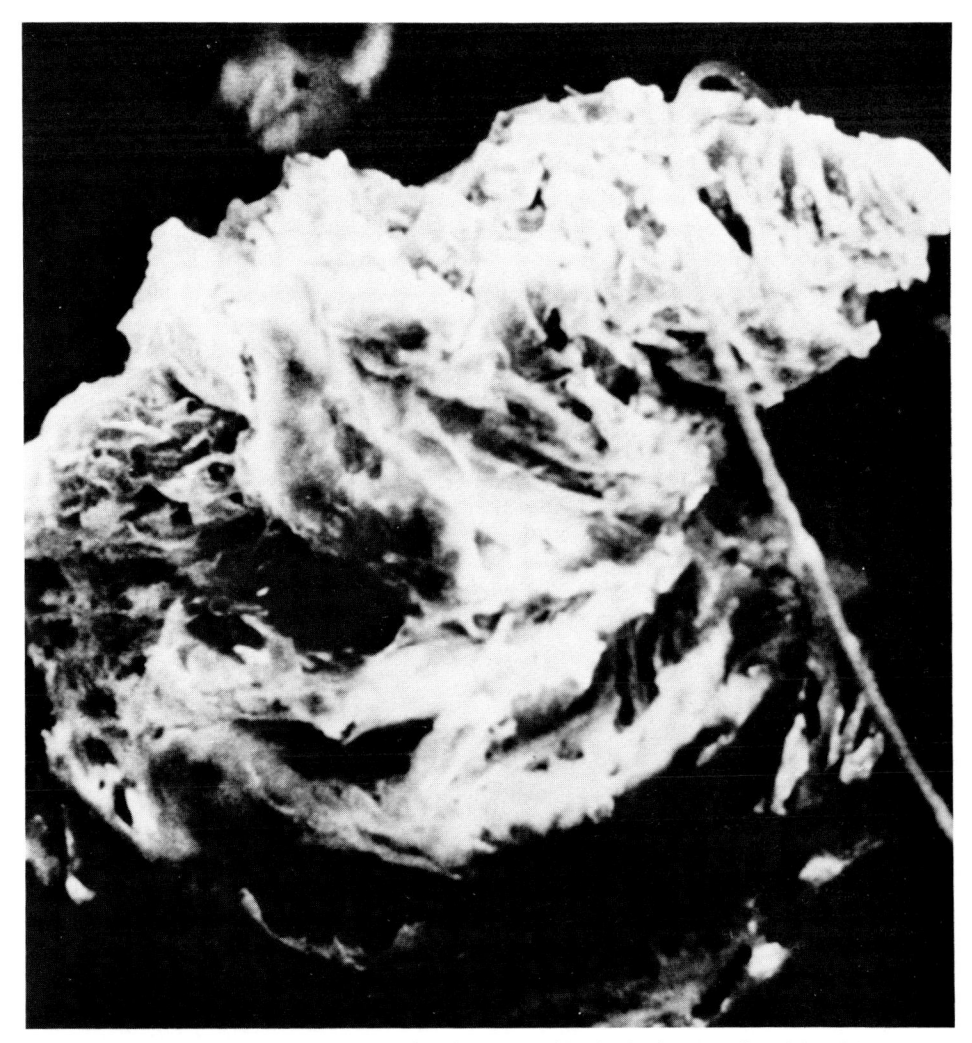

Figure 4. Expulsion of comedo after 2 weeks of tretinoin therapy. Event is clinically apparent to patient as one of the earliest, encouraging signs that medication is working. Nearby hair from another follicle is seen over comedonal mass (reduced from ×100).

ACCOMMODATION TO TRETINOIN

While the described effects on the lesions indicate the action of tretinoin on the follicular epithelium, it must be remembered that similar changes are occurring within the interfollicular skin. If one follows the events on the back, where the follicles are not so closely packed, rather than on the facial skin, it becomes apparent that the follicle is the specific site of action. In the skin of a patient who is susceptible to the irritant effect, the erythema begins

126 TREATMENT

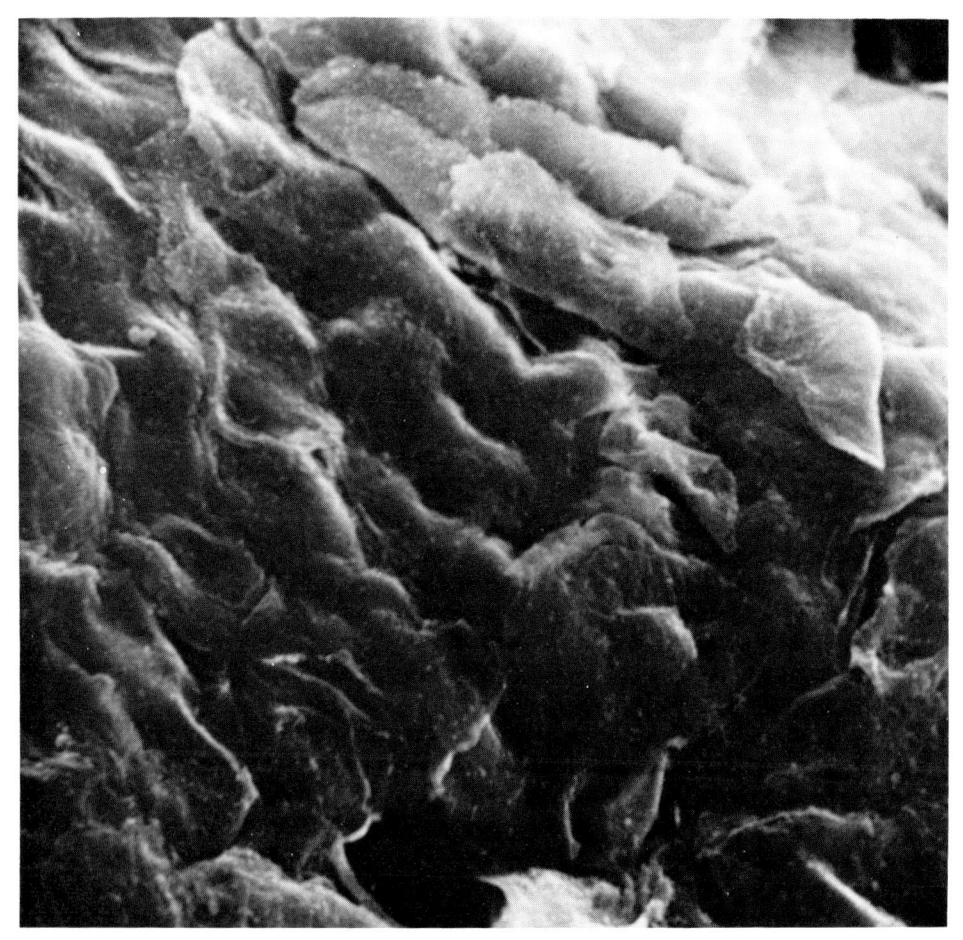

Figure 5. Intact, interfollicular stratum corneum before tretinoin treatment. Snuggly, abutted cells form an impenetrable barrier. Some of the surface greasiness of patient and many microorganisms are apparent (reduced from ×1000).

around the individual follicles, spreads centrifugally, becomes confluent at about one week, and then slowly recedes in exactly the opposite fashion: centripetally back to the follicle in the second week. The stratum corneum, which is normally a compact envelope of abutted, stratified squamae (Figure 5), transforms into a loose structure of cells which have not fully differentiated (Figure 6). During this initial phase, the skin is particularly susceptible to irritants and, in some patients, may become red and slightly scaly. Accommodation proceeds as the drug application is continued (Figure 7-10). The erythema and peeling fade, and a protective stratum corneum again forms. Much of the irritation originally attributed directly to the tretinoin represents the effect of other irritants which readily penetrate the susceptible skin. The instructions to the patients are designed to minimize such discomfort. When the need for such temporary proscriptions are explained, patients willingly cooperate.

RESOLUTION OF DEEP LESIONS

Shortly after tretinoin starts to expel the comedones and the existing papules and pustules resolve, its effect on the deeper, often unseen lesions becomes manifest. A quick and simultaneous eruption of small papules and pustules may occur sometime between 2-4 weeks after initiating therapy. These resolve spontaneously in 1-2 weeks, although concomitant antibiotic therapy may be used to suppress the evolution of such lesions.[10]

This event can be considered as a propitious sign of effective therapy, if the patient is alerted to expect it (Figure 11-13). Therapy should not be interrupted at this critical stage, since this will only delay the resolution. The apparent exacerbation occurs when tretinoin alters the permeability of the sebaceous capsule and follicular wall, allowing the trapped contents to gain access to the dermis and thus incite the inflammatory response.[3] Tretinoin augments the reaction by increasing the local blood flow and, consequently, the delivery of leukocytes (see Chapter 14). Tretinoin may also directly stimulate the cellular immune response.[11]

Maintenance Therapy

After 8-11 weeks of using tretinoin alone, about 75% of the treated patients will have a 50-100% reduction in total acne lesions. Tretinoin, however, does not cure acne. Continued treatment brings further improvement and, more importantly, prevents recurrence of the disease by inhibiting production of new comedones (Figure 14). Meanwhile, the accommodated skin, with an intact stratum corneum (Figure 15), functions normally, and the patient's skin is not overly sensitive to irritants.

Maintenance therapy is best achieved by keeping patients on daily treatment with the mildest preparation, rather than advocating alternate-day therapy. Once spacing intervals are recommended, the patient has a tendency to increase the time between applications until the drug no longer has its desired effect. At that point, the patient must return to the original regimen and will react as if the drug had been applied for the first time.

Selection of Dosage Form

The variety of topical tretinoin preparations available allows for treatment to be tailored to the individual's needs. Therapeutic potency, mildness (*ie*, freedom from irritancy), and drug concentration *per se* are not directly related. The carrier vehicle greatly influences the pharmacologic activity. While all the preparations provide similar benefits, a rank order of

128 TREATMENT

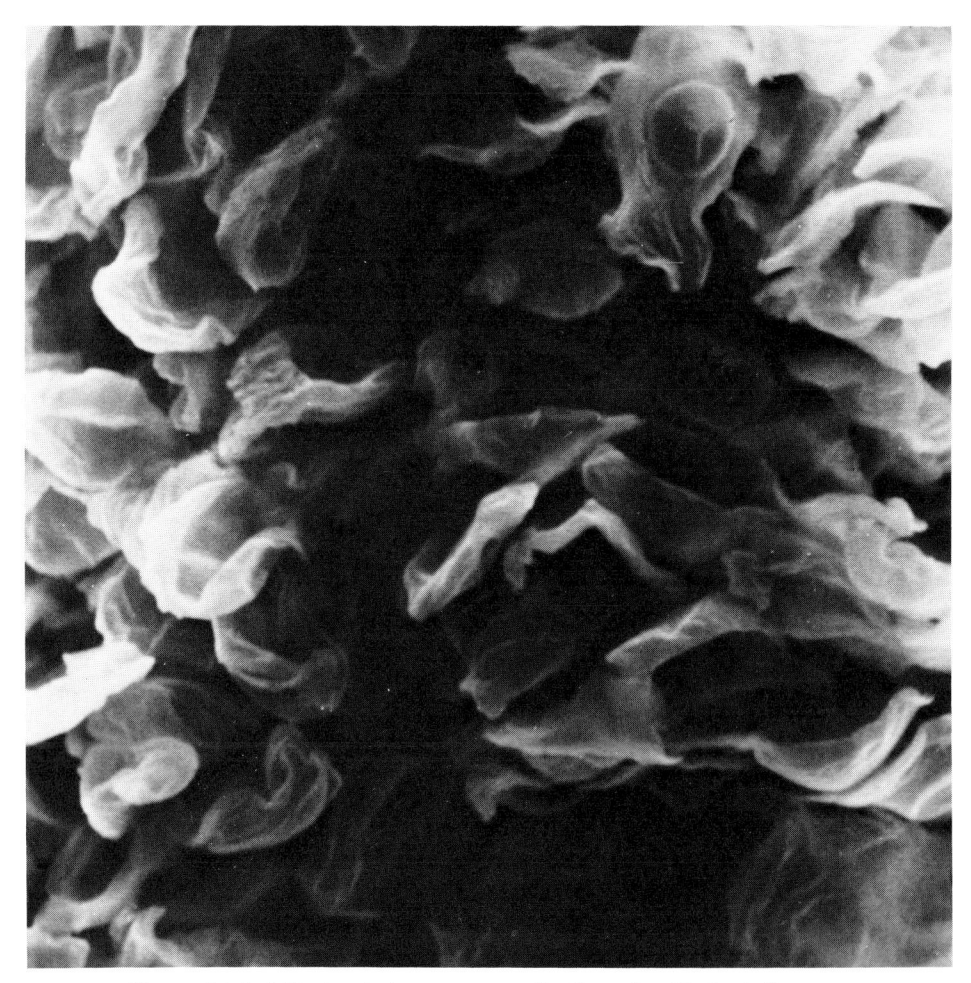

Figure 6. Interfollicular stratum corneum after 2 weeks of tretinoin therapy. As a result of increased epidermopoiesis, cells are not fully differentiated and do not form functioning, protective barrier (reduced from x1000).

potential irritancy shows alcoholic-polyethylene glycol solution at 0.05% concentration to be the harshest, followed by 0.025% alcoholic gel, with 0.05% and 0.1% creams being the mildest preparations. Again, simple reliance on drug concentration would be quite misleading in this matter.

Choice of the vehicle should be governed by the nature of the patient's skin and his physical environment, as well as the severity of the acne and its anatomic site. The solution, for example, works well and covers large areas such as the back or chest, but is quite irritating to the face. Patients with oilier, swarthy complexions appreciate the more drying gel formulation, particularly when the weather is hot and humid. The fair-skinned, sensitive individual will better tolerate the cream forms.

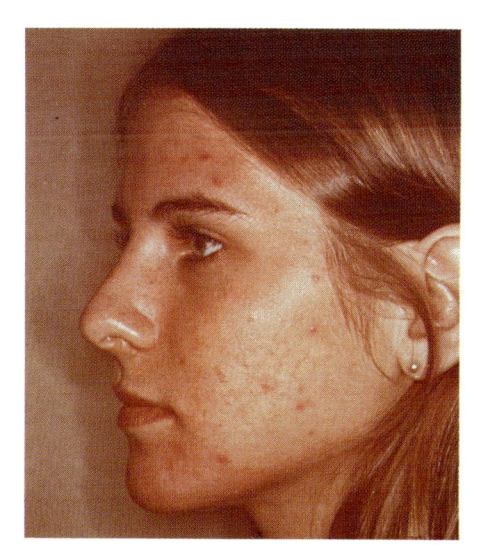

Figure 7. Pre-tretinoin therapy. Fair-skinned girl already has some erythema from using over-the-counter treatments. Photographs courtesy E. B. Stahl, MD.

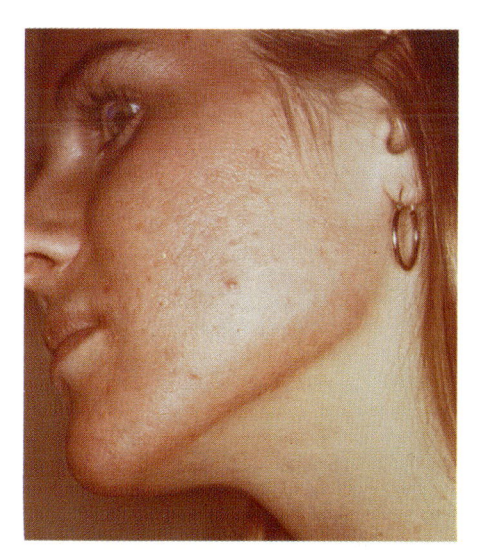

Figure 8. After 2 weeks of tretinoin therapy, a sharply circumscribed erythema with minimal scaling appears where tretinoin was applied.

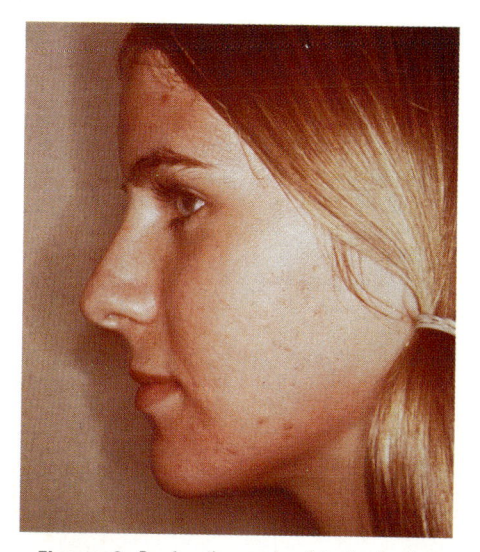

Figure 9. By fourth week of tretinoin therapy, there is accommodation to the drug. Erythema is less visible and patient is comfortable. Some of the "apparent exacerbation" appears as new inflammatory papules, while original lesions have disappeared.

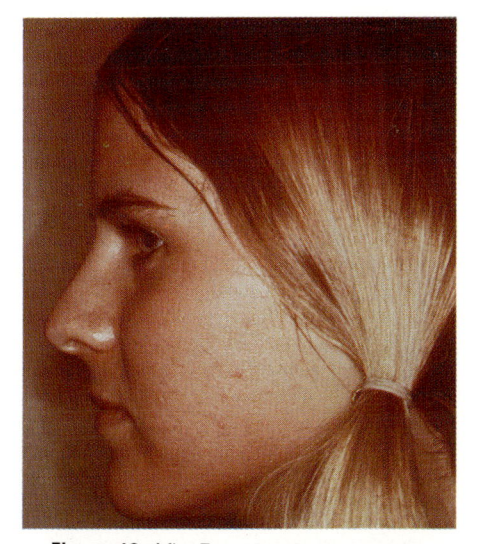

Figure 10. After 7 weeks of tretinoin therapy, acne is gone and patient continues with a fine "blush," which she considered an added cosmetic benefit.

130 TREATMENT

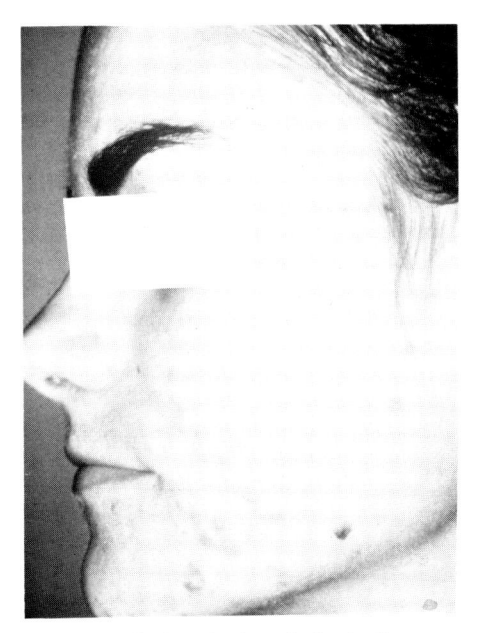

Figure 11. Patient before tretinoin therapy. Nevus near her mandible is convenient marker to note position of original inflammatory lesions. Photographs courtesy L. Montes, MD.

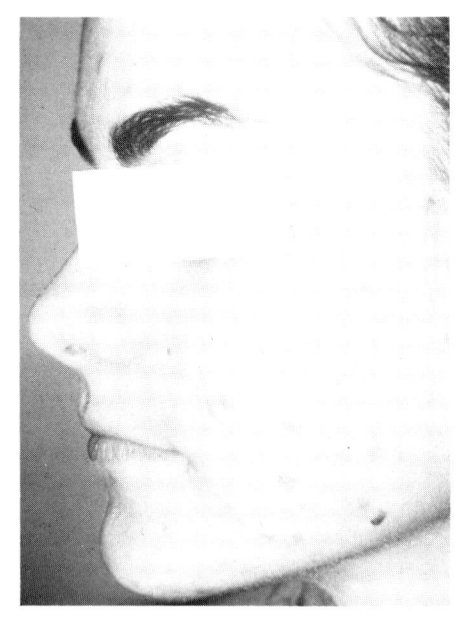

Figure 12. After 6 weeks of tretinoin therapy, initial lesions are gone. New pustules, inflammatory papules are "apparent exacerbation."

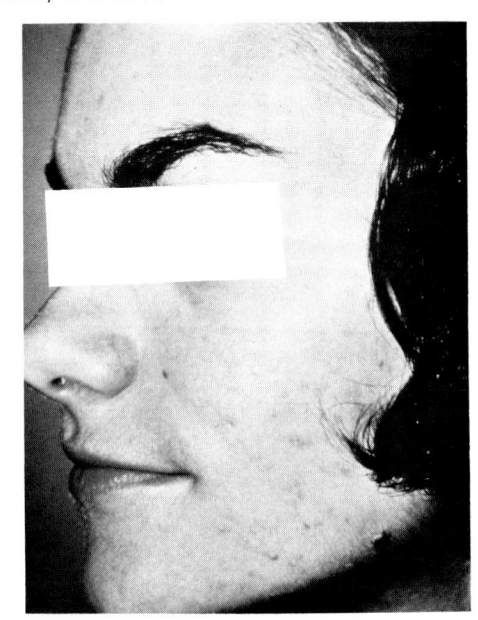

Figure 13. After 12 weeks of tretinoin therapy without any concomitant treatments, all lesions, except nevus, are gone.

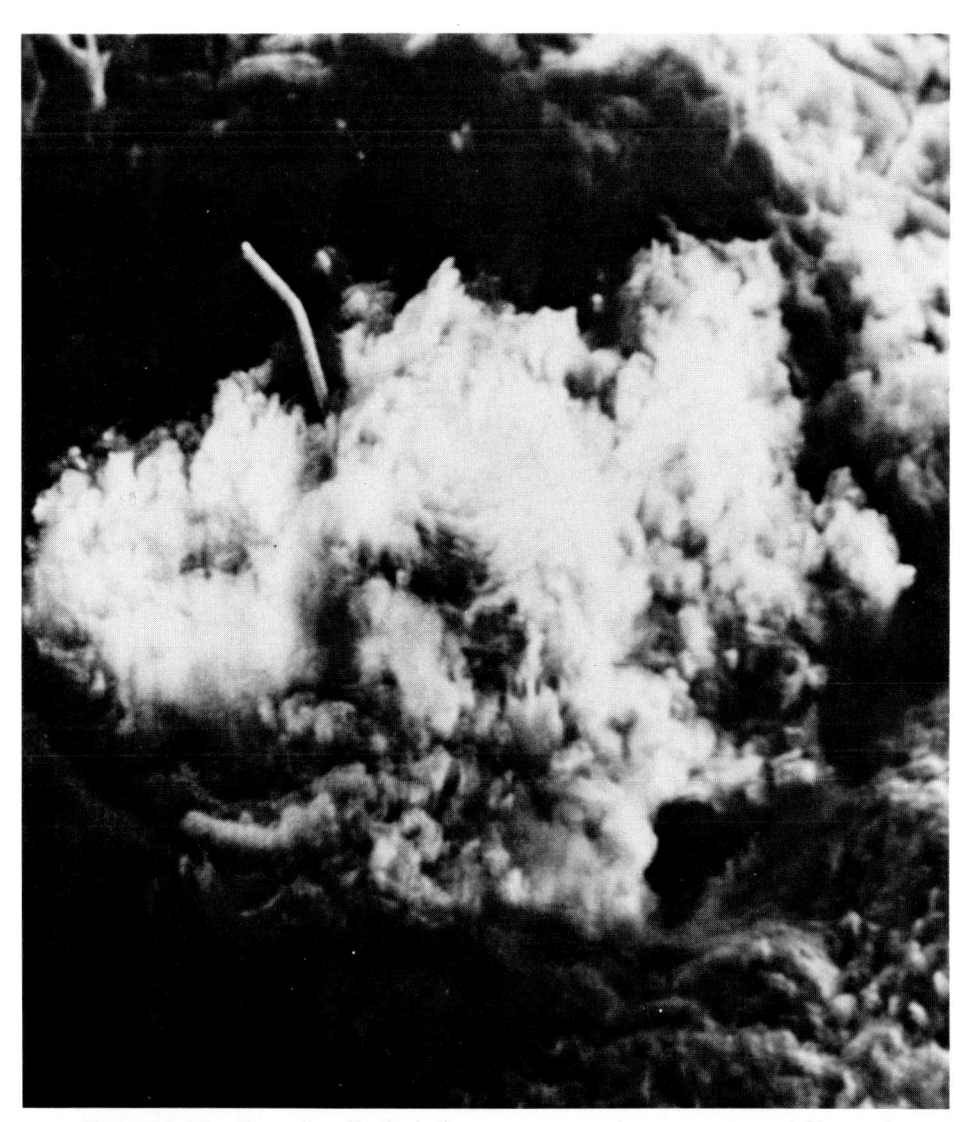

Figure 14. After 18 months of tretinoin therapy, no comedones were present. Biopsy of large follicular "pore" shows that cells shed into the lumen are small, noncohesive, and evidently incapable of forming a genuine comedonal mass (reduced from ×100).

Patient Instructions

Care should be taken to show the patient how to gently apply just enough of the product to cover the entire affected area. Uninstructed patients may simply dot the material on active lesions. Others may use the solution-impregnated swabs as abrasive rubbing pads. The medication should be spread away from, not toward, the eyes, nasolabial folds, or corners of the

132   TREATMENT

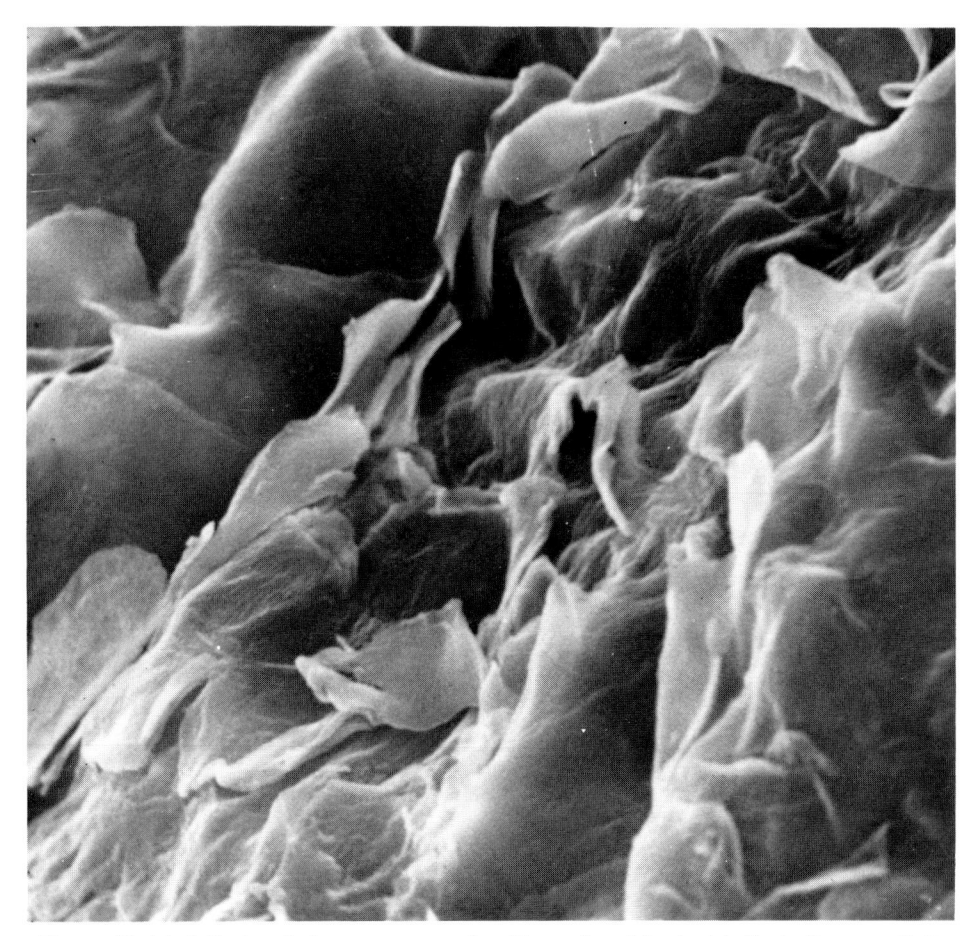

Figure 15. Interfollicular stratum corneum after 18 months of topical tretinoin therapy. Cells have returned to their thin, flat morphology and form competent barrier (reduced from ×1000).

mouth, where it is likely to pool and produce severe local irritation. A single daily application is all that is required.

The specification that the product be applied at bedtime is logical, since there follows the longest period between skin washing. Additionally, tretinoin undergoes degradation with ultraviolet light exposure, making its use during the day of questionable merit. If the tretinoin is applied at bedtime, however, there is less chance that the face will be scratched or otherwise manipulated while the patient sleeps; also, the patient may not even be aware of any possible minor discomfort at this time. Most importantly, bedtime application eliminates the patient's worry that the medication will be visible.

Instructions to avoid other irritants is vital. The misguided habits of frequent face washings and scrubbings with harsh, drying soaps must be altered. The patient should apply tretinoin to thoroughly dried skin 15 minutes after washing, since wet skin enhances penetration and increases the potential for irritation.

Always inquire into over-the-counter remedies. Patients do not necessarily regard these as medications and are likely to continue using them in addition to the tretinoin. Other potential irritants are found in "medicated" makeups, shaving creams, and after-shave lotions. Those containing menthol, lime, and spices are best avoided.

Concomitant Therapy

While tretinoin does work on the papules, pustules, and comedones of acne when used alone, there are occasions when other drugs may be added to the regimen. Systemic tetracycline or erythromycin, for example, may be used to supplement tretinoin during the first 1-2 months of therapy to reduce the "apparent exacerbation" which occurs. Thereafter, the patient is weaned from the antibiotic and continued on tretinoin alone.[10] Patients with severe, cystic, inflammatory acne are apt to do better with prolonged combination therapy.[12]

The concurrent use of topical benzoyl peroxide and tretinoin has been recommended to provide extra benefits[13] (see Chapter 16). The two should not be mixed in a single solution or applied directly on top of one another, because they are chemically incompatible and neutralize each other. Preferably, the tretinoin should be applied at bedtime and the benzoyl peroxide after the face is washed the next morning. To minimize the additive irritant effects of these preparations, it would seem advisable to introduce the benzoyl peroxide only after accommodation to the tretinoin.

Cutaneous Safety

Judicious use of topical tretinoin is possible without eliciting local side effects other than the mild, temporary inflammation which occurs during the initial 1-2 weeks of therapy. True allergic reactions rarely occur,[14] and tretinoin is neither a phototoxic nor a photoallergic agent. Early reports of "photoirritant" reactions, as well as temporary hypo- or hyperpigmentation, attended inappropriate use of the drug. They are nothing more than postinflammatory events, and are thus avoidable.[14] Black skin may be safely treated, and fair-skinned patients need only to avoid excessive sunlight, if the drug is used correctly and irritation is minimized or avoided. Patients with atopic eczema appear to be particularly sensitive to tretinoin. The drug should never be used on obvious eczematous skin.

The effect of topical tretinoin on ultraviolet tumorigenesis was studied in hairless albino mice.[15,16] The results are conflicting, showing either acceleration or retardation of epitheliomas in these special animals. Although the relevance of the information to humans is uncertain, the precautions to minimize sun and ultraviolet exposure while using tretinoin is prudent. Topical tretinoin, however, is reported to ameliorate premalignant and malignant epitheliomas in humans.[17,18]

Summary

The available tretinoin acne treatments have presented no problems of systemic toxicity or hypervitaminosis-A effects. Topical tretinoin has proven effective for the treatment and prevention of acne. As with other potent drugs, the physician must understand its pharmacologic properties, and the patient must be educated as to its appropriate use. These are small efforts, given the potential benefits of such therapy.

REFERENCES

1. Plewig G, Fulton JE: Autoradiographesche Untersuchungen an Epidermis und Adnexan nach Vitamin A-Säure-Behandlung. *Hautarzt* 23:128, 1972.
2. Christophers E, Wolff HH: Differential formation of desmosomes and hemidesmosomes in epidermal cell cultures treated with retinoic acid. *Nature* 256:209, 1975.
3. Kligman AM, Fulton JE, Plewig G: Topical vitamin A acid in acne vulgaris. *Arch Dermatol* 99:469, 1969.
4. Cullen SI: Evaluation of tretinoin in the treatment of acne vulgaris. *Cutis* 10:751, 1972.
5. Gunther S: Vitamin A acid in acne vulgaris: association between peeling effect and improvement. *Dermatol Monatsschr* 160:215, 1974.
6. Christiansen J, Holm P, Reymann F: Treatment of acne vulgaris with the retinoic acid derivative Ro 11-1430: a controlled clinical trial against retinoic acid. *Dermatologica* 153:172, 1976.
7. Christiansen J, Holm P, Reymann F: The retinoic acid derivative Ro 11-1430 in acne vulgaris: a controlled multicenter trial against retinoic acid. *Dermatologica* 154:219, 1977.
8. Woo-Sam PC: A quantitative study of membrane-coating granules in follicles undergoing experimental comedo formation. *Br J Dermatol* 99:387, 1978.
9. Retin-A® Brand Tretinoin Product Monograph, in *Physician's Desk Reference*, ed 31, p 864. Oradell, New Jersey: Medical Economics Co, 1977.
10. Kligman AM, Mills OH, Leyden JJ: Acne vulgaris: a treatable disease. *Postgrad Med* 55:99, 1974.
11. Levis WR, Emden R: Enhancing effect of vitamin A on *in vitro* antigen-stimulated lymphocyte proliferation. *Proc Am Assoc Can Res* 17:112, 1976.
12. Leyden JJ, Marples RR, Mills OH, et al: Tretinoin and antibiotic therapy in acne vulgaris. *South Med J* 67:20, 1974.
13. Hurwitz S: The combined effect of vitamin A acid and benzoyl peroxide in the treatment of acne. *Cutis* 17:585, 1976.
14. Papa CM: The cutaneous safety of topical tretinoin. *Acta Derm Venereol [Suppl] (Stockh)* 74:128, 1975.
15. Epstein JH: Chemicals and photocarcinogenesis. *Aust J Dermatol* 18:57, 1977.
16. Papa CM: Tretinoin: ultraviolet radiation tumorigenesis in hairless albino mice ("Dear Doctor" letter). New Brunswick, NJ: Johnson & Johnson Dermatologic Div, August 23, 1978.

17. Belisario JD: "Recent Advances in Topical Cytotoxic Therapy of Skin Cancer and Precancer," in *Melanoma and Skin Cancer: Proceedings*, pp 349-365. International Cancer Conference, Sydney, Australia, 1972.
18. Barranco VP, Olson RL, Everett MA: Response of actinic keratoses to topical vitamin A acid. *Cutis* 6:681, 1970.

Chapter 14

Vitamin A Acid Topical Therapy: Ultrastructural Effects

HELMUT H. WOLFF, MD
GERD PLEWIG, MD

Vitamin A acid (tretinoin, retinoic acid) is widely used in the treatment of acne. The drug is able to effectively expel comedones. Its mode of action differs from that of traditional peeling agents. The following is a brief illustrated discussion of the effects of vitamin A acid on the sebaceous follicles and comedones during treatment (see Chapter 13 and 16).

After vitamin A acid was applied to the skin of acne patients 1-3 times a day in a routine fashion, excisional biopsies were studied from the face (cheek and forehead) or upper trunk. The electron microscopical techniques are described elsewhere.[1]

The upper portion of the follicular channel of the sebaceous follicle is the acroinfundibulum; the lower portion is the infrainfundibulum. Even in light microscopy, differences in keratinization are evident (see Chapter 11). The acroinfundibulum forms a coherent stratum corneum; the infrainfundibulum does not.[2-4] When a comedo is treated with vitamin A acid, the living epithelium changes. The specific ultrastructural markers of keratinized epithelium (tonofilaments, desmosomes, and keratohyalin granules) begin to disappear (Figure 1). Abundant lipid material appears in the uppermost layers of the stratum spinosum and stratum granulosum (Figure 2). There are consequently marked alterations within the corneocytes formed by such epithelium. The horny cells are irregular, do not adhere, and are filled with lipids and foamy material (Figure 3 and 4). Finally, the comedonal core is expelled with vitamin A acid, and normal sebaceous follicles again form. Only

VITAMIN A ACID: ULTRASTRUCTURAL EFFECTS **137**

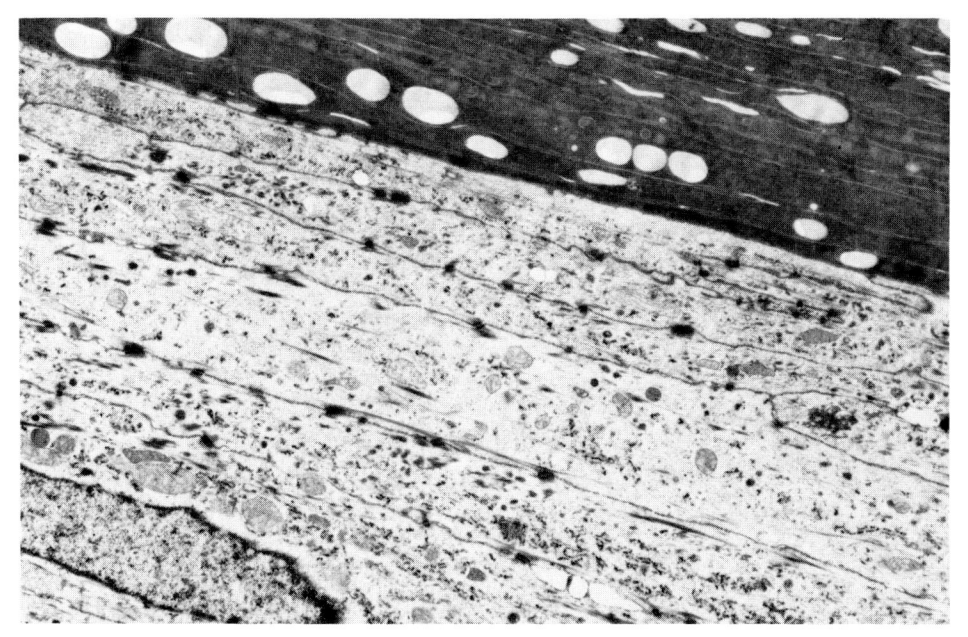

Figure 1. Comedonal core (upper portion) and comedonal wall (lower portion) after 4 weeks of vitamin A acid treatment. Decrease of specific indicators of keratinization is noted in the living cells (reduced from ×12,000).

Figure 2. Lipid inclusions in upper layers of living epithelium and corneocytes after 4 weeks of vitamin A acid treatment (reduced from ×10,000).

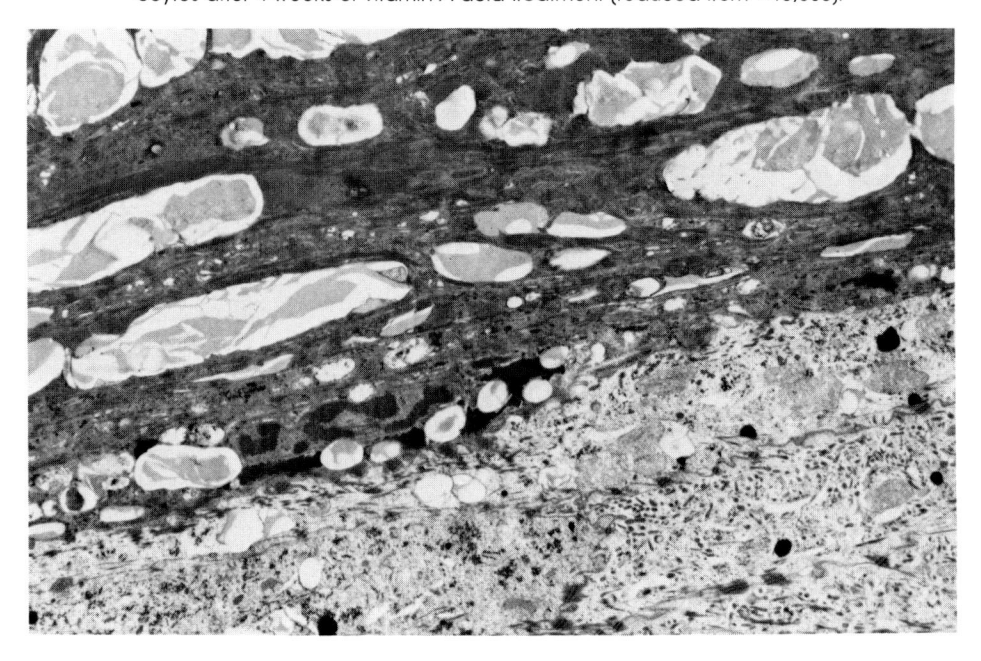

138 TREATMENT

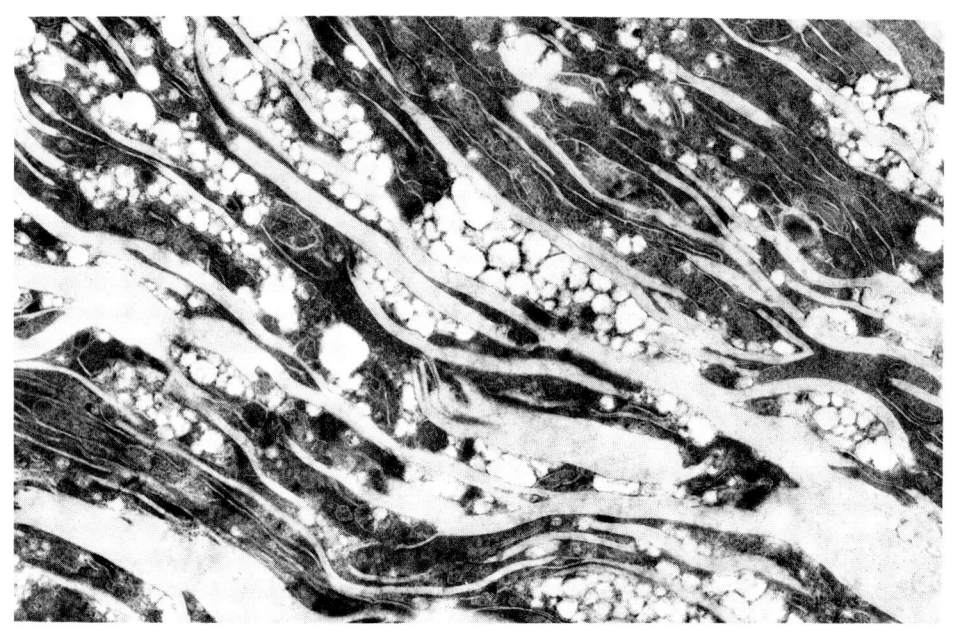

Figure 3. Horny framework of a comedo treated for 6 weeks with vitamin A acid. Corneocytes are irregular, noncoherent, and laden with lipid material (reduced from ×38,000).

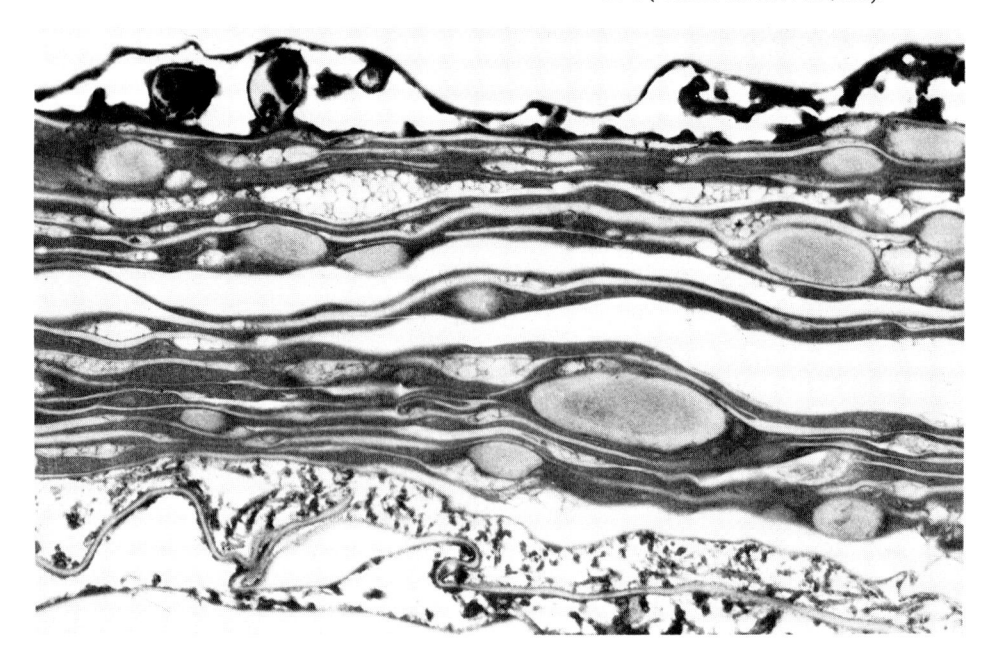

Figure 4. Intracellular accumulation of lipid and foamy material in corneocytes from a comedo treated for 6 weeks with vitamin A acid (reduced from ×22,000).

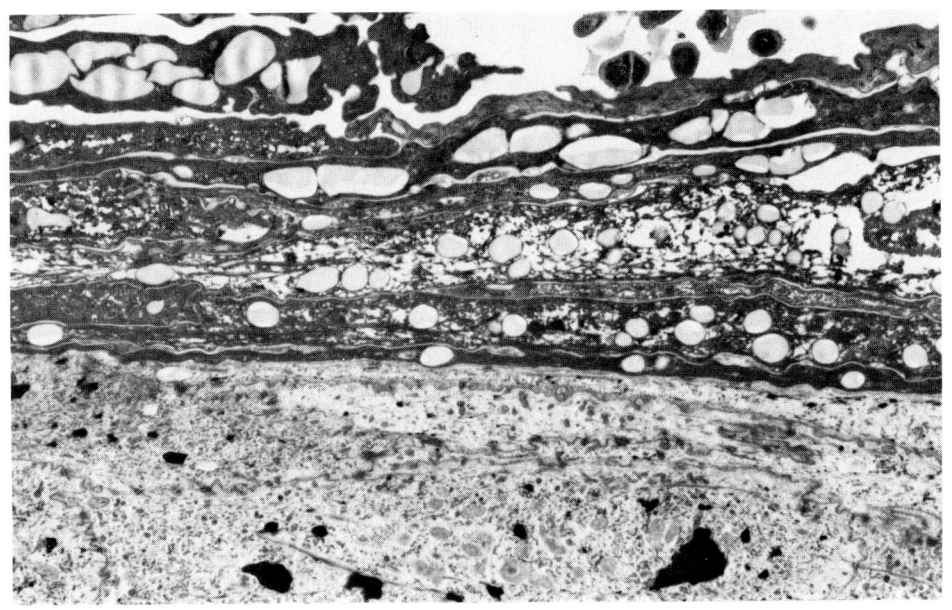

Figure 5. A former comedo which disintegrated after 6 weeks of vitamin A acid treatment. Original comedonal epithelium is now the follicular wall of sebaceous follicle. A thin layer of corneocytes sheds constantly; thus, the reformation of a comedo is prevented. *P. acnes* are present in follicular canal (reduced from ×9000).

Figure 6. Inflammatory changes that are occasionally seen in epidermis during vitamin A acid treatment. Scaling was present at time of biopsy. *left:* Extracellular edema (spongiosis) is present in epidermis. Basal lamina is below (reduced from ×7500). *right:* Note invasion of inflammatory cells into epidermis (exocytosis) (reduced from ×5000).

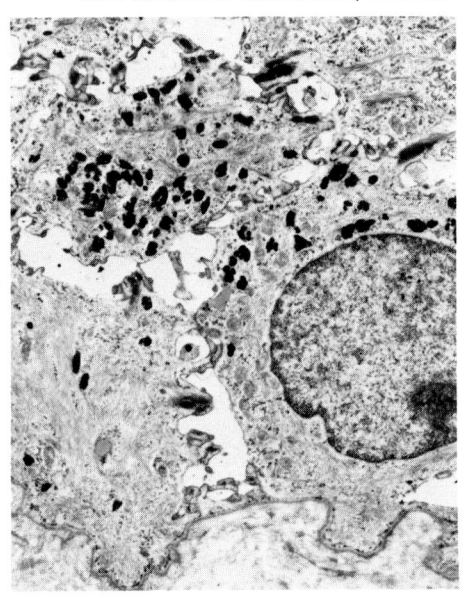

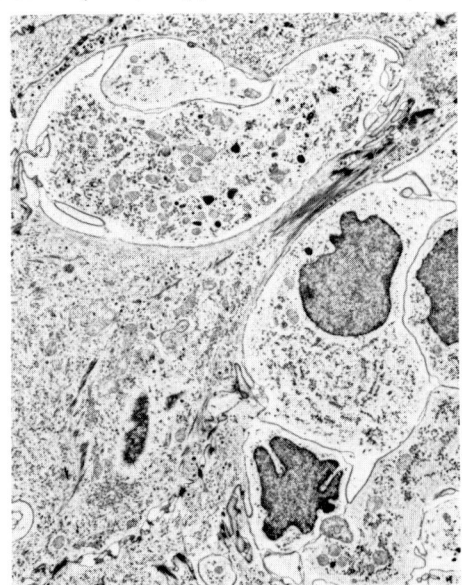

a few corneocytes line what was formerly the comedonal epithelial lining and is now the infundibular canal (Figure 5).

One of the common side effects of vitamin A acid treatment is a worsening of the clinical picture with the appearance of inflammation. Ultrastructurally, spongiosis (microacantholysis) and migration of inflammatory cells into the epithelium (exocytosis) are the changes seen (Figure 6).

The mode of action of vitamin A acid can be explained by the accelerated proliferation of the follicular and comedonal epithelium. This phenomenon was also demonstrated by autoradiography.[3,5] At the same time, the very compact, adherent, and thickened horny layer of the comedo is transformed into a disintegrating, loosened, thin layer. These circumstances combine to promote the extrusion of the primary lesion in acne, the comedo.

REFERENCES

1. Wolff HH, Plewig G, Braun-Falco O: Ultrastructure of human sebaceous follicles and comedones following treatment with vitamin A acid. *Acta Derm Venereol [Suppl] (Stockh)* 74:99, 1975.
2. Knutson DD: Ultrastructural observations in acne vulgaris: the normal sebaceous follicle and acne lesions. *J Invest Dermatol* 62:288, 1974.
3. Plewig G, Kligman AM: *Acne: Morphogenesis and Treatment.* New York: Springer-Verlag, 1975.
4. Wolff HH, Plewig G, Januschke E: Ultrastruktur der Mikroflora in Follikeln und Komedonen. *Hautarzt* 27:432, 1976.
5. Christophers E, Wolff HH: Effects of vitamin A acid in skin: *in vivo* and *in vitro* studies. *Acta Derm Venereol [Suppl] (Stockh)* 74:42, 1975.

Chapter 15

Benzoyl Peroxide Topical Therapy

JAMES E. FULTON, JR, MD, PhD
ANTOINETTE SCHENK

The days of standard tetracycline therapy for acne are over. Not only is the drug so inconsistently effective that only half the investigators can separate active drug from placebo,[1] but increased consumerism among patients and families has resulted in less reliance on oral therapy of any kind. Fortunately, more effective regimens are readily available which include the use of the newer gels of benzoyl peroxide, either with or without the addition of sulfur or the combined use of vitamin A acid. This Chapter reviews the mechanism of the peroxides and their proper use in acne therapy.

The Chemistry of Benzoyl Peroxide, a Diacyl Peroxide

The chemistry of benzoyl peroxide and its reaction with skin is quite interesting, although not yet fully understood. Benzoyl peroxide is among the group of diacyl peroxides which have the following general formula:

$$R-\overset{O}{\underset{\|}{C}}-OO-\overset{O}{\underset{\|}{C}}-R$$

To be effective, it is imperative that these diacyl peroxides decompose on skin contact, forming free radicals. These free radicals are generated during catalytic cleavage of the following type:

$$\text{R-}\overset{\overset{O}{\|}}{\text{C}}\text{-OO-}\overset{\overset{O}{\|}}{\text{C}}\text{-R} \rightarrow 2\text{R}\overset{\overset{O}{\|}}{\text{C}} + 2\text{O}^{\bullet} \rightarrow 2\text{R}\overset{\overset{O}{\|}}{\text{C}}\,[\text{protein, }etc] + O_2$$

$$\text{R-}\overset{\overset{O}{\|}}{\text{C}}\text{-OO-}\overset{\overset{O}{\|}}{\text{C}}\text{-R} \rightarrow 2\text{RCO-O}^{\bullet} \rightarrow 2\text{R}\overset{\overset{O}{\|}}{\text{C}}\,[\text{protein, }etc] + O_2$$

Catalysts for this decomposition can be physical factors, such as heat or ultraviolet radiation; or they can be chemical factors, such as oxidizing and reducing agents or the presence of metals or abstractable hydrogens.

Diacyl peroxides such as benzoyl peroxide have a wide use in industry as efficient cross-linking agents for polyolefins such as polyethylene and ethylene vinyl acetates; as vulcanizing agents for elastomers such as ethylene propylene copolymers and terpolymers; as curing agents for polyester resins; and, as synergists for flame-retardant polymers. Benzoyl peroxide and other analogues in the diacyl group have use in dermatology for similar reasons. Benzoyl peroxide decomposes on skin contact, forming free radicals of oxygens. However, the catalysts in the skin are unknown. Once the free radical is formed, these highly reactive molecules will react with any exposed proteins in their vicinity, including both those of bacterial and mammalian origins. The result is an extensive oxidation, or "bleaching" reaction, leading to a complete sterilization of bacterial skin flora within the first 2 months of application.[2]

Not only does benzoyl peroxide kill bacteria when applied topically, but it also has a vitamin A acid-like effect in causing follicular desquamation, thus reversing the formation of follicular impactions. As benzoyl peroxide penetrates the pores, a concomitant irritation that produces burning and slight erythema occurs. It seems impossible to completely eliminate these side effects and still maintain therapeutic effectivity. In short, the more peroxide decomposition, the more effective the formulation. Successful topical therapy can be simply reduced to how soon one desires therapeutic results.

The Art of Formulating Benzoyl Peroxide

During early investigations with vitamin A acid, the authors inadvertently came across an improved formulation of benzoyl peroxide. While comparing benzoyl peroxide to vitamin A acid in clinical trials using the same solvent, an ethanolic base, the authors found that, although benzoyl peroxide was not soluble in ethanol and the preparation required shaking before use, the clinical results were impressive. With a small amount of pruritus and desquamation, the inflammatory lesions disappeared. Comedones were also affected, but less dramatically. In addition, patient acceptance was better with benzoyl peroxide than with vitamin A acid, as the latter produces prostaglandin release[3] and concomitant erythema and burning; also, the acne condition often flares during the initial one month "start-up" period with vitamin A acid. These problems are much less severe with benzoyl peroxide. The simple ethanolic "shake-lotion" was not cosmetically pleasing, however, and it was suggested (H. Blank, personal communication, 1973) that the newer carboxy copolymer gels be used to suspend the insoluble benzoyl peroxide. This formulation has been extremely successful. Unfortunately, part of the efficacy is often lost in preparations subsequently modeled after this formulation. Studies conducted by the authors over the last 2 years demonstrated several reasons for this lack of uniformity in peroxide preparations.

The compound benzoyl peroxide is not new; it has been used as an antibacterial and as a moderate keratolytic agent for the last 70 years. Classically, benzoyl peroxide is dissolved in a volatile solvent (eg, chloroform), and then mixed with nonaqueous ingredients, such as petrolatum or the polyethylene glycols, for cutaneous use. The efficacy and stability of the benzoyl peroxide in this solubilized state is poor, and, after several months, the product does not retain the amount of active agent necessary to produce the desired effect. The release of the agent from these oily vehicles is inadequate. In studies made by the authors to find a better vehicle, it was found that the decomposition of benzoyl peroxide was dramatically different in various solvents. Thus, the choice of the solvent base is vital in formulating benzoyl peroxide. The dispersion of insoluble benzoyl peroxide in an aqueous gel of carboxy vinyl copolymer enhances its stability and efficacy. The combination or variation within this aqueous gel of the percentages of polar and nonpolar solvents can produce different curves of decomposition. Thus, for example, the decomposition of benzoyl peroxide in ethanol is more rapid than in distilled water, while the addition of glycerin or detergents inhibits benzoyl peroxide decomposition.

Clinical Responses to Benzoyl Peroxide

The development of benzoyl peroxide for use in the treatment of acne can be paralleled to the development of insulin for use in the treatment of another genetic disease, diabetes. The crude "shake-lotions" consisting of lower concentrations of benzoyl peroxide can be compared to the crude ethanolic extracts of the pancreas. The next phase was the progression to the solvent gels of higher concentrations with limited stability and an efficacy which was difficult to predict. These were accompanied by side effects comparable to those seen during the developmental stages of NPH and regular insulin, when many pharmaceutical companies were rushing into the market.

As in the case of insulin, the research and technology has not yet advanced to provide an ultimate cure for acne. As it now stands, 80% of the patients seen by the authors have conditions which can be controlled; these patients can attain a clear complexion within 2 months. The 20% whose conditions do not benefit from treatment are the real concern, and ongoing research to develop a topical treatment for these patients is imperative.

In the last several years, the over-the-counter market has grown in leaps and bounds. The efficacy of the commercial preparations is dependent upon the type of formulation. The least effective are lotions; the most effective are the highly organic solvent gels. The most potent formulation commercially available is PanOxyl®. However, this is the most unstable and most irritating formula. Desquam-X® is perhaps second to PanOxyl® in potency. Persa-Gel™ is the least potent, but it has the fewest side effects; it may be advantageous to start the patient on this preparation and eventually replace it with PanOxyl® as needed. Any of the formulations can be improved by the addition of sulfur (2-10%). The authors[4] were unable to substantiate the claim made by Kligman that sulfur is comedogenic. Sulfur *per se* is bacteriostatic for *Propionibacterium acnes*, and it potentiates the therapeutic effectivity of benzoyl peroxide.

The most serious drawback of the various commercial products is their unpredictable and sporadic decomposition during shelf storage. In random testing of these products, it was found that decomposition rapidly occurred. In addition, samples of various commercial preparations were tested prior to the expiration dates. The results showed a dramatic decrease in the amount of benzoyl peroxide remaining in the preparations. A few, with more than a year to go on the expiration date, had as little as 3% of the active agent remaining from the original 10% stated on the label. Obviously, the expiration dates can be misleading. The lack of consistency in the formulation may explain why clinicians do not see a uniform response to benzoyl peroxide. Also troublesome are the commercial additives, such as 6% polyoxyethylene 4-lauryl ether, which are more irritating than therapeutically helpful.

These facts become more important to the patient who is not progressing and therefore becomes discouraged. Both physician and patient should be aware of product inadequacies, especially if the patient is not responding to treatment as well as might be expected. Studies are now in progress to produce more dependable formulations. The results of these studies will be reported elsewhere.

It is sometimes difficult to determine which patients can be started on the stronger benzoyl peroxide formulations and which patients should be initiated on milder ones. Several criteria should help the clinician: 1) Does the patient have chronic debilitating Grade III-IV acne vulgaris? (These patients will tolerate almost anything—use stronger formulations); 2) Does the patient have mild acne which is complicated by premenstrual flares induced by stress? (Increase the therapy during the last 10 days of the menstrual cycle, or during times of stress); 3) Has the patient used the peroxides or vitamin A acid before? (If these were well-tolerated, consider a more potent formulation); 4) Is the skin quite oily? (Stronger formulations may be used); 5) Black skin is unusually sensitive to the peroxides. (Use milder formulations.)

Therapy with benzoyl peroxide should be commenced slowly (*eg*, 3-4 hours a day). The initial burning sensation subsides rapidly after the first few weeks, and exposure time can then be increased. Any excessive toxic irritation is rapidly reversible with 1-2 days of rest. Therapy can then be restarted. As the patient's skin becomes more accustomed to the benzoyl peroxide, the concentration and frequency of application can be gradually increased to the level required to maintain control.

Combining Vitamin A Acid with Benzoyl Peroxide for Resistant Cases

The new era of topical acne preparations really began with the discovery of vitamin A acid. This compound is more than just another irritant; it is a unique, highly potent dermatological, effective in the micromolecular range similar to that of topical corticosteroids or 5-fluorouracil. The exact mechanism of vitamin A acid in any tissue is unknown, but most current investigators are focusing on its effect on keratinosomes. These granules are alkaline phosphatase-positive, and they may be the key to the keratinization-desquamation process. During vitamin A acid therapy, these granules increase in the granular layer of the epidermis and appear to reduce the cohesiveness of the keratinocytes. As a result, the normal stratum corneum is reduced from 14 dead cell layers to 4-5.[5,6] The same loss of adhesion is apparent in the follicle wall, and the genetic predisposition to "retention hyperkeratosis" in acne-prone families is reversed (see Chapter 13).

The difficulties with vitamin A acid are not always with the compound. The inappropriate selection of patients, as well as the preparations and formulations presently available for clinical use, often create problems in themselves. As vitamin A acid is soluble only in lipids, it is frequently formulated in ethanolic solutions. After several days of use, these ethanolic solutions burn like after-shave lotion on raw skin. Even the new gel of vitamin A acid (Retin-A®) contains 90% ethanol. It would seem much wiser to formulate vitamin A acid in nonirritating vehicles. Also, concentrations such as 0.1% are way too far in excess of minimally effective therapeutic doses. These highly irritating alcoholic formulations as used on improperly selected patients have given this new and exciting compound a bad image.

Vitamin A acid is highly effective in patients with many closed comedones. It is also effective, in resistant cases, when combined with benzoyl peroxide. For the best response, vitamin A acid is applied to the skin and allowed to dry for 10-15 minutes before benzoyl peroxide is applied directly over the vitamin A acid. Although, from a biochemical point of view, this regimen would seem improbable, the effect is dramatic in some patients, producing an augmented vitamin A acid response. This is especially beneficial for treating acne on the back and chest, where penetration is limited.

Allergic Reactions to Benzoyl Peroxide

The continuing problem with benzoyl peroxide is the contact allergic reactions. It is sometimes difficult to separate the cases of toxic, overexposure to benzoyl peroxide from those cases in which reactions are truly contact allergic responses to the benzoyl radical. Apparently, during the decomposition of benzoyl peroxide with the release of reactive free radicals, these particles combine with the skin protein to produce a complete allergen, which in turn may stimulate a contact hypersensitivity reaction. Over the years, this reaction rate has remained at approximately 1-2% of those patients exposed to benzoyl peroxide.[7] It is interesting to note that the vast majority of these patients are females. In order to document this problem, the authors have been using a 6-item patch test kit in their clinics. Patch tests consist of 1% benzoyl peroxide, 1% polyoxyethylene 4-lauryl ether (Brij 30®), 10% propylene glycol, 1% sulfur, and 1% carboxymethylene polymers (Carbopol 940®) in petrolatum. In addition, the authors used 10% benzoyl peroxide in a cream vehicle.

From those patients whom the authors suspected of allergy, a more detailed history was taken to separate the possible reactions into 4 types: 1) the toxic reactions from overexposure; 2) extensive pruritus in the areas of application of benzoyl peroxide; 3) pruritus plus blotchy erythema in the areas of exposure to benzoyl peroxide; and 4) a classic contact dermatitis with pruritus, blotchy erythema, and small vesicles. During a 4-month period, it was deemed necessary to patch-test 41 patients: 36 females and 5 males. Of those, 16 had a Type 1 history, a history corresponding to a toxic overexposure; 7 had a Type 2 history, that of excessive pruritus; 6 had a Type 3 history, excessive pruritus plus blotchy erythema; and 4 had Type 4 history, a classic contact dermatitis reaction pattern to benzoyl peroxide. Twenty-five of these patients were patch test-positive to 10% benzoyl peroxide; 11 were patch test-positive to 1% benzoyl peroxide; and 3 were patch test-positive to propylene glycol. No reactions occurred with Brij 30®, Carbopol 940®, or sulfur.

This survey of allergic reactions to benzoyl peroxide leads to several interesting points. First, a patch test kit should be available for those patients experiencing an apparent overexposure to benzoyl peroxide; excessive pruritus and/or erythema often heralds early onset of benzoyl peroxide allergy. The patch tests were often positive in this group before flagrant contact allergic reactions with frank vesicles developed. Second, the incidence of allergic reactions was predominant in female patients: 60% of the authors' patients are women, but 88% of the reactions occurred in women, even though the exposure was similar in both male and female patients. Why this reaction rate was so much higher in women is unknown, although the pre-exposure to other types of peroxides (*eg*, hair bleach) is possible, or perhaps the protein involved in complexing with the free radical hapten is estrogen-dependent.

In reviewing the histories of the 41 patients, several interesting details were noted. In addition to the cutaneous reaction of delayed hypersensitivity, one patient complained of a tightening of the throat and difficulty in breathing every time she used the benzoyl peroxide on her face. Another patient broke out in hives every time she used the benzoyl peroxide. Similar reactions of immediate-type allergies associated with classic delayed contact dermatitis were reported by Maibach (personal communication, 1975). Many patients complained of allergic reactions to sulfur. However, on further questioning, this relates to "sulfa," ie, sulfonamide. Many patients misinterpret this allergy for elemental sulfur. All of the "sulfa"-allergic patients were patch test-negative to sulfur, and the authors have not seen an allergic reaction to elemental sulfur. The patients should be told about this mispronunciation; elemental sulfur is universally present in the body and is not a frequent allergen.

It was necessary to use a benzoyl peroxide 10% cream in this study to produce positive reactions in the majority of cases. Benzoyl peroxide 1% in petrolatum was inadequate, as patients allergic to benzoyl peroxide may go unnoticed if the patch tests are limited to the 1% concentration. The authors recommend that any patch test kit contain the 10% benzoyl peroxide in a cream vehicle. The gel vehicle should be avoided, as it also produces false-positive reactions. Also of interest are the positive reactions to propylene glycol, a solvent present in most formulations. Apparently, propylene glycol can be an allergen and may be a problem in dermatologic vehicles.

Summary

The topical treatment of acne has been revitalized with the use of the newer benzoyl peroxide gels with or without sulfur, or in combination with vitamin A acid. These formulations permit us to effectively treat acne without the use of systemic tetracycline, ultraviolet light, or alterations in the diet.

REFERENCES

1. Systemic antibiotics for treatment of acne vulgaris: efficacy and safety. Ad Hoc Committee Report. *Arch Dermatol* 111:1630, 1975.
2. Fulton JE Jr, Farzad-Bakshandeh A, Bradley S: Studies on the mechanism of action of topical benzoyl peroxide and vitamin A acid in acne vulgaris. *J Cutan Pathol* 1:191, 1974.
3. Ziboh VA, Price B, Fulton JE Jr: Effects of retinoic acid on prostaglandin biosynthesis in guinea-pig skin. *J Invest Dermatol* 65:370, 1975.
4. Fulton JE Jr, Bradley S, Aquendez A, et al: Non-comedogenic cosmetics. *Cutis* 17:344, 1976.
5. Kligman AM, Fulton JE Jr, Plewig G: Topical vitamin A acid in acne vulgaris. *Arch Dermatol* 99:469, 1969.
6. Fulton JE Jr: Vitamin A acid—the last five years. *J Cutan Pathol* 2:155, 1975.
7. Pace W: A benzoyl peroxide-sulfur cream for acne vulgaris. *Can Med Assoc J* 93:252, 1965.

Chapter 16

Combined Vitamin A Acid and Benzoyl Peroxide Topical Therapy
SIDNEY HURWITZ, MD

The treatment of acne was hindered for years by mythical concepts of etiology, a lack of concern for the physical and psychological trauma of those afflicted with severe forms of this disorder, and ineffective therapeutic regimens based on misconceptions and misinformation. Although the basic cause of acne vulgaris remains unknown, considerable data accumulated in recent years concerning its pathogenesis allows a rational and therapeutically successful approach to the management of this disease. To date there is no single treatment for acne. The choice of therapy must be individualized with appropriate variations and modifications as the activity of the disease fluctuates. This Chapter describes the clinical results of a simple, yet uniquely effective, topical treatment of acne vulgaris. Under proper management, this treatment can produce dramatic results in a relatively short period of time for patients with even the most severe forms of pustulocystic acne.[1]

Pathogenesis

A clear understanding of the pathogenesis of acne vulgaris can simplify one's therapeutic attitude towards this disorder. Acne usually begins at puberty, due to androgenic stimulation of the sebaceous glands and to a faulty keratinization process which results in obstruction of the pilosebaceous unit. The cause of this abnormal keratinization is as yet unknown, although patients with a predisposition to acne seem to have a tendency for irritation to the follicular wall by free fatty acids.[2] The result is a retention of keratinocytes and the impaction of horny cells within the lumen of the sebaceous follicle. The epithelial lining of the follicle becomes distended, and a comedo is formed.[3] Comedones appear to result from two abnormalities in keratinization: increased formation of horny cells, and increased adhesion among those cells.[4] Follicular hyperkeratinization produces two types of comedones: the open comedo, or "blackhead," and the closed comedo, or "whitehead."

Acne lesions arise principally from closed comedones. Once the follicular wall is breached, sebum escapes from the sebaceous follicle into the dermis and is responsible for much of the inflammatory response that occurs in acne.[5-7] Sebum is comprised of a mixture of triglycerides, wax esters, squalene, and sterol esters. Free fatty acids are currently believed to play an important role in comedogenesis and in the formation of inflammatory lesions.[8] Free fatty acids, however, are not present in the lipids found within the sebaceous canal. Their release appears to be the result of hydrolysis within the pilosebaceous follicles by bacterial lipases, principally those of the anaerobic diphtheroid, *Propionibacterium acnes*.[9,10] Free fatty acids, particularly those with short chains (C_8 to C_{14}), are the most irritating components of sebum, and may be the primary cause of the inflammatory reaction in acne vulgaris.[11]

The goal of acne therapy is to arrest the development of lesions.[7] Effective therapy, therefore, depends on the ability to prevent follicular hyperkeratosis, to lower the level of *P. acnes* and free fatty acids, and to deter the formation of comedones and the resulting papules, pustules, cysts, and nodules. Today this goal can be achieved with the proper selection of available medications, and with the cooperation of the patient.

Therapy

For years, various drying and exfoliating agents (*eg*, abrasive soaps, astringents, ultraviolet light, sulfur, resorcin, and salicylic acid), alone or in various combinations, were the mainstays of acne therapy. Controlled clinical experiments demonstrating the efficacy of these agents are lacking.[12] Although such preparations may indeed promote drying and peeling, remove oils from the surface of the skin, and suppress individual lesions to a limited degree, they fail to prevent the development of new lesions, and they actually impede the effectivity of topical pharmaceutical agents currently available for the treatment of acne vulgaris.

Systemic antibiotics suppress *P. acnes* and inhibit bacterial lipases, causing a reduction of free fatty acids, the primary irritant of sebum. For years, broad-spectrum antibiotics have been invaluable in the treatment of inflammatory pustules, nodules, and cystic lesions. Today, however, the use of systemic antibiotics can be decreased and often eliminated; the proper use of the new and more effective topical agents is fast replacing the old methods. Of the topical pharmacologic agents available today, benzoyl peroxide and vitamin A acid (tretinoin, retinoic acid), although potentially irritating, appear to be the most effective. Based on our current understanding of the pathogenesis of acne, these two agents, used alone or in combination, offer a highly effective therapeutic regimen that can be tailored to each patient. Although success in the management of acne vulgaris can be achieved by the use of topical vitamin A acid or benzoyl peroxide alone, it now appears that, under proper management, the therapeutic effect can be increased substantially by the use of the two agents in combination.[13]

BENZOYL PEROXIDE

In 1934, encouraging results were reported[14] from the use of topical benzoyl peroxide in the treatment of acne vulgaris and follicular pyoderma of the beard (sycosis barbae). During the 1960's, this chemotherapeutic agent was reintroduced as an adjunct in the topical therapy of acne vulgaris.[15-18] Studies[19-21] suggested that benzoyl peroxide acts as an irritant and as a keratolytic agent, and that it may also possess a bacteriostatic or bactericidal effect on *P. acnes*. Whether the therapeutic success of benzoyl peroxide is related to its keratolytic or possible antibacterial effect, or to a combination of the two, remains open to conjecture.

Although benzoyl peroxide in lotion form is helpful in the topical management of acne vulgaris, the newer gel formulations appear to be more potent[22] (see Chapter 15). In these newer vehicles, the benzoyl peroxide appears to penetrate the pilosebaceous follicle more effectively, and has a more substantial antibacterial effect in suppressing *P. acnes* and lowering free fatty acids.[21] While benzoyl peroxide may be used alone in mild to moderate inflammatory acne, it appears to be most effective in combination with systemic antibiotics and/or vitamin A acid.[12,13,19,20] The side effects of topical benzoyl peroxide are largely due to overzealous or improper application. A relatively low incidence of allergic contact dermatitis (1-2.5%) suggests, however, that a certain degree of caution should be taken in its use.[23]

VITAMIN A ACID (TRETINOIN)

Oral vitamin A has been administered for years to patients with acne vulgaris to reduce hyperkeratosis of the sebaceous follicle. Unfortunately, therapeutic effect requires dosages in the toxic range of 400,000-700,000 units a day. In 1969, in an effort to deliver a substantial dose of this drug to the target area without involving systemic toxicity, the use of topical vitamin A acid in acne therapy was proposed[24] (see Chapter 13 and 14).

This agent (tretinoin, retinoic acid) appears to have several beneficial effects on the skin of acne patients. Included among these benefits are an increased cell turnover within the pilosebaceous ducts and a decreased cohesiveness of epidermal cells due to a reduction in the number of desmosomes. This stimulates a dehiscence of horny cells with resulting thinning of the horny layer, and appears to decrease the formation of solid plugs within the comedones, with an associated sloughing and expulsion of existing comedones from their sebaceous follicles.[24] Vitamin A acid therefore appears to reverse comedo formation, thus reducing the number of inflammatory lesions which arise from these comedones.[25] It is unfortunate that, while vitamin A acid is perhaps the single most effective topical remedy for acne, it is potentially irritating, and is often used improperly by many physicians.

THE COMBINATION OF VITAMIN A ACID AND BENZOYL PEROXIDE

In 1972, the combined use of vitamin A acid and benzoyl peroxide was suggested for the topical therapy of acne vulgaris (see Chapter 15). It was proposed that, in addition to its keratolytic effect, benzoyl peroxide could suppress *P. acnes*, inhibit triglyceride hydrolysis, and lower the free fatty acids of sebum; vitamin A acid would thin the epidermis, lessen follicular hyperkeratosis and enhance the transepidermal penetration of benzoyl peroxide. It was theorized that this combination of two potent topical medications could produce an additive, and possibly a synergistic, effect, and result in a more effective method for the management of acne vulgaris.[19]

To test this hypothesis, 404 patients with varying degrees of acne vulgaris were started on a regimen of topical vitamin A acid and benzoyl peroxide.[13] Two hundred and six men and 198 women, all between 10-29 years of age, were included in this study. Of these, 317 (77%) had moderate to severe cases of acne vulgaris, many of which were unresponsive to previous conventional therapeutic measures (Table I). Of the 404 patients, 227 (56.2%) were

Table I — Severity of Acne Vulgaris Prior to Benzoyl Peroxide and Vitamin A Acid Therapy

	Mild	Moderate	Severe	Total
Men	28	140	38	206 (51.0%)
Women	59	104	35	198 (49.0%)
Total	87	244	73	404

Table II — Patients Treated with Antibiotics in Addition to Topical Benzoyl Peroxide and Vitamin A Acid

Antibiotics	# Patients	%
Tetracycline	191	47.3
Erythromycin	17	4.2
Minocycline	14	3.5
Clindamycin	5	1.2
None	177	43.8
Total	404	100.0%

treated simultaneously with systemic antibiotics; 177 patients (43.8%) received no antibiotics (Table II).

Although a double-blind study would be the most scientific method for determining the efficacy of this therapeutic method, the nature of the agents under study and the reactions associated with their topical application made this impossible. Therefore, in order to document results, lesion counts were performed and clinical photographs were taken at regulated intervals with a Nikon F camera with a micro-Nikkor 55 millimeter lens, using Kodachrome II daylight X-135 film. All photographs were taken at approximately the same focal distance, under similar lighting conditions, and with the same lens aperture.

Method—Most patients were seen at 2-4 week intervals initially, and then less frequently as their acne responded to therapy. Education of the patient prior to the initiation of this therapy was essential. Careful history was taken, the nature of the disease was explained, potential pitfalls were discussed, and treatment was described in detail.

Vitamin A acid. This was applied in the form of Retin-A® Swabs (0.05%) or Retin-A® Cream (0.05% or 0.1%), depending on the complexion of the patient and tolerance of the medication. For persons with sensitive and easily irritated skin (light-complexioned blonds and redheads, particularly women), vitamin A acid cream, as opposed to the liquid or swab form of the medication, was recommended. Because of its known capacity to cause severe irritation and peeling, topical vitamin A acid therapy was initiated conservatively, on an alternate-day or, occasionally, an every-third-day regimen. As satisfactory tolerance was demonstrated (generally within the first 10-14 days of treatment), the frequency of administration was increased to daily application of the medication.

In order to minimize possible adverse cutaneous reactions, all recommended precautions for vitamin A acid therapy were carefully emphasized and strictly implemented.[26] Patients were instructed to wash with a mild soap, no more than 2-3 times a day, and to wait at least 30 minutes after washing (to insure that the skin was completely dry) before applying vitamin A acid. Patients were also advised to avoid all other local medications; only oil-free cosmetics were allowed, and excessive sun exposure was limited. If prolonged sun exposure was anticipated, patients were cautioned to use a protective sunscreen (*eg*, PreSun®, Paba-Gel®, SunDown®).

Benzoyl peroxide. A gel formulation in a 10% concentration (*eg*, 10-Benzagel®, Desquam-X 10®, PanOxyl® 10, or Persa-Gel™ 10%) was used, but not before testing for possible benzoyl peroxide allergy by open patch tests on the volar aspect of the wrist. Since it was suggested[19] that benzoyl peroxide might oxidize vitamin A acid if the two preparations were applied simultaneously, all patients were instructed to apply the two medications separately (one in the morning and the other at night).

Systemic antibiotics. These were prescribed for those with pustular or

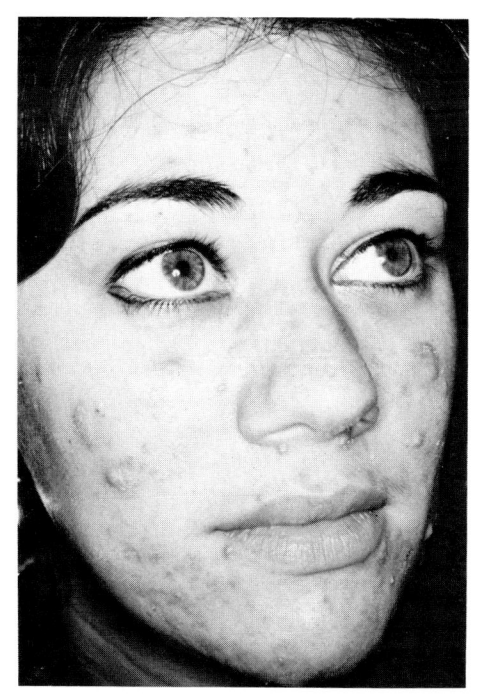

Figure 1. Twenty-three-year-old woman with Grade III-IV acne (large papules, pustules, and numerous indurated cystic lesions) before vitamin A acid and benzoyl peroxide treatment.

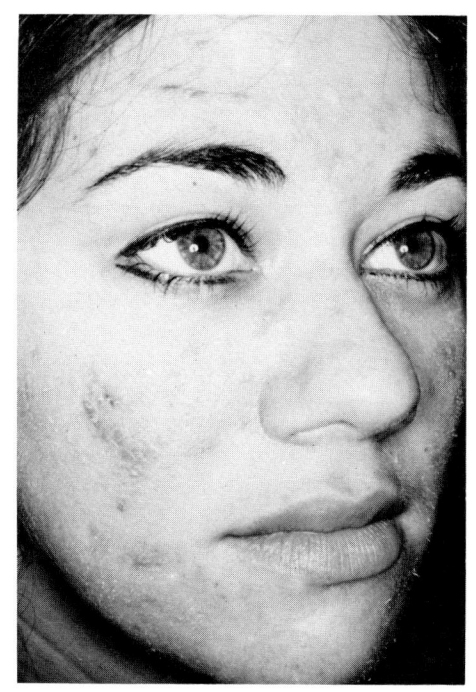

Figure 2. Same patient after 5 weeks of treatment with vitamin A acid cream (0.1%) in the morning and benzoyl peroxide gel (10%) in the evening.

cystic forms of acne vulgaris (Table II). Once the inflammatory aspect improved, antibiotics were tapered and, whenever possible, completely discontinued.

To assure a minimum of complications, patients were instructed to maintain close telephone communication, particularly during the first weeks of treatment. At each office visit, therapy was reviewed, comedones were extracted, liquid nitrogen was applied to hasten the resolution of inflammatory lesions, and pustulocystic lesions were treated with intralesional corticosteroids. When irritation occurred, treatment was discontinued for several days, and a moisturizer was used for 1-2 days, after which treatment was slowly and cautiously reinstated. Careful evaluation at each visit revealed that side effects of vitamin A acid and/or benzoyl peroxide, when present, generally were associated with excessive application or failure to follow instructions.

Results—Although success in the management of acne vulgaris can often be achieved by the use of topical vitamin A acid or benzoyl peroxide alone, the therapeutic effect is substantially increased by the use of the two potent topical agents in combination (Figure 1-8). Within a period of 6-8 weeks, 88.1% of the 404 patients treated with this combination showed good

154 TREATMENT

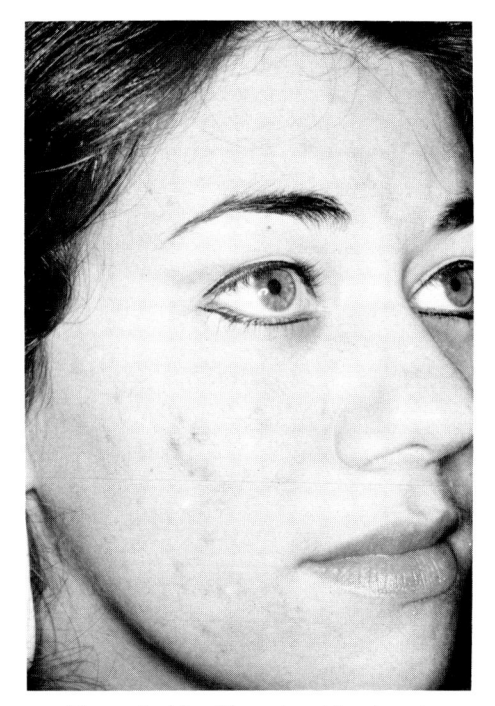

Figure 3. After 14 weeks of treatment.

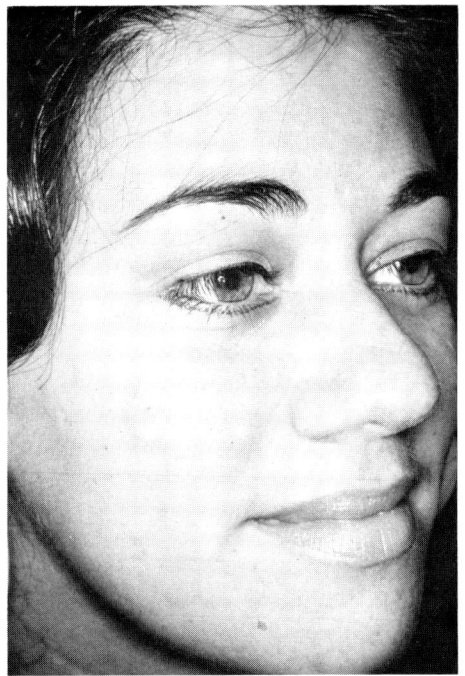

Figure 4. After 6 months of treatment. Patient received systemic minocycline (100 mg, 2 times a day initially, with gradual reduction and discontinuation after 6 months).

to excellent results: 67.3% had excellent results (over 90% clearing of lesions), and 20.8% had good results (80-90% clearing) (Figure 1-8); 7.4% demonstrated fair results (60-80% clearing), and 4.5% exhibited poor results (less than 60% clearing), or were lost to follow-up (Table III).

Vitamin A acid, used alone, can be irritating to the skin and may be poorly tolerated by many patients (Figure 9). Benzoyl peroxide appears to toughen the epidermis against this cutaneous reaction. When the two agents were used in combination in this study, there was better tolerance of vitamin A acid, and irritation was substantially reduced (Figure 10).

Systemic antibiotics are often required for the effective treatment of inflammatory lesions of acne vulgaris; however, in this study of 404 patients, 43.8% of the cases were controlled solely by the combined use of topical vitamin A acid and benzoyl peroxide (Table II). Although some patients with severe pustular or pustulocystic acne (Grade III and IV) did require antibiotics to control their disease, antibiotics could be decreased or eliminated for many patients.

Since this study was completed, the number of patients using the combination of vitamin A acid and benzoyl peroxide was increased from 404 to 1200, and the use of antibiotics was further reduced from 56.2% to 15.0%.

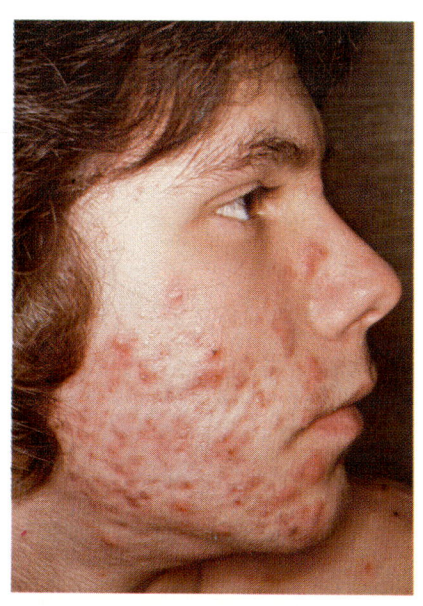

Figure 5. Sixteen-year-old boy with Grade III-IV acne (large papules, pustules, and cystic lesions) before vitamin A acid and benzoyl peroxide treatment.

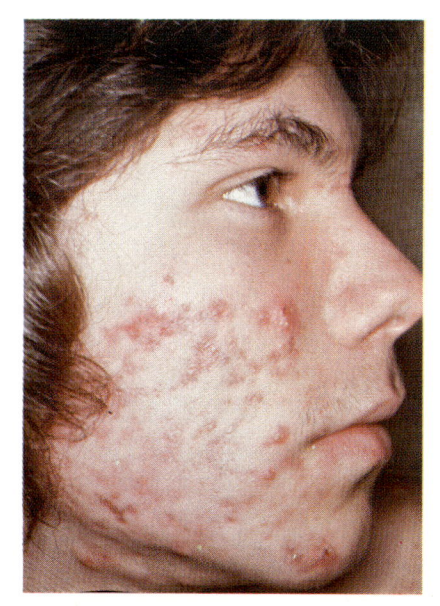

Figure 6. Same patient after 6 weeks of treatment with vitamin A acid gel (0.025%) in the morning and benzoyl peroxide (10%) in the evening.

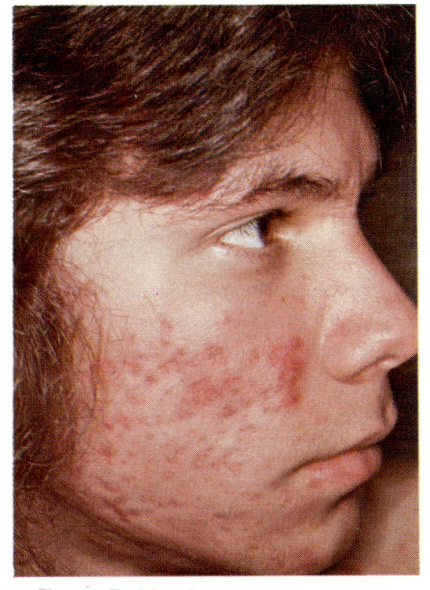

Figure 7. After 9 weeks of treatment.

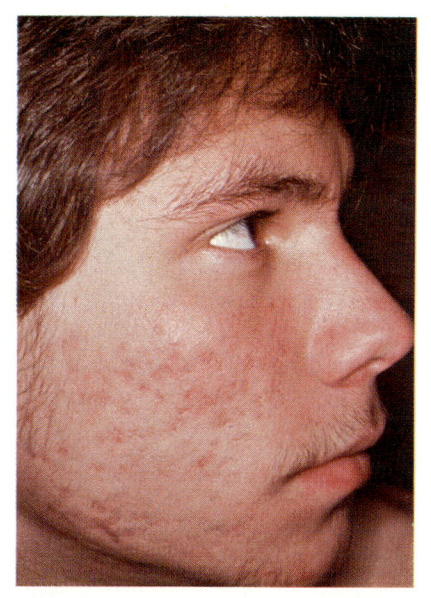

Figure 8. After 16 weeks of treatment. Patient received systemic tetracycline (500 mg, 2 times a day initially, with gradual reduction and eventual discontinuation).

Table III — Response to Benzoyl Peroxide and Vitamin A Acid Therapy

Results	#Patients	%
Excellent	272	67.3
Good	84	20.8
Fair	30	7.4
Poor	4	1.0
	390	96.5
Lost to follow-up	14	3.5
Total	404	100.0%

Excellent: 90% clearing of comedones, papules, pustules, nodules, and cysts
Good: 80-90% clearing
Fair: 60-80% clearing
Poor: less than 60% improvement

In this series, an additional 48 patients (3.8%) were found to be sensitive to or irritated by the benzoyl peroxide gel (Figure 11 and 12). These patients were treated with a combination of vitamin A acid and topical erythromycin. The topical erythromycin used was prepared as a 2% solution of erythromycin base in ethanol-propylene glycol, or as a 2.0-2.7% solution of erythromycin base dissolved in E-Solve® Lotion. When used in combination with vitamin A acid, both topical erythromycin formulations were found to be effective and cosmetically acceptable. The erythromycin in E-Solve® solution appeared to be less drying and offered greater flexibility in preparation and concentration. The response to this combination, although good, did not appear to be as rapid or as effective as that achieved with 10% benzoyl peroxide gel.

Summary

The art of medicine is predicated on the physician's ability to balance side effects against the potential benefits of various pharmacologic agents. Although a double-blind study would undoubtedly be the most scientific method for determining the efficacy of this treatment, the nature of the agents under study and the reactions associated with their topical application made this impossible. Nevertheless, a study of 1200 patients with varying degrees of acne vulgaris clearly demonstrated that: 1) the combination of vitamin A acid and benzoyl peroxide, when used properly, offers a well-tolerated, extremely effective therapeutic method for the topical management of acne vulgaris; 2) this combination of two potent topical chemotherapeutic agents is better tolerated than is vitamin A acid when used alone; 3) the use of systemic antibiotics can often be decreased or eliminated (an antibiotic-sparing effect) and replaced by the use of these two agents in combination; 4) education of the patient and careful monitoring of therapy is essential; 5) dramatic thera-

COMBINED VITAMIN A ACID AND BENZOYL PEROXIDE 157

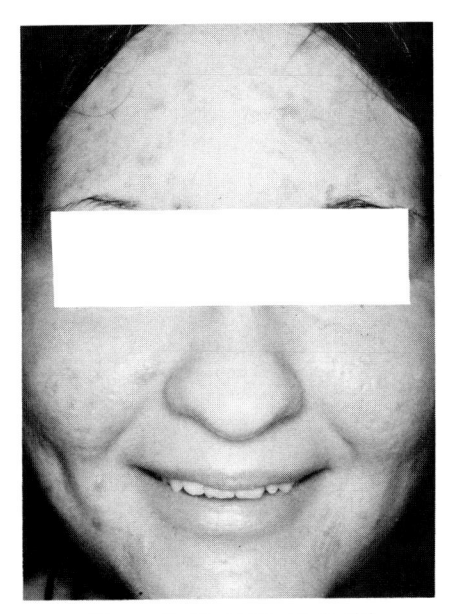

Figure 9. Nineteen-year-old woman with erythema due to improper use of vitamin A acid.

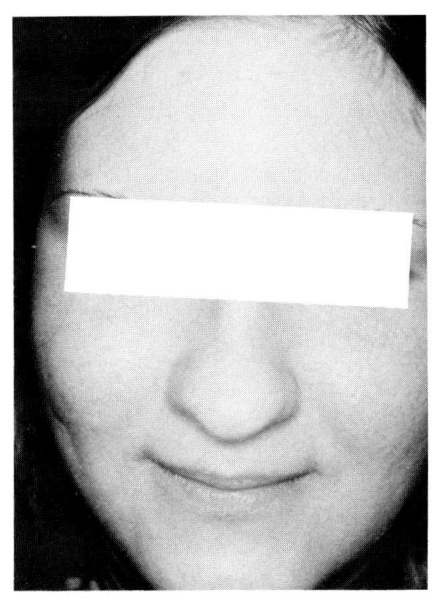

Figure 10. Same patient after treatment with vitamin A acid cream (0.1%) in the morning and benzoyl peroxide gel (10%) at night, with proper precautions taken for use of each preparation.

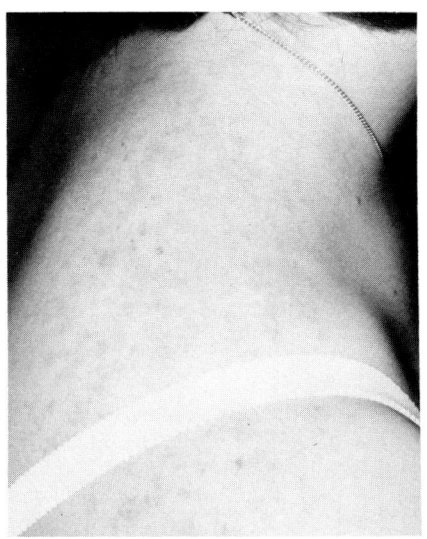

Figure 11. Fifteen-year-old girl with contact allergy to benzoyl peroxide who was subsequently treated with vitamin A acid cream (0.1%) in the morning and 2% solution of erythromycin base in ethanol-propylene glycol at night, with excellent results.

peutic results can be achieved in a relatively short time in a high percentage of patients, even in those with severe pustulocystic forms of this disorder.

REFERENCES

1. Hurwitz S: "Diseases of the Sweat and Sebaceous Glands—Acne," in Gellis SS, Kagan BM (Eds): *Current Pediatric Therapy*, vol VI. Philadelphia: WB Saunders, 1973.
2. Plewig G, Fulton JE Jr, Kligman AM: Cellular dynamics of comedo formation in acne vulgaris. *Arch Dermatol Forsch* 242:12, 1971.
3. Kligman AM: An overview of acne. *J Invest Dermatol* 62:268, 1974.
4. Plewig G: Follicular keratinization. *J Invest Dermatol* 62:308, 1974.
5. Knutson DD: Ultrastructural observations in acne vulgaris: the normal sebaceous follicle and acne lesions. *J Invest Dermatol* 62:288, 1974.
6. Strauss JS, Kligman AM: The pathologic dynamics of acne vulgaris. *Arch Dermatol* 82:779, 1960.
7. Orentreich N, Durr NP: The natural evolution of comedones into inflammatory papules and pustules. *J Invest Dermatol* 62:316, 1974.
8. Shalita AR: Genesis of free fatty acids. *J Invest Dermatol* 62:332, 1974.
9. Kellum RE, Strangfeld K, Ray LF: Acne vulgaris: studies in pathogenesis: triglyceride hydrolysis by *Corynebacterium acnes* in vitro. *Arch Dermatol* 101:41, 1970.
10. Marples RR, Kligman AM, Lantis LR, et al: The role of aerobic microflora in the genesis of fatty acids in human surface lipids. *J Invest Dermatol* 55:173, 1970.
11. Kellum RE: Acne vulgaris: studies in pathogenesis: relative irritancy of free fatty acids from C_2 to C_{16}. *Arch Dermatol* 97:722, 1968.
12. Shalita AR: Acne vulgaris: not curable but treatable. *Mod Med* 43:66, 1975.
13. Hurwitz S: The combined effect of vitamin A acid and benzoyl peroxide in the treatment of acne. *Cutis* 17:585, 1976.
14. Peck SM, Chargin L: Sycosis vulgaris: a new method of treatment. *Arch Dermatol Syphilol* 29:456, 1934.
15. Frank L: Active oxygen in acne therapy. *Cutis* 1:306, 1965.
16. Edelstein AJ: Synergism in recalcitrant acne vulgaris. *Penn Med* 69:26, 1966.
17. Frank L, Petrou P: Active oxygen plus chlorhydroxyquinoline in acne and pyodermas. *Cutis* 3:256, 1967.
18. Witkowski JA, Parish LC: Chlorhydroxyquin-benzoyl peroxide lotion in the treatment of acne. *Cutis* 5:1481, 1969.
19. Fulton JE Jr: Acne—pathogenesis and treatment. *Postgrad Med* 52:85, 1972.
20. Fulton JE Jr, Farzad-Bakshandeh A, Bradley S: Studies on the mechanism of action of topical benzoyl peroxide and vitamin A acid in acne vulgaris. *J Cutan Pathol* 1:194, 1974.
21. Anderson AS, Galdys GJ, Green RC, et al: Improved reduction of cutaneous bacteria and free fatty acids with new benzoyl peroxide gel. *Cutis* 16:307, 1975.
22. Fulton JE Jr, Bradley S: The choice of vitamin A acid, erythromycin, or benzoyl peroxide for the topical treatment of acne. *Cutis* 17:560, 1976.
23. Eaglstein WH: Allergic contact dermatitis to benzoyl peroxide—report of cases. *Arch Dermatol* 97:527, 1968.
24. Kligman AM, Fulton JE Jr, Plewig G: Topical vitamin A acid in acne vulgaris. *Arch Dermatol* 99:469, 1969.
25. Strauss JS, Pochi PE, Downing DT: Acne: perspectives. *J Invest Dermatol* 62:321, 1974.
26. Kligman AM, Mills OH Jr, Leyden JJ, et al: Postscript to vitamin A acid therapy for acne vulgaris (letter to the editor). *Arch Dermatol* 107:296, 1973.

Chapter 17

Topical Tetracycline Therapy

HARRY L. WECHSLER, MD
JACQUELYN KIRK, MD

Broad-spectrum antibiotics, particularly tetracycline, have gained wide acceptance as effective agents in the treatment of acne. Administration of these has been, with rare exception, by oral route. However, assuming the action of these antibiotics to be local, it would seem logical that topical application would be preferable. Topical application has particular merit in acne therapy since, although the tetracyclines have been given with very few deleterious effects, the tendency has been to shy away from systemic administration of drugs that are to be taken over prolonged periods. Probably the failure to move towards percutaneous use has been due to lack of confidence in the stability of preparations and in the deliverance of the active agent within the pilosebaceous apparatus. However, clinical trials have shown that tetracycline,[1-7] erythromycin,[8,9] and clindamycin[10] are as effective topically as they are systemically. Despite wide use of antibiotics and much investigative study, there is far from general agreement as to what the beneficial action of the antibiotic is.[4,9-17] It is purported to be due to a direct or indirect lowering of the free fatty acids of sebum.[11-16] What is generally accepted is that the beneficial effect is due to the antibiotic's local action.[16] This Chapter discusses the possible effect of topical tetracycline on the pathogenesis of acne and its action on the clinical course of the disease.

Preparations

Various preparations consisting of creams, pastes, and solutions with concentrations of tetracycline varying from 0.5-5.0% have been suggested for topical use in acne therapy. Kanter and Šaško[1] first suggested applying 2% tetracycline HCl in a soft zinc oxide paste. Gloor et al[2] used a 5% tetracycline cream with and without 40% dimethyl sulfoxide (DMSO). Kraus[12] added n,n-dimethylacetamide to enhance tetracycline absorption of a 2% solution. He used this only for the purpose of studying its effect on the free fatty acid content of skin sebum, and not for treatment of acne. Mills et al[9] had limited experience with 2% tetracycline in an ethanol-propylene glycol base.

What was used extensively in clinical trials, and appears to be a relatively stable solution with an effective enhancer of percutaneous absorption, is the following: tetracycline HCl 0.22% and 4-epitetracycline HCl 0.28%, in a 40% ethanol/60% water solution with n-decyl methyl sulfoxide 0.125%, sucrose esters 0.125% and sodium bisulfite 0.1%.[3-7] The epitetracycline was added to stabilize the tetracycline concentration, so that a therapeutic level would be assured throughout the product's use. The sucrose monooleate affords antilipolytic action, and the sodium bisulfite provides for anti-oxidant action. N-decyl methyl sulfoxide enhances percutaneous absorption of the aqueous soluble material.[18] According to Blaney and Cook,[6] the active components are tetracycline, n-decyl methyl sulfoxide, and sucrose monooleate. Elimination of any one seems to lower therapeutic effectiveness. In clinical trials by the authors[7] which extended over a period of one year, it was evident that the preparation was stable for at least one month, as fresh solution was given every 4 weeks. Chalker et al[19] reported potency to be unchanged after aging of solutions up to 11 weeks prior to use.

Mode of Action

The most popular explanation of the action of oral tetracycline in acne treatment has been that there is reduction in the irritating free fatty acids of sebum, due either to suppression of the lipase-secreting *Propionibacterium acnes*[11,14-16] or to inhibition of the free fatty acids *per se*.[12,13] Fulton,[8] in a comparative study, found that oral and topical tetracycline, benzoyl peroxide, and erythromycin effectively lowered the free fatty acids of sebum. Since erythromycin had no antilipolytic action, the reduction in free fatty acids was attributed to suppression of *P. acnes*. Kraus,[12] after applying tetracycline with a percutaneous enhancer to the faces of patients with normal skin, noted a drop in free fatty acids, comparable to that reported by Freinkel et al[11] after administering oral tetracycline. Gloor et al,[2] adding DMSO to a topical tetracycline preparation, also noted a marked reduction in free fatty acids. However, Anderson et al[4] failed to observe any change in the number of free fatty acids in acne patients who were treated with topical tetracycline. They pointed out that the conflicting results may have been due in part to variable techniques in collecting lipid samples. Mills et al,[9] although they observed beneficial results in the skin of acne patients using topical erythromycin, did not find suppression in growth of *P. acnes*. Resh and Stoughton[10] reported that clindamycin lotion suppressed growth of diphtheroids in open comedones; erythromycin and tetracycline did not. However, all three antibiotics were effective therapeutically. Fulton[17] later found that reduction of free fatty acids is not a prime requisite of effective acne treatment. He showed that applying a potent lipase inhibitor (a pyridyl phosphate compound) to the skin of acne patients did not alter the course of the disease. These studies add further evidence that the benefical effect in treatment of acne is not primarily due to suppression of lipase-secreting bacteria or to direct lowering of free fatty acids.

The beneficial effect of topical tetracycline is a local one. It was estimated[5] that only 5-6 mg of tetracycline are applied to the skin when patients use the preparation 2 times a day. Storrs et al (personal communication, 1976) separately determined serum levels of tetracycline in a group of patients taking topical tetracycline and in another taking oral tetracycline. The latter group received 500 mg a day. None of the 23 individuals on topical treatment had detectable serum levels ($> 0.1 \mu g/ml$) after 6-8 weeks of treatment; one of 12 had detectable amounts after 11-13 weeks. In an essentially comparative number receiving oral medication, 17 of 19 patients had detectable serum levels at 6-8 weeks, and 10 of 14 at 11-13 weeks. Based on this, it would be difficult to imagine that topical application would have any systemic effect.

Therapeutic Effectiveness

Although good results have been reported with topical tetracycline in acne treatment, it was not until a stable preparation and an effective percutaneous enhancer were available that significant clinical trials were attempted (Table I). Double-blind studies conducted over a 3-month period showed that the results of topical application were comparable to those of oral administration of 500 mg of tetracycline.[4-6,19] Smith et al[5,19] reported some improvement in the control groups as well. Cook et al[4,6] noted similar results, but did not observe any improvement in their placebo groups. Frank[3] confirmed the effectiveness of topical treatment. In a large, collaborative, open clinical trial numbering 300 patients, Frank reported that, on a 0-8 grading scale, at the end of a 13-week study period, the average reduction in severity grade was 1.83 grade points. This represented a 44% drop in severity.

As an extension of Frank's study, Wechsler et al[7] continued treatment and observations for a total of 12 months, from midwinter to midwinter, to determine if the beneficial effects of topical tetracycline were altered by the often observed seasonal variations in acne. That the overall severity grade of 4.37 in 105 patients had fallen to 1.57 in the same season a year later (Figure 1 and 2), without any evidence of exacerbation at any time during the course of the study, would tend to rule out a seasonal variable (Figure 3).

A fortuitous spin-off of the Wechsler et al study occurred in the year

Table I — Therapeutic Effectiveness of Topical and Oral Tetracycline*

Investigators	# Patients	Type of Study	Duration in weeks	Results
Smith et al[5]	135	double-blind: topical, oral, and placebo	13	topical and oral equally effective; placebo improved
Blaney and Cook[6]	75	double-blind: topical, oral, and placebo	13	topical and oral equally effective; better than placebo
Anderson et al[4]	60	double-blind: topical, oral, and placebo	13	topical and oral equally effective; better than placebo
Frank[3]	300	open study: topical	13	significant improvement
Wechsler et al[7]	105	open study: topical	48-55	significant improvement
Chalker et al[19]	223	double-blind: topical, oral, and placebo	10	topical and oral equally effective; placebo improved

*Methods of Procedure—Patients applied topical solution to face twice a day. Degree of acne severity was scored according to the grading of Blaney and Cook.[6] Depending on duration of study, patients were evaluated every 2 weeks; then every 3 weeks for 13 weeks; then monthly. Photographs were taken on each visit. These were graded by impartial observers, and results were compared with clinical observations.

after the study was completed. There were 9 patients who had persistent Grade 2 or 3 acne and who elected to continue under treatment with traditional methods, and there were 2 more who were removed from the study midway because of a poor response to topical tetracycline. Ten of these were started on oral tetracycline at 750 mg a day; the eleventh, a boy with severe cystic acne, was placed on erythromycin, 750 mg a day. All were given local keratolytics. In only one of the 11 did the patient and the examiner feel that systemic treatment was demonstrably better than topical tetracycline over a 3-6 month follow-up period.

On the other hand, one female patient who had removed herself from the topical tetracycline study when her acne cleared from a Grade 6 to a Grade 1 in less than 3 months returned several months later with a flare which responded dramatically in 2-3 months with systemic treatment. These observations, while limited to a very small group, support the findings[4-6,19] that the responses to local tetracycline and systemic tetracycline are comparable.

Advantages

It is apparent that topical tetracycline can be applied over a prolonged period with sustained effect, and without any of the complications caused by

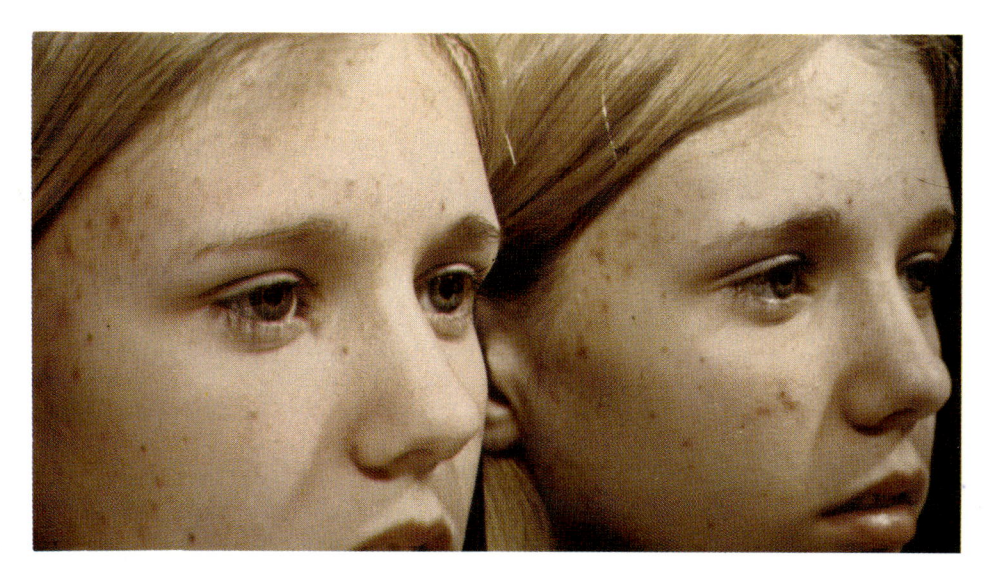

Figure 1. *above:* Thirteen-year-old girl with Grade 6 acne prior to treatment. *below:* After 9 months of topical tetracycline treatment, patient's acne improved to Grade 1.

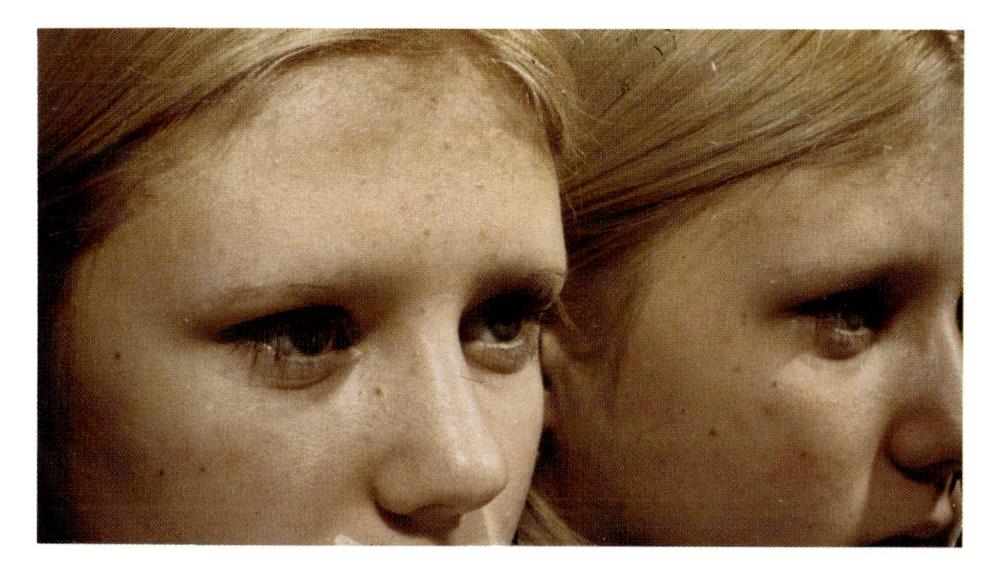

oral administration. Gastrointestinal disturbances and vaginal candidiasis, the most common problems encountered with the oral route[20,21] were, of course, avoided with the topical treatment. Although the gut bacterial flora were not studied when topical tetracycline was used, resistent strains, such as those Valtonen et al[22] reported occurring in individuals who had taken oral tetracycline for a 2-month period, would hardly be expected to develop. Such

164 TREATMENT

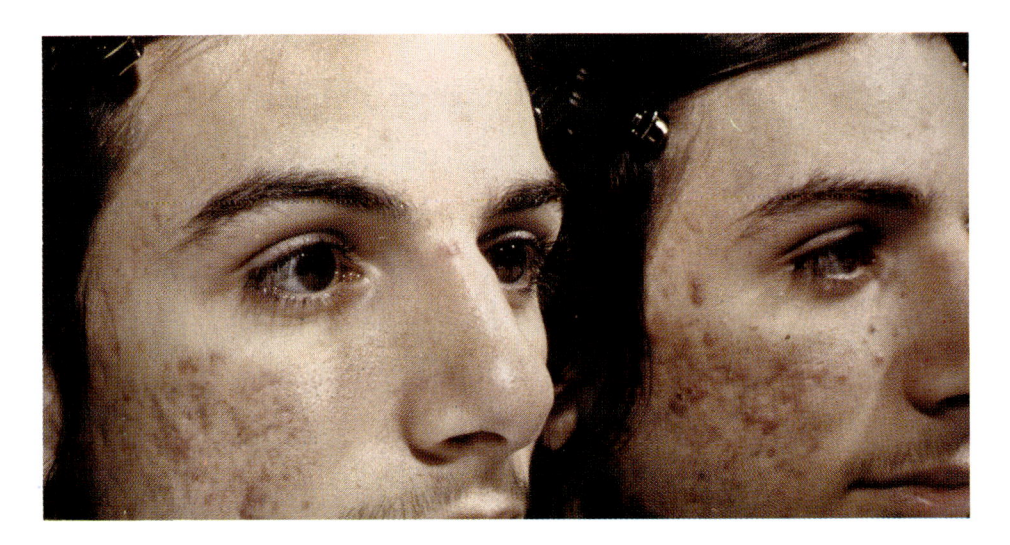

Figure 2. *above:* Eighteen-year-old boy with Grade 8 acne prior to treatment. *below:* After 11 months of topical tetracycline treatment, patient's acne improved to Grade 2.

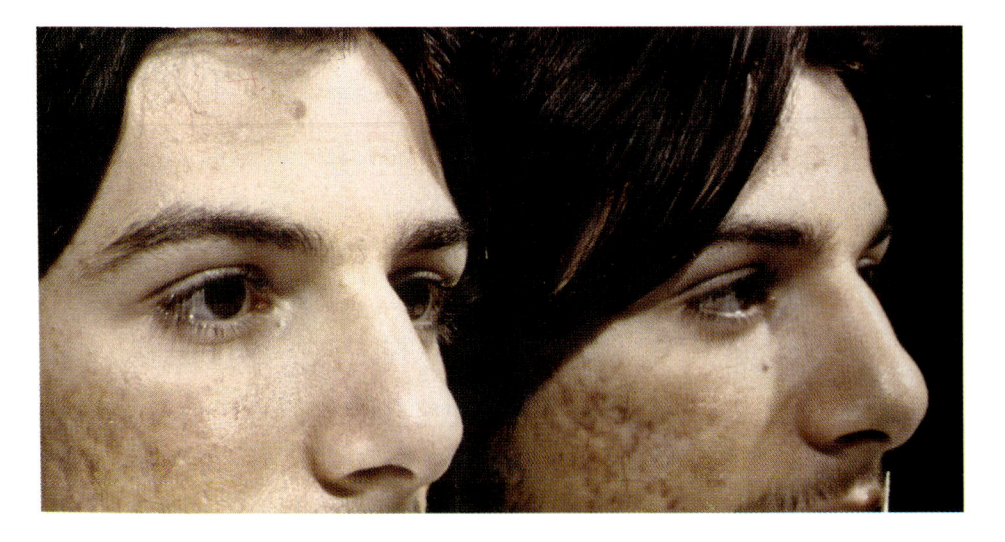

a deduction seems logical, as 5-6 mg of tetracycline applied topically[5,6] does not produce any significant serum levels, as does oral treatment (Storrs et al, personal communication, 1976). In fact, such a small dose, if completely absorbed systemically, would not cause deleterious effects in any systemic condition, with the possible exception of an allergic reaction. Experience, although limited, suggests that topical tetracycline can be used in the presence of underlying disease when systemic administration may be contraindicated. Results were beneficial without adverse side effects when a young man

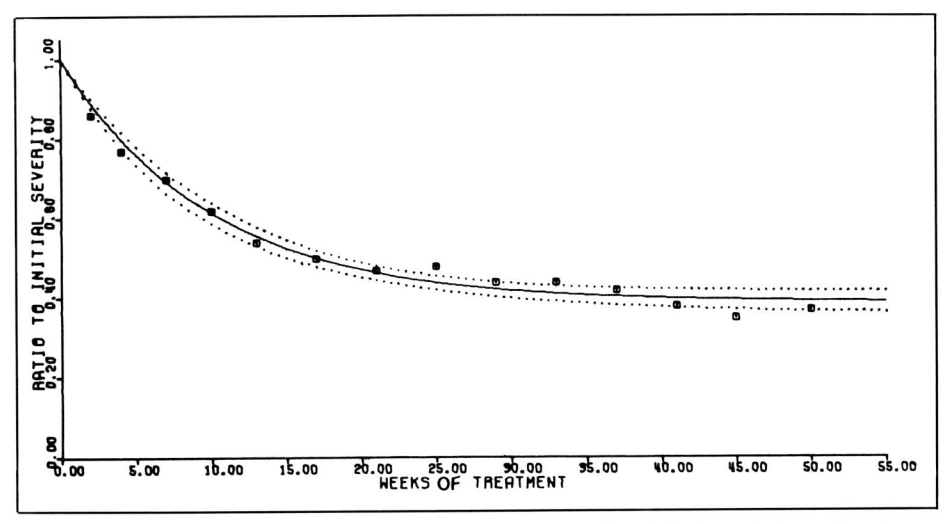

Figure 3. Asymptotic curve shows ratio to initial severity plotted against weeks of treatment. Dotted contours are 95% confidence limits of true means. Results show sustained beneficial effect without seasonal variation. Reproduced with permission from Wechsler HL, Kirk J, Slone J: Acne treated with a topical tetracycline preparation for a period of one year: results of a multi-group study. *Int J Dermatol* 17:237, 1978.

with juvenile diabetes and one with congenital nephritis were treated with topical tetracycline.[7] There was no mention in these reports[1-7] of photoreactivity or of development of contact sensitization to any of the components in the preparation. Neither was there any irritation or dryness of the skin that occurs at times with the use of topical retinoic acid, bleaches, and other surface agents.

Disadvantages

The most common complaints which arose from application of topical tetracycline were immediate but transitory stinging, and yellow discoloration of the skin. This occurred in respectively 28% and 20% of the individuals in the early part of the 12-month study conducted by Wechsler et al.[7] Few registered complaints after 3 months. The stinging was mitigated by having the patient wipe the face dry one hour after applying the solution. At no time was yellowing such a problem that it was cosmetically unacceptable.

Topical tetracycline was most effective in those individuals with the papular and pustular form of the disease. There was little evidence of improvement in individuals with cystic acne or with a predominance of comedones. In fact, comedones appeared to become more prominent in some patients as the pustular component cleared. It was suggested[3,7] that the therapeutic effectiveness of the topical tetracycline preparation could be enhanced by adding retinoic acid or benzoyl peroxide to the regimen.

Summary

Topical tetracycline is an effective agent in the treatment of pustular acne, particularly when the vehicle is stable and contains an enhancer of percutaneous absorption. Results with topical treatment suggest that the mode of action is local, although not primarily due to suppression of *P. acnes* or to direct lowering of free fatty acids of sebum. There have been no deleterious side effects observed in individuals taking topical tetracycline such as those seen in individuals receiving oral medication. In fact, there is indication that topical treatment can be used in patients with systemic disease when the oral route may be contraindicated. The yellowing and stinging of the skin noted in some patients after tetracycline applications were of minor consequence, and did not deter use of the preparation. There was only slight benefit in cystic and comedonal types of acne. The addition of retinoic acid and benzoyl peroxide and other anti-acne measures may increase the benefit.

REFERENCES

1. Kanter S, Saško E: Topical effects of oxytetracycline in acne vulgaris. *Cesk Dermatol* 45:45, 1970.
2. Gloor M, Hübscher M, Friederich HC: Untersuchungen zur externen Behandlung der Acne vulgaris mit Tetracyclin und Ostrogen. *Hautarzt* 25:391, 1974.
3. Frank SB: The topical treatment of acne with a tetracycline preparation: results of a multi-group study. *Cutis* 17:539, 1976.
4. Anderson RL, Cook CH, Smith DE: The effect of oral and topical tetracycline on acne severity and on surface lipid composition. *J Invest Dermatol* 66:172, 1976.
5. Smith JG Jr, Calker DK, Wehr RF: The effectiveness of topical and oral tetracycline for acne. *South Med J* 69:695, 1976.
6. Blaney DJ, Cook CH: Topical use of tetracycline in the treatment of acne: a double-blind study comparing topical and oral tetracycline therapy and placebo. *Arch Dermatol* 112:971, 1976.
7. Wechsler HL, Kirk J, Slone J: Acne treated with a topical tetracycline preparation for a period of one year: results of a multi-group study. *Int J Dermatol* 17:237, 1978.
8. Fulton JE Jr, Pablo G: Topical and antibiotic therapy for acne. *Arch Dermatol* 110:83, 1974.
9. Mills OH Jr, Kligman AM, Stewart R: The clinical effectiveness of topical erythromycin in acne vulgaris. *Cutis* 15:93, 1975.
10. Resh W, Stoughton RB: Topically applied antibiotics in acne vulgaris: clinical response and suppression of *Corynebacterium acnes* in open comedones. *Arch Dermatol* 112:182, 1976.
11. Freinkel RK, Strauss JS, Yip SY, et al: Effect of tetracycline on the composition of sebum in acne vulgaris. *N Engl J Med* 273:850, 1965.
12. Kraus S: Reduction in skin surface free fatty acids with topical tetracycline. *J Invest Dermatol* 51:431, 1968.
13. Beveridge GW, Powell EW: Sebum changes in acne vulgaris treated with tetracycline. *Br J Dermatol* 81:525, 1969.
14. Marples RR, Downing DT, Kligman AM: Control of free fatty acids in human surface lipids by *Corynebacterium acnes*. *J Invest Dermatol* 56:127, 1971.
15. Hassing GS: Inhibition of *Corynebacterium acnes* lipase by tetracycline. *J Invest Dermatol* 56:189, 1971.

16. Mills OH Jr, Marples RR, Kligman AM: Oral therapy with tetracycline and topical therapy with vitamin A. *Arch Dermatol* 106:200, 1972.
17. Fulton JE Jr: Lipases: their questionable role in acne vulgaris. *Int J Dermatol* 15:732, 1976.
18. Sekura DL, Scala J: "The Percutaneous Absorption of Alphyl Methyl Sulfoxides," in Montagna W, et al (Eds) *Pharmacology and the Skin*, pp 257-269. New York: Appleton-Century-Crofts, 1972.
19. Chalker DK, Smith JG Jr, Wehr R: The effect of storage or aging upon the efficacy of topical tetracycline in treating acne vulgaris. Presented at the 69th Annual Scientific Meeting of the Southern Medical Association, Section on Dermatology, Miami Beach, Florida, November, 1975.
20. Clendenning WE: Complications of tetracycline therapy. *Arch Dermatol* 91:628, 1965.
21. Gilgor RS: Complications of tetracycline therapy for acne. *NC Med J* 33:331, 1972.
22. Valtonen MV, Valtonen VV, Salo OP, et al: The effect of long-term tetracycline treatment for acne vulgaris on the occurrence of R factors in the intestinal flora of man. *Br J Dermatol* 95:311, 1976.

Chapter 18

Topical Erythromycin Therapy
ALAN R. SHALITA, MD

Systemic therapy with broad-spectrum antibiotics plays an important role in the treatment of acne vulgaris. This type of therapy is effective primarily because of the ability of these drugs to reduce the follicular population of *Propionibacterium acnes*. In over 20 years of use, broad-spectrum antibiotics have achieved a remarkable record of safety and efficacy.[1] Nevertheless, there has been intense interest in the development of antibacterial agents which would be effective when applied topically. This interest is due in part to the frequent problems, including patient compliance and side effects, (*eg*, vaginal candidiasis and gastrointestinal upset), which are encountered with the use of systemically administered antibiotics. The logic inherent in delivering drugs directly to the target organ is another reason for the increased interest in developing effective topical antibacterial agents.

Benzoyl peroxide is an effective antibacterial agent; it suppresses *P. acnes*, and it is clinically effective in the treatment of acne. This compound is discussed in greater detail elsewhere (see Chapter 15 and 16). Attention has been directed more recently towards the investigation of the use of topical antibiotics in the treatment of acne. Fulton and Pablo[2] reported on both the clinical efficacy of topically applied solutions containing 2% erythromycin and their efficacy in reducing the free fatty acids of skin surface lipids. The latter is an indirect measurement of the effect on *P. acnes*, since this organism is believed to be primarily responsible for the generation of free fatty acids in skin surface lipids.[3] Mills et al[4] also reported favorable results with the use of topical erythromycin in the treatment of acne vulgaris.

Method of Investigation

The ability of erythromycin to reduce the inflammatory lesions of acne was tested by comparing the results of the use of a commercially prepared 2% erythromycin base in a hydroalcoholic vehicle to those of the vehicle used alone. The investigations reported in this Chapter were obtained in double-blind studies with 70 patients. All of the patients had moderate papulopustular acne, had not received other therapy for their disease for one month prior to entering the study, and were in good health. Patients were assigned, in a random fashion, to either the test medication or to the vehicle alone, and were instructed to apply the medications 2 times a day. All of the patients were observed for at least 8 weeks.

Results

The results indicated an average reduction of 50% in inflammatory lesions in the patients treated with the 2% erythromycin solution, as compared to only an approximate 30% reduction in those treated with the vehicle alone (Figure 1). This data correlates very well with the results of a national cooperative study which will be reported elsewhere (J. Bernstein, personal communication, November 1977).

This author has had the opportunity to follow a portion of the patients on the active lotion for an additional 4 months beyond the formal study period. Continued improvement was noted in all of the patients.

Summary

The results suggest that topical solutions of erythromycin are effective in the treatment of inflammatory acne. It is this author's impression that these results are comparable to those achieved with benzoyl peroxide gel, but that topical solutions of erythromycin are less effective than systemically administered antibiotics. Of interest, however, is the observation of this author that many patients experienced less local irritancy with the erythromycin solution than with the vehicle alone. This perhaps suggests that erythromycin may possess certain anti-inflammatory properties, as noted by Plewig.[5] Indeed, preliminary experiments in this author's laboratories suggest that both erythromycin and tetracycline may inhibit neutrophil chemotaxis *in vitro*. Thus, topical erythromycin may provide an alternative to benzoyl peroxide therapy when the latter proves too irritating, when the patient has become sensitized to benzoyl peroxide, or when more frequent application is desired.

This author has also had the opportunity to evaluate a variety of

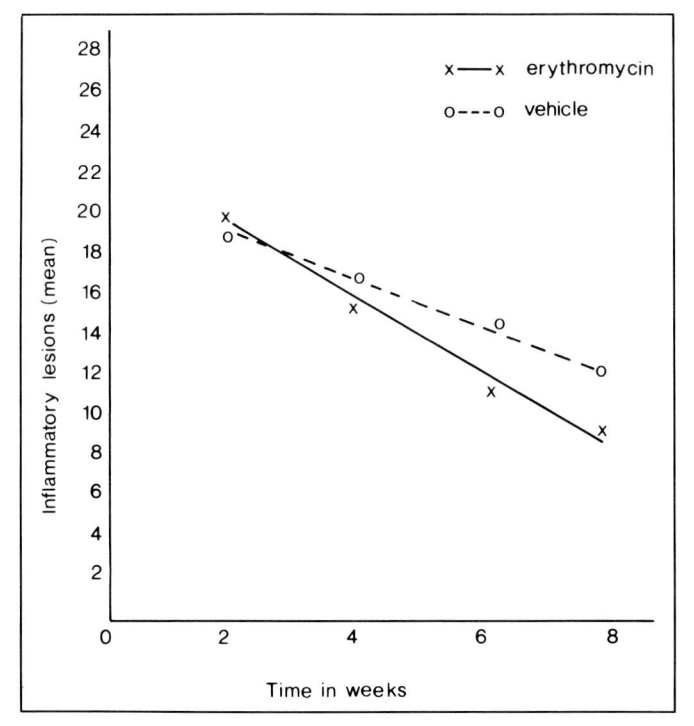

Figure 1. Comparison of effects of 2% erythromycin solution with vehicle alone in 70 patients.

extemporaneous formulations containing erythromycin tablets, and found them to be most unsatisfactory. A lotion consisting of erythromycin-base tablets dissolved in E-Solve® Lotion appears to be effective. It should be noted that erythromycin base is extremely pH- and temperature-labile, and that considerable care is required to make a relatively stable and active formulation.

In conclusion, topically applied solutions of erythromycin base appear to be effective and safe for use in the treatment of acne vulgaris.

REFERENCES

1. Systemic antibiotics for treatment of acne vulgaris: efficacy and safety. Ad Hoc Committee Report. *Arch Dermatol* 111:1630, 1975.
2. Fulton JE Jr, Pablo G: Topical antibacterial therapy for acne: study of the family of erythromycins. *Arch Dermatol* 110:83, 1974.
3. Shalita AR: Genesis of free fatty acids. *J Invest Dermatol* 62:332, 1974.
4. Mills OH, Kligman AM, Stewart R: The clinical effectiveness of topical erythromycin in acne vulgaris. *Cutis* 15:93, 1975.
5. Plewig G, Schopf E: Anti-inflammatory effects of antimicrobial agents: an *in vivo* study. *J Invest Dermatol* 65:532, 1975.

Chapter 19

Topical Clindamycin Therapy

RICHARD B. STOUGHTON, MD
WILLIAM RESH, MD

Some important facts are now known regarding topical antibiotics used in the treatment of acne. It is not difficult to significantly decrease the amount of bacteria which colonize on the surface of the skin.[1] It is just as evident that those agents which are capable of decreasing surface growth do not necessarily play a role in the treatment of acne vulgaris. It therefore appears that it is the organisms growing within the follicles and comedones which are important, and that the topical germicides or antibiotics which essentially sterilize the surface may have little or no effect on organisms in the comedones and follicles. Thus, the primary goal should be to find agents which prevent the growth of organisms (*Propionibacterium acnes* in particular) in the follicles rather than on the skin's surface.

In reviewing the literature, it is evident that practically no work has been done that measures the effect of germicides and antibiotics on the bacterial content of follicles and comedones. It is a reasonable supposition that, to be effective in the treatment of acne vulgaris, the given antibiotic must penetrate the comedo or follicle.

For the past few years, the authors have been exploring the topical use of clindamycin phosphate in the treatment of acne vulgaris. In this Chapter, the authors present their reasons for exploring this area, the *in vitro* studies which led to the selection of a few specific agents for *in vivo* testing, and the clinical results of the use of clindamycin phosphate lotion in acne therapy.

Many years ago, our group tried to detect the presence of tetracycline in

Table I – Effect of Antibiotics on *P. acnes in vitro*

	\multicolumn{4}{c}{Growth Inhibition of P. acnes in mm}
	\multicolumn{4}{c}{Antibiotic Concentration in Disc}
	0.1%	0.01%	0.001%	0.0001%
Erythromycin base	35	23	9	0
Erythromycin estolate	33	25	10	0
Clindamycin PO$_4$	31	20	4	0
Lincomycin	32	22	5	0
Tetracycline HCl	17	10	0	0
Bacitracin	14	7	2	0
Chloroxine	4	2	0	0
Sodium fusidate	0	0	0	0

* All antibiotics dissolved in N-methyl-2-pyrrolidone

follicles after topical application of dimethyl sulfoxide (DMSO). This was *in vitro* work, and it involved attempts to detect radiolabeled tetracycline by radioautographs of frozen sections, as well as those to detect fluorescence in follicles with fluorescence microscopy. We were unable to detect any tetracycline in follicles using these techniques. We recently repeated these experiments with equally unrewarding results.

The next step was to determine if there was any penetration of antibiotics as measured by a bioassay system,[2] which determines the amount of antibiotic in the corium at various periods after topical application. This *in vitro* assay using human skin was conducted using only potent antibiotics. The ability of the antibiotic to inhibit *P. acnes* was demonstrated when discs were soaked in concentrations of less than 0.1% of the antibiotic, thus enabling us to determine which agents were most potent (Table I). We concluded that clindamycin and erythromycin were very active in the bioassay system using human skin *in vitro*. Tetracycline was not as active, but did show some evidence of ability to penetrate into the corium (Table II).

Our next major consideration was whether a drop could be detected in the *P. acnes* count in comedones of acne patients treated with agents shown to be active in the *in vitro* assays. These results were published[3] in detail, and what we found was that 1% clindamycin phosphate lotion will sterilize the open comedones 6-10 weeks after initiation of topical treatment. Curiously, tetracycline and erythromycin had no measurable effect on the population of *P. acnes* in open comedones of acne patients (Table III).

Because of the surprising and very interesting finding that 1% clindamycin phosphate lotion could sterilize open comedones, we then conducted a double-blind study with 60 acne patients, using two forms of clindamycin

Table II — Bioassay Based on Penetration into Corium of Human Skin *in vitro*

	Corium Discs of Treated Skin # Samples	Average Inhibition of *P. acnes* in mm
Clindamycin PO$_4$		
N-methyl-2-pyrrolidone vehicle	20	16
Hydroalcoholic vehicle	10	8
Propylene glycol vehicle	10	12
Erythromycin base		
N-methyl-2-pyrrolidone vehicle	10	12
Hydroalcoholic vehicle	10	6
Erythromycin estolate		
N-methyl-2-pyrrolidone vehicle	10	11
Hydroalcoholic vehicle	10	4
Tetracycline HCl		
N-methyl-2-pyrrolidone vehicle	10	3
Hydroalcoholic vehicle	10	1
Bacitracin		
N-methyl-2-pyrrolidone vehicle	10	0
Hydroalcoholic vehicle	10	0
Benzoyl peroxide	10	0

(clindamycin phosphate and clindamycin base) and two vehicle preparations (hydroalcoholic vehicle and hydroalcoholic vehicle plus N-methyl-2-pyrrolidone), so that there were 4 groups of 15. The N-methyl-2-pyrrolidone was used with FDA approval, and is not available for general use, as it has not been officially approved by the FDA. A 1% clindamycin phosphate or base solution can be prepared by dissolving the aqueous injectable form of Cleocin® Phosphate in equal parts of water and 95% ethanol. Again, these preparations of clindamycin phosphate for topical use have not been officially approved by the FDA.

    The number of erythematous papules decreased substantially in all treated groups (Table IV), but was most marked in the group using clindamycin phosphate in the pyrrolidone vehicle, where an 80% improvement was seen within the 8-week period. The clindamycin phosphate in the hydroalcoholic vehicle gave a 55% improvement. Clindamycin base gave a 50% improvement in the hydroalcoholic vehicle and a 75% improvement in the pyrrolidone vehicle (Table V indicates the number of patients in each group showing sterility of the open comedones in regard to *P. acnes*). It was evident that clindamycin phosphate in the pyrrolidone vehicle was superior to all the other preparations, and that all the other preparations totally inhibited *P. acnes* within 8 weeks in less than half the patients. We concluded from these studies that clindamycin phosphate in the pyrrolidone vehicle is superior to

Table III – Comparison of Antibiotics with regard to Effect on Growth of *P. acnes* in Open Comedones

	# Patients	# Patients with Sterile Comedones Before Treatment	# Patients with Sterile Comedones After Treatment (8 weeks or longer)
Clindamycin PO$_4$ (pyrrolidone vehicle)	20	0	17
Clindamycin HCl (hydroalcoholic vehicle)	18	0	10
Clindamycin PO$_4$ (hydroalcoholic vehicle)	15	0	6
Erythromycin (pyrrolidone vehicle)	8	0	0
Tetracycline (pyrrolidone vehicle)	3	0	0

the other preparations, but that the others also demonstrate definite activity in controlling acne vulgaris.

A parallel group of acne patients was treated with a conventional regimen including oral tetracycline and topical agents such as benzoyl peroxide, an abradant soap, and topical sulfur preparations. This group was graded (by the same evaluators of the other study) according to the number of inflammatory papules over an 8-week period of observation. These patients were college students, as were the patients in the clindamycin study, but attended a different college in the same city. All groups were followed in the same year and at the same time of year (Table VI shows the results of the group receiving conventional oral tetracycline acne therapy as compared with results of the group receiving topical clindamycin). No bacterial studies were done on this parallel group. This cannot be considered a strict control group, since it was observed in a different college, but it does give some indication of the degree of difference in conventional treatment *vs* topical clindamycin phosphate.

In late 1976, a questionnaire regarding the use of topical antibiotics in the treatment of acne was sent, in a random sample, to 600 dermatologists in the United States (Figure 1). The results, in which 54.5% of those surveyed responded, are presented in Table VII-XII.

It is evident that the use of topical antibiotics is widespread, and that such antibiotics have favorable therapeutic applications in the management of patients with acne vulgaris. However, all of the use at this time is based on "homemade" formulations which are crude and untested with regard to bioavailability of the antibiotic in these assorted vehicles, stability, shelf life, safety, *etc.*

Some formulations of clindamycin, tetracycline, and erythromycin are now being tested under supervision of pharmaceutical companies and the

Table IV — Comparison of 4 Separate Groups Receiving Clindamycin*

	# Patients	Before Treatment	# Inflammatory Papules (Average) After 2 Weeks	(% Improvement)	After 8 Weeks	(% Improvement)
1% Clindamycin PO$_4$ in pyrrolidone vehicle	15	25	14	(44%)	5	(80%)
1% Clindamycin PO$_4$ in hydroalcoholic vehicle	14	22	15	(32%)	10	(55%)
1% Clindamycin base in pyrrolidone vehicle	15	22	13	(41%)	5	(75%)
1% Clindamycin base in hydroalcoholic vehicle	15	22	16	(27%)	11	(50%)

* Clinical improvement based on number of inflammatory papules (average)

Table V — Sterilization of Open Comedones in 8 Weeks with regard to *P. acnes*

	# Patients	Sterilized	Not Sterilized
1% Clindamycin PO$_4$ in pyrrolidone vehicle	14	11	3
1% Clindamycin PO$_4$ in hydroalcoholic vehicle	13	6	7
1% Clindamycin base in pyrrolidone vehicle	15	6	9
1% Clindamycin base in hydroalcoholic vehicle	12	5	7

Table VI — Comparison of Clinical Response of Acne Vulgaris in 3 Different Treatment Groups

	# Patients	Before Treatment	# Inflammatory Papules (Average) After 2 Weeks	(% Improvement)	After 8 Weeks	(% Improvement)
1% Clindamycin PO$_4$ in pyrrolidone vehicle	15	25	14	(44%)	5	(80%)
1% Clindamycin PO$_4$ in hydroalcoholic vehicle	14	22	15	(32%)	10	(55%)
Conventional regimens including oral tetracycline	14	22	18	(18%)	16	(27%)

176 TREATMENT

Dear Colleague:
For a coming talk to the American Academy of Dermatology in December, I would like to learn about the extent of the use of topical antibiotics in the treatment of acne. Will you help me? This should take no more than 1-2 minutes. Many thanks.

Richard B. Stoughton, MD

1) Do you use topical antibiotics to treat acne? Yes _____ No _____
   If yes, please complete questions below.
2) Which topical antibiotic do you use the most? Cleocin® _____
   Erythromycin _____ Tetracycline _____ Other _____
3) What percent of your acne patients get one of the above topical antibiotics that you use most?
   0-15% _____ 15-30% _____ 30-45% _____ 45-60% _____
   60-75% _____ 75-100% _____
4) Results compared to all other treatments including oral tetracycline:
   Same _____ Better _____ Worse _____
5) Side effects noted and incidence (topical therapy only):
   _____ Irritation—What % of users _____
   _____ Sensitization—What % of users _____
   _____ Vaginitis—What % of users _____
   _____ Candidiasis—What % of users _____
   _____ Gram-negative folliculitis—What % of users _____
   _____ Diarrhea—What % of users _____
   _____ Staining of the skin—What % of users _____
   Other _____
6) If you have time, would you please indicate the type of vehicle you use and the specific form of the antibiotic (eg, Cleocin® Phosphate (injectable) 1% hydroalcoholic solution)? _____

Any additional comments are welcome:

_____
Signed (optional)

Figure 1. A questionnaire regarding the use of topical antibiotics in acne therapy.

FDA. It is hoped that satisfactory formulations will be developed for general use by dermatologists, and that these formulations will ultimately be proven safe and effective.

It is known that erythromycin is very unstable and probably has a short period of activity in most of the "homemade" formulations being used. Clindamycin HCl (Cleocin®) and clindamycin PO$_4$ (Cleocin® Phosphate) are quite stable and have a satisfactory shelf life (3-6 months) in most of the hydroalcoholic preparations prescribed. The clindamycin HCl is less expensive than clindamycin phosphate, and is probably as effective and as stable, particularly if the pH of the vehicle is kept between pH 6.0-7.0. The ideal vehicle and concentration have not been established for Cleocin® HCl, but we

Table VII – Percentage of Dermatologists Using Topical Antibiotics

Using topical antibiotics	57
Not using topical antibiotics	43

Table VIII – Primary Topical Antibiotic % Used by Dermatologists

Clindamycin HCl	56.0
Erythromycin	42.0
Tetracycline	1.5
Others	0.5

Table IX – Percentage of Patients Receiving Topical Antibiotics as Reported by Dermatologists

	% Dermatologists Reporting	
% Patients	Erythromycin	Clindamycin HCl
0-15%	68	61
15-30	17	23
30-45	6	8
45-60	8	4
60-75	0	3
75-100	1	1

Table X – Comparison of Topical Antibiotics with Oral Tetracycline

	(90 Dermatologists) Clindamycin HCl	(58 Dermatologists) Erythromycin
Same	51%	44%
Better	23%	17%
Worse	26%	39%

have found the following to be clinically effective and stable for at least 6 months, when kept at room temperature:

Cleocin® Capsules (4)   600 mg
70% isopropyl alcohol   48 ml
Distilled water   6 ml

Stir well for 10 minutes and filter with coarse filter paper. Then add 6 ml propylene glycol.

The lotion should be applied with the fingers in the morning and in the early evening to all affected areas after washing.

Table XI – Side Effects of Topical Antibiotics

Clindamycin HCl	Erythromycin
Irritation – 41% of dermatologists report mild irritation in 10-15% of cases (probably secondary to hydroalcoholic vehicle)	Irritation – 36% of dermatologists report mild irritation in 10-15% of cases (probably secondary to hydroalcoholic vehicle)
Sensitization – None	Sensitization – None
Vaginitis – None	Vaginitis – None
Diarrhea – None*	Diarrhea – None
Staining – None	Staining – None
Gram-negative folliculitis – None	Gram-negative folliculitis – None

* Since this questionnaire was sent, 6 cases of diarrhea have been reported

We have not had any significant experience with the use of Cleocin® lotion in combination with other topical therapeutic agents, primarily because most of our patients do very well with the Cleocin® lotion alone.

Regarding the occurrence of side effects from the topical application of clindamycin, the authors are now aware of 6 cases of diarrhea associated with the use of Cleocin® lotion. These all cleared rapidly when use of the lotion was discontinued. No cases of pseudomembranous colitis have been reported with the use of topical Cleocin® lotion.

REFERENCES

1. Lowbury EJL: "Removal of Bacteria from the Operation Site," in Maibach HI, Hildick-Smith G (Eds): *Skin Bacteria and Their Role in Infection.* New York: McGraw-Hill, 1965.
2. Stoughton RB: Bioassay of antimicrobials. *Arch Dermatol* 101:160, 1970.
3. Resh W, Stoughton RB: Topically applied antibiotics in acne vulgaris: clinical response and suppression of *Corynebacterium acnes* in open comedones. *Arch Dermatol* 112:182, 1976.

Chapter 20

Oral Antibiotics
WILLIAM A. AKERS, MD
HOWARD I. MAIBACH, MD

An informal survey was recently conducted among 17 members of the National Acne Association and the Ad Hoc Committee on the Use of Antibiotics in Dermatology, Division of Research, National Program for Dermatology of the American Academy of Dermatology.[1] Each participant had published on clinical or laboratory investigations concerning cutaneous infections or acne vulgaris. The purpose of the survey was not to develop statistical data, but to obtain recommendations on the use of oral antimicrobial agents for the treatment of acne. The questionnaire consisted of 202 questions and statements, and provided room for comments on antibiotics and sulfonamides used in acne therapy. The responses to this survey are summarized in this Chapter, as an outline for the use of oral antibiotics in the treatment of acne.

Since all the participants did not answer every question, the following terms are used to express a degree of agreement among those who did respond to a particular question or statement: *unanimous*—everyone responding; *all*—95%, all but one person; *most*—around 75%; *majority*—around 60%; *divided*—around 45-55%; *some*—around 40%; and *few*—around 15%. Given the small sample size, unwarranted precision should not be attached to the percentages. The responses usually represent a percentage of 17 (or less) respondents. One of the group surveyed stated that, with the advent of more efficacious topical agents, he rarely uses systemic antibiotics in his practice.

Indications

SCARRING

Although the questionnaire did not include the subject of scarring, numerous comments were made about the scarring, however minimal, that results from acne lesions. This was a major indication for using oral antibiotics. At a later meeting of the Ad Hoc Committee, the group agreed unanimously that scarring is one of the indications for employing oral antibiotics, but that pain, disfigurement, and interference with function are also major indications.

SEVERITY

Pillsbury et al[2] have classified acne lesions in terms of severity. Using this classification, the physicians responded that they use oral antibiotics as follows: the majority did not recommend the use of oral antibiotics for treating mild (Grade I) acne vulgaris; most recommended the use of oral antibiotics for treating moderate (Grade II) acne vulgaris; all recommended the use of oral antibiotics for treating severe (Grade III) acne vulgaris; the group unanimously recommended the use of oral antibiotics for treating severe (Grade IV) acne vulgaris; two doubted the efficacy of antibiotics in the most severe cases, but believed a trial of antibiotics is warranted.

TYPES OF ACNE

As to the diagnostic categories of acne vulgaris, the participants responded: all agreed that the use of oral antibiotics is not indicated for noninflammatory comedogenic acne; the group unanimously agreed that the use of oral antibiotics is indicated for pustular, papular, and papulopustular acne vulgaris; the group unanimously agreed that the use of oral antibiotics is warranted for treating cystic acne and acne conglobata, although one respondent had doubts concerning the efficacy of antibiotics in severe cases.

Other Therapy

As to questions regarding the use of antibiotics alone for treating acne, the respondents replied: most (87%) agreed that oral antibiotics are seldom employed as the sole therapy in acne vulgaris. The majority (67%) agreed that oral antibiotics are adjunctive or supplemental therapy in the management of patients with moderate to severe inflammatory acne vulgaris; the rest believed that antibiotics are the major therapy, while other treatments are supplemental.

Contraindications

The group offered the following contraindications for using an antibiotic for treating an acne patient. Absolute contraindications are: hypersensitivity to the drug, and pregnancy in the second and third trimesters (during the first trimester, 78% do not prescribe antibiotics).

Relative contraindications are, depending on the type and severity of the disease: liver disease, and renal disease.

Other contraindications are: a history of gastrointestinal upsets to the drug (usually temporary); severe vaginal candidiasis; parental concern over the use of antibiotics; and, staining of the teeth by use of the tetracyclines in patients below 8 years of age. (The staining of the molars by the tetracyclines in older children and adolescents is considered a minor matter.)

Age Limits

The group unanimously agreed that there is no upper age limit when treating patients with acne vulgaris. The group did not agree on the lower age limit. Eighty-five percent recommended 10-13 years of age (age 10, four responses; age 13, two responses) as the lower age limit to initiate antibiotic therapy. One recommended age 7, while another recommended age 14.

Duration

All agreed that there is no limit to the duration of antibiotic treatment for acne vulgaris, but that the physician should try to reduce the dose and stop the use of antibiotics when possible. Some recommended discontinuing use of the drug during the summer, if the patient's condition is stable. One recommended trying to stop use of the drug every 3 months.

Laboratory Tests

INITIAL

Should routine laboratory tests be done prior to starting an acne patient on antibiotics therapy? Most (69%) recommended no screening laboratory tests unless indicated. A few do a complete blood count and urinalysis. No one performs a battery of blood chemistry tests (*eg*, SMA-12), stool culture, or vaginal culture for *Candida albicans*. One recommended an initial blood urea nitrogen (BUN), liver function, and renal function tests, and two perform bacteriology and antibiotic-sensitivity tests for investigative purposes only.

FOLLOW-UP

For acne patients on long-term, low-dosage antibiotics, some do the following: one-third do a complete blood count at 6 months, then yearly; one-fourth recommended urinalysis at 6 months, then yearly; and, several do a multiphasic blood chemistry analyses (SMA-12) yearly. All agreed that laboratory tests should be done when clinically indicated. Some (43%) do follow-up laboratory tests.

The authors' personal preference is to perform an initial complete blood count, urinalysis, BUN, and SGOT on a patient who may possibly require long-term antibiotic treatment. The tests are then repeated at 6 months, 12 months, then yearly. If other patients later require long-term administration of antibiotics, the authors test at 6 months; one year; then yearly, or sooner, if indicated.

Frequency of Follow-up

Since acne vulgaris varies in severity and in its response to therapy, general recommendations as to frequency of follow-up are difficult. Early after initiating antibiotic therapy, one physician checks his patients every 2 weeks; nine see their patients at monthly intervals; and five follow their patients every 6 weeks. If the acne improves, most examine the patient at increasing intervals from 2-3 months. Only two examine the patient at 4-6-month intervals after the disease has been controlled.

The authors' personal preference is to check the patient every 3-4 weeks until response to the antibiotic is obtained (usually 6-8 weeks), then re-examine the patient at 6-8-week intervals. When the patient's acne is clinically stable, the follow-up frequency is decreased.

Refills

How frequently are prescriptions for antibiotics to be refilled? The group diverges in its recommendations: four stated that refills are indicated every 4 weeks; four at 2-month intervals; and six at 3-month intervals. One recommended refills once every 6 months. As the course of the patient's disease is determined and as the patient becomes knowledgeable as to proper usage, the interval between refills is increased.

Are refills ever justified without seeing the patient? Most believed that there are such instances. Some recommended refills as follows: 1) after observing a reliable patient for several months; 2) limit the prescription to 3 months only; and 3) if the patient is doing well. Those who disagreed stated that the practice is rarely indicated, or that the need for continued antibiotics cannot be determined in advance.

Ceasing Therapy

The group listed indications for the cessation or modification of antibiotic therapy. These include: complete remission of acne; pregnancy; the development of a concurrent illness; and, poor response to the drug. Other indications are: when the family physician requests stopping the drug, or when the patient becomes distressed over taking the drug.

The occurrence of various side effects requires individual corrective therapy. The following recommendations were offered: if *hypersensitivity reaction* occurs, stop drug; if *photosensitivity* occurs, substitute another, nonphotosensitizing, antibiotic; if *diabetes insipidus syndrome* occurs, reduce the dose or stop the drug; if there is *significant change in complete blood count or liver function tests,* stop drug and do repeat follow-up tests; when *high milk intake is needed,* change to another drug. If side effects are temporary (*eg,* vaginitis; pruritus ani; diarrhea; esophageal distress; nausea; flatulence; black hairy tongue), reduce drug or stop therapy.

Concomitant Therapy

All recommended that concomitant therapy should be employed. All use systemic vitamin A in the treatment of some patients; four use oral contraceptive agents in the treatment of some patients; four use systemic corticosteroids in the treatment of severe cases. Half always employ topical agents, while the other half frequently use topical agents such as benzoyl peroxide, tretinoin, resorcinol-sulfur, and salicylic acid preparations. Most use physical modalities (acne surgery, carbon dioxide slush, liquid nitrogen, ultraviolet light) on many patients. Some inject intralesional corticosteroids into severe lesions.

Dosage

Ordinarily, the dose of antibiotics initially ranges between 2-4 capsules or tablets a day, and is reduced, usually after 4-8 weeks of observation, to 3, 2, or even one capsule a day, depending on the patient's response. Higher doses may be prescribed for patients whose conditions are refractory.

Two schedules are practiced for initiating oral antibiotic therapy in a patient: high-dosage and low-dosage. For the patient with severe acne, most physicians begin with the higher dose. For mild to moderate acne, some employ the low-dosage schedule.

TETRACYCLINE HYDROCHLORIDE

This is the antibiotic most frequently prescribed, while oxytetracycline and chlortetracycline are employed by a few.

High dose—250 mg, 4 times a day, one hour before meals and at bedtime, for 3 weeks (66%) or 6 weeks (33%); then the dose is revised upward or downward by 250 mg every 2-4 weeks (60%) or 6-8 weeks (40%), depending on the patient's response. Some recommended dosages of 2 times a day as simpler for the patient.

Low dose—250 mg, once a day, one hour before or 2 hours after a meal, for 4-8 weeks; then the dose is adjusted every 4-8 weeks, depending on the patient's response. Those physicians advocating low dosage noted that many patients, especially those with papular and pustular acne, respond well to this regimen.

Some of the group's comments were: 1) start with a low dose if the patient has had side effects to the drug in the past; and 2) prescribe an initial dosage of 2000 mg a day for some severe cases.

The package insert (and the *Physician's Desk Reference*) lists severe acne vulgaris as an indication for adjunctive therapy with tetracycline, oxytetracycline, and chlortetracycline. Most find that the usual maintenance dose is 250-500 mg a day. Only one recommended 1000 mg a day for maintenance. The usual number of tablets or capsules prescribed initially is 100 (65%), 60 (20%), or 30 (15%). (Prescribing 100 tablets of tetracycline often saves money, since the drug is packaged in bottles of 100.)

ERYTHROMYCIN

This is the second most common antibiotic used for treating acne patients. No one in the group considered erythromycin to be the drug of choice, but all use it when the tetracyclines fail to help the patient, or when the patient does not tolerate tetracyclines. The drug can be used during pregnancy, although its safety has not been definitely established. Erythromycin appears to have no teratogenic effect on the human fetus.

High dose—250 mg, 3-4 times a day, one hour before meals and at bedtime, for 2-6 weeks; then the dose is adjusted every 4-6 weeks (recommendations ranged from 1-8 weeks), depending on the response.

Low dose—250 mg a day, one hour before meals or at bedtime, for 4-6 weeks; then the dose is adjusted every 4-6 weeks, depending on the patient's response. One respondent adjusts the dose weekly; another at 8-week intervals.

The group divided into three equal segments in recommending a daily dosage of 1000 mg for 4 weeks, 6 weeks, and 8 weeks as an adequate trial before switching to another antibiotic. All stated that they do not use erythromycin estolate because of the rare occurrence of hepatic dysfunction in sensitized persons.

DEMECLOCYCLINE

About half of the respondents use demeclocycline in treating some acne patients. One considered it the initial drug of choice. Three use the phototoxicity from demeclocycline to therapeutic advantage, since the phototoxicity can improve acne if carefully controlled. Problems with diabetes insipidus syndrome may arise in a third of the patients receiving 600 mg a day.

High dose—150 mg, 4 times a day, one hour before meals and at bedtime, for 3-6 weeks; then the dose is adjusted every 3-4 weeks, depending on the response.

Low dose—150 mg, once a day, one hour before a meal, for 6 weeks;

then the dose is adjusted every 6 weeks, depending on the response. The patient must be instructed as to the phototoxic potential of the drug.

MINOCYCLINE

One third of the respondents use minocycline in the treatment of acne patients, which is one of the conditions the package insert lists as an indication for employing the drug. Food or milk do not notably influence the absorption of minocycline.

High dose—100 mg, 2 times a day, for 3-6 weeks; then the dose is adjusted every 3-6 weeks, depending on the response. Vestibular symptoms were observed in less than 5% of patients on the high-dosage schedule only.

Low dose—50-100 mg a day, for 4-6 weeks; then the dose is adjusted every 6 weeks, depending on the response.

LINCOMYCIN AND CLINDAMYCIN

Neither lincomycin nor clindamycin were considered by most (87%) of the group to be the initial drug of choice in the treatment of acne vulgaris. Most (77%), at the time of the survey, used the drugs for moderate and severe cases of acne vulgaris not responsive to other antibiotics and refractory to other therapies.

One fourth of the respondents prescribe *lincomycin*, but none uses a high-dosage schedule of lincomycin.

Low dose—250 mg, 2 times a day, for 2-4 weeks; then the dose is adjusted every 4 weeks, depending on the response.

Half of the respondents prescribe *clindamycin*, usually by the low-dosage schedule.

High dose—150 mg, 3 times day, or 300 mg, 2 times a day, for 4 weeks; then the dose is adjusted every 4 weeks, depending on the response.

Low dose—75-150 mg, 2 times a day, for 2-4 weeks; then the dose is adjusted every 4 weeks, depending on the response.

All warn their patients that if diarrhea (not soft bowel movements) develops (more than 3 diarrheal stools in one day), they should call the physician and stop using the drug. One tells a patient to discontinue use of the drugs if abdominal cramps occur. Others suggested that these two drugs should not be prescribed for patients with known bowel problems.

Since it has been established that pseudomembranous colitis is associated with the oral use of these two antibiotics, it is now believed that these drugs, as taken orally, are not frequently prescribed for treatment of acne.

DOXYCYCLINE

One third of the group use doxycycline in the treatment of acne, while half do not prescribe the drug because it costs more than tetracycline HCl. A renal diabetes insipidus syndrome can occur at higher doses. Phototoxicity has been reported. This drug possesses no advantage over tetracycline. The package insert lists severe acne vulgaris as an indication for using doxycycline as adjunctive therapy.

High dose—200 mg, 2 times a day, for 2-4 weeks; then the dose is adjusted, depending on the response. Only one respondent favored the high dose. The others favored the low dose schedule.

Low dose—200 mg, once a day, for 6-8 weeks; then the dose is adjusted, depending on the response.

The usual maintenance dose varies between 50, 100, or 200 mg a day.

TRIMETHOPRIM-SULFAMETHOXAZOLE COMBINATION

No one in the group had had experience with the trimethoprim 80 mg-sulfamethoxazole 500 mg combination tablet. Controlled clinical trials in England attested to the efficacy of the medication in treating acne vulgaris. The recommended dose for initial therapy and maintenance is one tablet a day.

The toxicity for the combination is classified the same as sulfonamides with low toxicity. Good experimental evidence for safety and efficacy is available abroad, but there is little clinical experience in the United States for its use in acne therapy.

Rationale

The mechanisms offered by appropriate antibiotics which produce improvement in inflammatory acne lesions remain unidentified. Bacterial inhibition, reduction of lipase elaboration, reduction of free fatty acids, and chelation of enzymes and metallic ions were all demonstrated to occur with the use of antibiotics;[1] one or all are logical reasons for using antibiotics to treat acne.

Originally, the rationale for using antibiotics was based on the supposition that pus in acne lesions indicated secondary bacterial infection. Bacterial studies demonstrating the frequent recovery of coagulase-positive staphylococci from acne pustules supported this view.[3] Further examination revealed that the bacteria in acne lesions comprised only resident follicular organisms (primarily the anaerobic diphtheroid, *Propionibacterium acnes*, and *Staphylococcus epidermidis*, biotype 1), raising doubts about the action of antibiotics.

Penicillin and sulfonamides were the first commonly employed antimicrobial agents. Increasing clinical experience showed penicillin to be only marginally effective in the treatment of acne; sulfonamides, although widely prescribed, failed to correct the acne in many cases. Broad-spectrum antibiotics have proven to be more consistently beneficial than sulfonamides for treating acne. Many cases of acne can be controlled by doses of antibiotics lower than those usually required to suppress bacterial infections.

Orally administered tetracycline, even in doses as small as 250 mg a day, results in a significant (P=0.001) reduction of the free fatty acid concentration in sebum.[4] Free fatty acids are the most irritating components of sebum and are most likely responsible for the formation of the inflammatory lesions of acne.[5,6] This suggests that antibiotic therapy achieves its beneficial effect by lowering the concentration of inflammation-evoking free fatty acids.

Bacterial inhibition and consequent reduction in lipase elaboration are believed to be the mechanisms responsible for suppressing free fatty acid release from sebum triglycerides. The following lines of evidence support this view: *P. acnes* is sensitive to broad-spectrum antibiotics *in vitro*;[7] the oral administration of broad-spectrum antibiotics reduces the quantity of *P. acnes* organisms;[8-17] *P. acnes* releases free fatty acids from triglycerides *in vitro*,[4-13] and tetracycline can inhibit this effect; and, the activity of lipases of *P. acnes* origin can be reduced by broad-spectrum antibiotics *in vitro*.[15,16] This latter observation suggests that direct bacterial lipase inhibition may be a major effect of antibiotic treatment. However, erythromycin reduces free fatty acids in sebum but has no effect on lipases.[15] The combination of trimethoprim and sulfamethoxazole also significantly (P<0.01) reduces the surface free fatty acids.[17] Thus, direct suppression of lipase-elaborating bacteria is a more likely mechanism.

Presently, the concept that the beneficial effect from broad-spectrum antibiotics results solely from a decrease in free fatty acids has not been proven. No controlled studies have demonstrated an unequivocal cause-and-effect relationship between free fatty acid inhibition and clinical improvement.[18]

Efficacy

The Ad Hoc Committee on the Use of Antibiotics in Dermatology[1] recently reviewed critically the literature in the English language concerning the efficacy of certain antibiotics and sulfonamides. From the published evidence, in the Committee's judgment, tetracycline, chlortetracycline, oxytetracycline, minocycline, erythromycin, clindamycin, and lincomycin are all effective drugs for treating inflammatory acne vulgaris when each is given in doses equivalent to 1 gm a day or less of tetracycline HCl over long periods. Although proven effective in controlled studies, doxycycline and the trimethroprim-sulfamethoxazole combination require more clinical experience before they can be recommended without qualification.

The authors made a reasonable estimate, based on the best literature values available,[1] that the tetracyclines are 70% effective for treating acne vulgaris, and that the placebo response is 30%. To demonstrate that doxycycline would be 10% more effective than tetracycline HCl (80% vs 70% at a confidence level of 0.05 and at a power of 0.8, the traditional values for clinical trials) would require at least 332 patients in the new drug group and 332 patients in the tetracycline HCl group—a total of 664 patients! Conversely, to demonstrate the difference in effectivity between an antibiotic (70%) and placebo (30%) requires 33 patients in each group, or a total of 66, to prove that 40% difference—a study which is more likely to be done.[19] No wonder there are so few meaningful studies on the differences of efficacy between antibiotics as compared to an antibiotic *vs* a placebo for acne therapy.

Leyden[20] emphasized that deep nodular lesions and burrowing, epithelialized sinus tracts do not involute with antibiotic therapy. He also noted that failure of patients to take the drug, failure to follow directions, use of external comedogenic substances, aggravation by anticonvulsive and systemic corticosteroid medications, and repeated friction and pressure (acne mechanica) are all factors which can cause an apparent failure to respond to antibiotic therapy (see Chapter 21). Correcting the fault may allow for a response to the antibiotic.

Safety

Are oral antibiotics safe for long-term administration to acne patients? The authors define "long-term" use of an antibiotic as the administration of an antibiotic to an acne patient for more than 6 weeks.

Most patients with acne are otherwise healthy and are treated on an outpatient basis with low doses of antibiotics (equivalent to 1 gm a day or less of tetracycline HCl). Inpatient experiences with seriously ill or immunologically compromised patients, who constitute many of the drug reaction cases cited in the literature, are inappropriate standards for comparison. The most germane information concerning side effects has been derived from patients who have acne.[1,21]

Whenever a physician treats a patient with antimicrobial therapy, he applies the principle of selective toxicity and hopes the drug will interfere with the cellular metabolism of an offending organism without injuring the patient. No antibiotic is without toxicity.[22] To treat common conditions like acne, both the physician and the patient need to know the relative safety of the topical and systemic therapies prescribed. The authors use the term "relative safety" to imply that there is a risk in practically all human pursuits. Every risk cannot be known in every situation; but, if major risks are known, a reasonable decision can be made by the physician and patient as to the risk/benefit ratio. As yet, neither an operational definition for safety nor unequivocal standards for the clinical and laboratory abnormalities that are considered safe and those that are not have been established.[23]

Recently, the Ad Hoc Committee[1] reviewed the safety of oral antibiotics and sulfonamides used in treating acne vulgaris. The Committee analyzed only controlled studies of adverse effects. (The evaluation of drug reactions requires proper controls as in any other form of clinical investigation.[24]) Surprisingly, when these authors reviewed the literature, we found more

Table I — Complications of Tetracycline Therapy[25]

Irritation
  nausea
  vomiting

Suppression of Normal Flora
  diarrhea
  folliculitis
  candidiasis

Allergic Reactions
  rashes
  anaphylactoid reactions

Photosensitization
  exaggerated sunburn
  onycholysis

Chelation
  discoloration of teeth

Inhibition of Protein Synthesis
  enamel hypoplasias (children)
  bone growth retardation (infants)
  negative nitrogen balance

Renal — No Pre-existing Diseases
  symptomatic diabetes insipidus syndrome

Renal and Liver — Pre-existing Diseases
  exacerbation of renal or liver diseases

Other
  fixed drug eruption

---

controlled studies concerning the long-term use of tetracyclines for treating acne than for treating any other chronic disease.[21]

Adverse Drug Reactions

The authors define an "adverse drug reaction" as an unwarranted or undesirable drug effect of any severity that produces signs, symptoms, or changes in normal laboratory values in a patient taking the drug. Adverse reactions to the antimicrobial agents are related to the age of the patient, the disease treated, concomitant diseases, dosage, route of administration, duration of therapy, genetic defects of the patient, and the toxic effect (pharmacologic action) of the drug. Since the Ad Hoc Committee chose only controlled trials for statistical analysis of the antibiotics, this discussion will include other clinical trials which address the question of safety. We will consider that the acne-prone individuals are from 10-45 years of age (thereby excluding infants, young children, and the elderly), and that they are treated as outpatients, and are otherwise healthy.

This discussion focuses on several side effects which can occur with the use of antibiotics, especially those elicited by tetracyclines (Table I[25]). The physician is referred to Zelick[22] and Kucers[26] for more complete presentations.

GASTROINTESTINAL UPSETS

Despite the vast experience with antibiotics, the incidence of such common symptoms as nausea, cramps, diarrhea, and flatulence remains inadequately documented. Mild gastrointestinal complaints occur more frequently in a healthy population than previously recorded, and 4-8% of 670 people surveyed[24] reported nausea, vomiting, or diarrhea on any single day.

In another study, tetracycline and chlortetracycline, administered in oral doses of 500 mg a day or less to 208 acne patients, caused gastrointestinal disturbances in 5% of the patients. These disturbances subsided while patients were still taking the drug, or ceased promptly on discontinuation.[27] In a third report,[25] of 202 acne patients receiving tetracycline, 7 developed gastrointestinal symptoms within the first 6 weeks, but became asymptomatic on stopping the drug; 4 of the 7 resumed treatment without experiencing a recurrence of the gastrointestinal symptoms. Gastrointestinal upsets may occur with any antibiotic.

WEIGHT LOSS

Tetracyclines have an anti-anabolic effect because of their interference with protein synthesis in man.[26] How frequently weight loss due to tetracyclines occurs in acne patients is unknown, although there are no adverse reports indicating that this is a problem.

RENAL TOXICITY

Patients with stable, chronic renal failure may be precipitated into terminal renal failure when treated with tetracyclines.[28] In patients with impaired renal function, the tetracyclines (except doxycycline) may cause further rise in the blood urea nitrogen and creatinine. Whether this is a direct toxic effect, or is rather caused by the additional load of products of amino acid metabolism from tetracycline inhibition of protein synthesis, remains unresolved.[26] Direct renal cellular damage from tetracycline cannot be demonstrated experimentally.[22] In a metabolic ward, in 6 of 7 normal patients who were given 1 or 2 gm tetracycline a day, an average 2 gm% rise occurred in their BUN levels, but no rise occurred in their creatinine levels.[29] A long-term, controlled study[28] of 246 acne patients taking 250-500 mg a day of several different tetracyclines detected no abnormalities in the BUN levels before, during, or after treatment. Results of blood chemistry studies of 325 patients receiving low-dosage tetracycline HCl therapy continuously for 3 years or longer revealed insignificant changes in all patients.[30]

When severe kidney failure is present, the physician should prescribe antibiotics that are primarily metabolized in the liver, *eg*, erythromycin, chlortetracyline, and doxycycline.

DIABETES INSIPIDUS SYNDROME

After some acne patients developed polyuria, polydipsia, and weakness while taking demeclocycline, renal concentrating defects were found in 8 of 24 study patients. The syndrome occurred in all 5 receiving 1200 mg a day and in 3 of 9 receiving 600 mg a day, but in none of the 10 patients receiving 150 mg a day.[31] The dose dependence and the reversibility of the antidiuretic hormone unresponsiveness are probably due to inhibition of cyclic-AMP generation and action. One respondent to the survey reported that this syndrome occurred with high dosages of doxycycline.

HEPATIC TOXICITY

Abnormal liver function tests, including elevation of the SGOT, SGPT, and alkaline phosphatase, increased thymol turbidity, and BSP retention, have occurred from administering more than 1 gm a day of tetracycline intravenously to seriously ill women. Six women died; most of the women were pregnant; all had infections; and all had pre-existing renal functional impairment.[26] Hepatotoxicity is rare in patients receiving 1 gm a day or less of oral tetracycline.[28]

Hepatic dysfunction, with or without jaundice, has occurred chiefly in association with erythromycin estolate administration.[32] This syndrome seems to be a form of sensitization, occurs usually in adults, reappears within 48 hours of readministering the drug, and reverses when the medication is discontinued.

HEMATOLOGIC EFFECTS

Although anemia, neutropenia, and eosinophilia were observed during tetracycline therapy,[33] they rarely constitute problems. No toxic effects on the blood elements were demonstrated in 22 patients receiving 500 mg a day of tetracycline for 5 months.[34] Another author[30] reported no toxic effects from administering 250-500 mg a day of tetracycline HCl for 3-13 years to 325 patients with acne vulgaris and other chronic skin infections. An 18-year-old woman had megaloblastic anemia due to a mild folate-deficiency possibly associated with receiving 500 mg a day of tetracycline for 3 years for the treatment of acne.[35] These authors found no other similar reports. Impaired blood clotting has occurred only with high doses of intravenous tetracyclines.[26]

SUPRAINFECTION

"Suprainfection," rather than "superinfection," is a suggested term to describe secondary infections arising during treatment with antimicrobial drugs.[26] No overwhelming or debilitating bacterial, fungal, or viral infections have been reported from the emergence of resistant or nonsusceptible organisms in acne patients treated with tetracyclines or erythromycin.[27,36] However, two suprainfections do occur in acne patients on long-term antibiotics: 1) overgrowth of *Candida albicans,* and 2) gram-negative folliculitis of the face.

Of 202 acne patients who received 1 gm a day or less of tetracycline for 1-21 months and were followed at 2-6-week intervals, 16 women (13%) developed yeast vaginitis and 7 had gastrointestinal disturbances; none developed pruritus ani.[25] Vaginal candidiasis occurs with variable frequency. The mechanism involved was extensively studied;[37] tetracycline-related candidiasis generally responds promptly to anticandidal therapy. If the patient does not have a predisposition to candidiasis, tetracycline can usually be restarted some weeks after clearing. The authors start these patients at 250 mg a day, and gradually increase the dose to a therapeutic level. Some patients respond to anticandidal therapy while continuing tetracycline.

Gram-negative folliculitis of the face may follow colonization of the nose with gram-negative bacteria. Deep nodular and cystic lesions occur. More commonly, superficial pustules (usually grouped around the nose) are associated with a lactose-fermenting, gram-negative rod. In 4 years, 50 cases were identified among 1200 new cases of acne vulgaris.[38] Therapy remains under study. Gram-negative bacteria colonize the exterior nares of some healthy adults. In one study, 5 of 17 patients carried these organisms which constituted from 0.2-2.0% of their anterior nares flora. When they received cephalosporin antibiotic therapy, the gram-negative bacteria became the second dominating organism. The increase was seen principally in patients who had the organism prior to therapy. After stopping therapy, the bacteria of the anterior nares flora returned to baseline levels.[39] Gram-negative folliculitis occurs in patients receiving not only tetracycline but other broad-spectrum antibiotics as well. To assess the risk, more information is needed about the pathophysiology of the syndrome.

PHOTOTOXICITY

Phototoxicity reactions, including photo-onycholysis, have been reported to all the tetracyclines, but most frequently to demeclocycline. About 20% of persons taking demeclocycline develop photosensitivity both in clinical practice and by experimental induction.[40] The incidence for other tetracyclines is unknown, but it is far less than 1% in acne patients.

Two cases of onycholysis associated with tetracycline therapy for acne, but without phototoxicity, were reported.[41] The authors have observed enough additional examples to suggest that onycholysis is often not identified. It can occur early in therapy, or after months or even years. The extent of sun exposure is critical. The nail re-adheres to the bed upon cessation of therapy. The authors have seen second episodes of onycholysis when the patient inadvertently increased his sun exposure.

TETRACYCLINE BULLOUS DRUG ERUPTION ON THE HAND

Five women taking oral tetracyclines for acne developed bullae on the dorsum of the hand. When tetracycline therapy was continued, the hands developed skin fragility and milia morphologically similar to those seen in porphyria cutanea tarda. Porphyrin levels in blood, urine, and stool were normal. The histology and morphology led to the suggestion that this was a drug-induced porphyria-like eruption.[42]

After drug cessation, bullae stop developing within a period of weeks. Complete resolution may take months if the drug is not discontinued soon after the bullae develop.

ALLERGY

Allergic reactions to tetracycline are rare. They include fixed eruptions, urticaria, angioneurotic edema, erythema multiforme, exfoliative dermatitis, and anaphylactoid reactions. By 1967, 10 cases of anaphylaxis (none fatal) were reported.[43]

COLITIS

Lincomycin and its derivative, clindamycin, may cause severe and persistent diarrhea. The colitis begins during or shortly after therapy and can last for weeks, despite cessation of administration of the drug.[44,45] Antibiotic-related deaths from severe colitis and intestinal perforation were reported,[44] but the risk of fatal complications remains undetermined. One nonfatal case of severe colitis was reported in a patient with acne who was treated with clindamycin.[46] Cytopathic toxins elaborated by the usually suppressed clostridial species in the intestine have been implicated in this syndrome.[47]

VESTIBULAR SYMPTOMS

Vestibular symptoms in some patients taking minocycline have been reported. Lightheadedness, dizziness, and vertigo may develop, and the patients should be cautioned about driving or working with hazardous machinery. These symptoms may actually disappear during treatment; they do disappear rapidly upon discontinuing use of the drug. Respondents to the survey indicated that no patient on the minocycline low-dosage schedule had reported vestibular symptoms, although symptoms were observed in patients on the high-dosage schedule.

SULFONAMIDE ADVERSE REACTIONS

The trimethoprim-sulfamethoxazole combination showed the patterns and relative incidence to adverse reactions expected from a sulfonamide of low toxicity.[48] The combination is contraindicated during pregnancy and the nursing period,[49] and has been approved only for short-term use in the treatment of urinary tract infections.

Perspective

The authors wish to add their perspective to the use, whether short-term or long-term, of antibiotics in the treatment of acne.

In comments made before a United States Senate Committee, in remarks made in nationwide television newscasts, in charges made by consumer groups, and in editorials published by several medical journals, dermatologists have been accused of using toxic, risky, even deadly antibiotics indiscriminately, irrationally, and protractedly for a trivial disease—acne vulgaris. The authors counter that only an insensitive person views the suffering acne patient as having an inconsequential disease; furthermore, they assert that experiences with hospitalized, immunologically compromised, postsurgical, and seriously ill patients are inappropriate standards for comparison. To answer these critics, more information is needed on the use beyond 6 months of antimicrobial agents in acne therapy. How many acne patients receive antibiotics for one year or more? How many of these patients require continued antibiotics? Does the acne patient suffer weight loss from the long-term use of tetracyclines? Such a study would be difficult, although possible, in adolescents, because of their rapid growth; this could be done more easily in adults, providing age- and sex-matched control individuals (receiving no systemic acne therapy) were included in the study. Another intriguing question is why some acne patients fail to respond to antibiotics, while others benefit from such therapy.

Unfortunately, no satisfactory standard procedures exist for assessing the safety or efficacy of drugs.[23] Perhaps a cooperative reporting system with well-defined criteria, descriptions, and physician standardization which would enable practitioners to pool their information to provide hard data on safety and efficacy could be established. Since we know that no deaths and no serious sequelae have been attributed to tetracyclines prescribed for treating acne, we would search for milder, subtler side effects. In drug evaluations where no reactions occur or where horrible side effects do happen, no control patients are needed. But to find mild side effects requires the use of control patients of the same age and sex receiving no other acne therapy.

In weighing risk *vs* benefit in treating patients with acne, the physician must consider the outcome of *not* treating the patient with systemically administered antibiotics because of safety concerns. Failure to prescribe the most effective treatment will increase the number of patients who develop severe scarring, a complication that often has lifelong psychological, social, and economic consequences. No one can regard the pain and disfiguration suffered by acne patients as trivial; therefore, it is as much the physician's responsibility to provide maximally effective treatment as it is to avoid undesirable side effects.

Summary

After reviewing the available literature, the Ad Hoc Committee on the Use of Antibiotics in Dermatology[1] concluded the following: 1) tetracycline is a rational, effective, and relatively safe drug for use in the treatment of acne vulgaris when given in dosages of 1 gm a day or less for long-term therapy. The drug is not curative; not all patients respond; and the incidence of relapse, when therapy is discontinued, is unknown; 2) chlortetracycline and oxytetracycline are alternative choices; 3) minocycline and doxycycline may also be effective, but there is insufficient evidence on this point; 4) demeclocycline causes photosensitivity reactions in a substantial number of patients.

This must be considered when treating patients exposed to sunlight; 5) erythromycin, in the form of its base and ethylsuccinate and stearate salts, offers a reasonable, effective, and relatively safe alternative therapy; 6) the previously mentioned drugs are effective and relatively safe for treatment and suppression of the development of acne pustules, papules, and cysts. They are not effective for the treatment of comedones; 7) lincomycin and clindamycin appear to be effective drugs, although it would be prudent to avoid the use of these drugs for the treatment of acne until evidence shows that the risk of serious side effects is acceptably low; and 8) clinical experience has not yet adequately confirmed the efficacy and long-term safety of the trimethoprim-sulfamethoxazole combination for the treatment of acne.

These are the members who were invited to offer their recommendations for using antibiotics to treat acne: William A. Akers, San Francisco; Joseph W. Burnett, Baltimore; Samuel B. Frank, White Plains, New York; Ruth K. Freinkel, Chicago; James E. Fulton, Jr, Miami, Florida; Joseph H. Greenberg, San Francisco; Peter N. Horvath, Washington, DC; Robert E. Kellum, Seattle; Paul Lazar, Highland Park, Illinois; James J. Leyden, Philadelphia; Allan L. Lorincz, Chicago; Albert M. Kligman, Philadelphia; Howard I. Maibach, San Francisco; Richard R. Marples, London, England; Norman Orentreich, New York City; Peter E. Pochi, Boston; Ronald M. Reisner, Los Angeles; Alan Shalita, New York City; Edgar B. Smith, Albuquerque; John Strauss, Boston.

REFERENCES

1. Systemic antibiotics for treating acne vulgaris: efficacy and safety. Ad Hoc Committee Report. *Arch Dermatol* 111:1630, 1975.
2. Pillsbury DM, Shelley WB, Kligman AM: *Dermatology*, pp 806-811. Philadelphia: WB Saunders, 1974.
3. Cronk GA, Naumann DE, Garrison C: The effect of prolonged tetracycline therapy on the sensitivity of bacterial isolates from acne patients. *Antibiot Med* 2:153, 1956.
4. Freinkel RK, Strauss JS, Yip SY, et al: Effect of tetracycline on the composition of sebum in acne vulgaris. *N Engl J Med* 273:850, 1965.
5. Strauss JS, Pochi PE: Intercutaneous infection of sebum and comedones: histological observations. *Arch Dermatol* 92:433, 1965.
6. Kellum RE: Acne vulgaris: studies in pathogenesis: relative irritancy of free fatty acids from C_2 to C_{16}. *Arch Dermatol* 97:722, 1968.
7. Pochi PE, Strauss JS: Antibiotic sensitivity of *Corynebacterium acnes (Propionibacterium acnes)*. *J Invest Dermatol* 36:423, 1961.
8. Goltz RW, Kjartansson S: Oral tetracycline treatment on bacterial flora in acne vulgaris. *Arch Dermatol* 93:92, 1966.
9. Marples RR, Downing DT, Kligman AM: Control of free fatty acids in human surface lipids by *Corynebacterium acnes*. *J Invest Dermatol* 56:127, 1971.
10. Marples RR, Kligman AM: Ecological effects of oral antibiotics on the microflora of human skin. *Arch Dermatol* 103:148, 1971.
11. Reisner RM, Silver DZ, Puhvel SM, et al: Lipolytic activity of *Corynebacterium acnes*. *J Invest Dermatol* 51:190, 1968.
12. Kellum RE, Strangfeld K, Ray LF: Acne vulgaris: studies in pathogenesis: triglyceride hydrolysis by *Corynebacterium acnes in vitro*. *Arch Dermatol* 101:41, 1970.

13. Whiteside JA, Voss JG: Incidence and lipolytic activity of *Propionibacterium acnes* (*Corynebacterium acnes* group I) and *P. granulosum* (*C. acnes* group II) in acne and in normal skin. *J Invest Dermatol* 60:94, 1973.
14. Weaber K, Freedman R, Eudy WW: Tetracycline inhibition of a lipase from *Corynebacterium acnes*. *Appl Microbiol* 21:639, 1971.
15. Puhvel SM, Reisner RM: Effect of antibiotics on the lipases of *Corynebacterium acnes in vitro*. *Arch Dermatol* 106:45, 1972.
16. Shalita AR, Wheatley V: Inhibition of pancreatic lipase by tetracyclines. *J Invest Dermatol* 54:413, 1970.
17. Cotterill JA, Cunliffe WJ, Williamson B: The effect of trimethoprim-sulfamethoxazole on sebum excretion rate and biochemistry in acne vulgaris. *Br J Dermatol* 85:130, 1971.
18. Voss JG: Acne vulgaris and free fatty acids: a review and criticism. *Arch Dermatol* 109:894, 1974.
19. Fleiss JL: *Statistical Methods for Rates and Proportions*, pp 69, 193. New York: John Wiley, 1973.
20. Leyden JJ: Antibiotic-resistant acne. *Cutis* 17:593, 1976.
21. Akers WA, Maibach HI: Relative safety of long-term administration of tetracycline in acne vulgaris. *Cutis* 17:531, 1976.
22. Zelick R: "Antibiotics," in Moser RH (Ed): *Disease of Medical Progress: A Study of Iatrogenic Disease*, ed 3, pp 3-82. Springfield: Charles C Thomas, 1969.
23. Feinstein AR: Clinical biostatistics. IX. How do we measure "safety and efficacy?" *Clin Pharmacol Ther* 12:544, 1971.
24. Reidenberg MM, Lowenthal DT: Adverse non-drug reactions. *N Engl J Med* 279:678, 1968.
25. Gilgor RS: Complications of tetracycline therapy for acne. *NC Med J* 33:331, 1972.
26. Kucers A: *The Use of Antibiotics: A Comprehensive Review with Clinical Emphasis*, pp 271-300. London: William Heineman, 1972.
27. Sulzberger MB, Witten VH, Steagall RW Jr: Treatment of acne vulgaris: use of systemic antibiotics and sulfonamides. *JAMA* 173:1911, 1960.
28. Delaney TJ, Leppard B, MacDonald DM: Effects of long-term treatment with tetracycline. *Acta Derm Venereol (Stockh)* 54:487, 1974.
29. Shils ME: Renal disease and the metabolic effects of tetracycline. *Ann Intern Med* 58:389, 1963.
30. Sutton GC: Safety of long-term tetracycline therapy for acne. *Arch Dermatol* 112:1603, 1976.
31. Singer I, Rotenberg D: Demeclocycline-induced nephrogenic diabetes insipidus: *in vivo* and *in vitro* studies. *Ann Intern Med* 79:679, 1973.
32. "Erythromycin and its Derivatives," in *AMA Drug Evaluations 1971*, ed 1, pp 401-403. Chicago: American Medical Association, 1971.
33. Ory EM: The tetracyclines. *Med Clin North Am* 54:1173, 1970.
34. Osment LS, Hammack WJ: The long-term use of tetracycline in acne vulgaris; effect on blood elements. *South Med J* 63:1156, 1970.
35. Jones CC: Megaloblastic anemia associated with long-term tetracycline therapy: report of a case. *Ann Intern Med* 78:910, 1973.
36. Björnberg A, Roupe G: Susceptibility to infections during long-term treatment with tetracyclines in acne vulgaris. *Dermatologica* 145:334, 1972.
37. Seeling M: Mechanisms by which antibiotics increase the incidence and severity of candidiasis and alter the immunologic defenses. *Bacteriol Rev* 30:442, 1966.
38. Leyden JJ, Marples RR, Mills OH Jr, et al: Gram-negative folliculitis—a complication of antibiotic therapy in acne vulgaris. *Br J Dermatol* 88:533, 1973.
39. Aly R, Maibach HI, Strauss WG, et al: Effects of a systemic antibiotic on nasal bacterial ecology in man. *Appl Microbiol* 20:240, 1970.

40. Weigand DA: Tetracycline photosensitivity. *Cutis* 8:267, 1971.
41. Kestel JL Jr: Tetracycline-induced onycholysis unassociated with photosensitivity. *Arch Dermatol* 106:766, 1972.
42. Epstein JH, Seibert JS: Porphyria-like cutaneous changes induced by tetracycline hydrochloride photosensitization. *Arch Dermatol* 112:661, 1976.
43. Barnett CF Jr: Anaphylactoid reaction to orally administered tetracycline. *South Med J* 60:963, 1967.
44. Viteri AL, Howard PH, Dyck WP: The spectrum of lincomycin-clindamycin colitis. *Gastroenterology* 66:1137, 1974.
45. Tedesco FJ, Barton RW, Alpers DH: Clindamycin-associated colitis: a prospective study. *Ann Intern Med* 81:429, 1974.
46. Wolfe MS: Clindamycin-associated colitis. *JAMA* 229:266, 1974.
47. Bartlett JG, Chang TW, Gurwith M, et al: Antibiotic-associated pseudomembranous colitis due to toxin-producing clostridia. *N Engl J Med* 298:531, 1978.
48. Frisch JM: Clinical experience with adverse reactions to trimethoprim-sulfamethoxazole. *J Infect Dis* 128(suppl):607, 1973.
49. "Sulfonamides," in *AMA Drug Evaluation 1971*, ed 1, pp 413-421. Chicago: American Medical Association, 1971.

Chapter 21

Choice of Antibiotics: Management of Antibiotic-resistant Acne

JAMES J. LEYDEN, MD

The evidence for a microbial factor in the pathogenesis of acne vulgaris has been reviewed in previous chapters. Formidable evidence exists to implicate the anaerobic diphtheroid, *Propionibacterium acnes*. This organism resides in the deeper recesses of the sebaceous follicle, and therein lies the difficult problem of antibiotic therapy. Although *P. acnes* is extremely sensitive[1] to all antibiotics, with the exception of the aminoglycosides and the sulfonamides, its residence beneath the skin surface shields it from topical therapy. Systemic agents which are capable of penetrating the sebaceous follicles and reaching *P. acnes* are effective, while those incapable of this *in vivo* penetration are not, even though they may perform superbly in *in vitro* testing.

The ideal antimicrobial approach would be to use a topical agent of low-contact sensitization and irritation potential which is capable of penetrating the depths of the sebaceous follicles and eliminating *P. acnes*. To date, the only agents officially cleared by the FDA for use in local antimicrobial therapy are the benzoyl peroxide formulations and a topical tetracycline. There are numerous reports[2-4] demonstrating the formidable effects of benzoyl peroxide on *P. acnes*. The data of these reports suggest that the benzoyl peroxide formulations are superior even to systemic agents, although this is not the experience of some clinicians.

This apparent paradox now seems explainable by recent experiments in the author's laboratories. Past methodologies for evaluating an agent's effect on *P. acnes* involved collection by a surface detergent scrub method, which samples only the uppermost tip of the anaerobic *P. acnes* population. In more recent experiments in which the skin surface was first delipidized and sterilized and was then sampled one and three hours later, this author found that the striking reductions in *P. acnes* previously reported with benzoyl peroxide preparations were far less dramatic. Similar experiments with the newer topical antibiotic preparations (*eg*, 2% erythromycin base in alcohol and water, 1% clindamycin in hydroalcoholic or pyrrolidone vehicle, or the topical tetracyclines) are needed to determine whether they are capable of more efficient penetration.

The weight of experimental and clinical evidence, however, does indicate that benzoyl peroxide and topical antibiotics are useful in acne therapy. These agents are often used alone for the treatment of mild to moderately inflammatory acne, and are generally combined with systemic antibiotics and/or topical retinoic acid for the management of more severe cases. Future research will undoubtedly lead to better formulations which will penetrate the skin more efficiently and produce better results in the deeper recessess of the sebaceous follicles. At present, no available topical preparation, by itself, is as effective as systemic antibiotic therapy, in this author's opinion. In combination with retinoic acid, which exerts a primary anti-acne effect by its action on follicular keratinization and which also enhances penetration, benzoyl peroxide and topical antibiotics appear to approximate systemic antibiotic effects on *P. acnes*, and in clinical improvement.

It is generally agreed that systemic antibiotics are highly successful in the management of inflammatory acne. Agents such as tetracycline, erythromycin, lincomycin, and clindamycin, which are capable of penetrating the sebaceous follicles[5] and reducing *P. acnes*, are generally judged to be clinically effective; penicillin and the sulfonamides, which do not reach the lumen of the sebaceous follicles, are not clinically effective. To date, no published studies exist in which dosage response effects on *P. acnes* and clinical benefit have been correlated. This author attempted such a study, although the work is yet unpublished. Variability in patient compliance, intestinal absorption of antibiotics and, most importantly, the fact that acne is a multifactorial disease in which bacteria are central but by no means the only factor, combined to produce variable results. However, a rank correlation between *P. acnes* reduction and clinical improvement was determined. While occasional patients achieved excellent clinical results with corresponding suppression of *P. acnes* at low doses of demeclocycline (150 mg a day), in general, higher doses (600-1200 mg a day) led to more rapid reduction of *P. acnes* as well as to speedier clinical improvement. Until more is learned about the pharmokinetics of systemic antibiotics, particularly in regard to penetration of the sebaceous follicles, hard and firm guidelines of dosage remain elusive. The general approach of starting a patient off with 500-1000 mg a day of tetracycline or erythromycin and then titrating the dose according to clinical response remains the most effective.

Despite its widespread acceptance, antibiotic therapy is not uniformly successful. A significant number of patients do not achieve complete suppression of inflammatory lesions even with prolonged therapy, and some exhibit little or no improvement. Plewig et al[6] found that only 34% of patients achieved a good to excellent response in a controlled study of doxycycline; 23% actually worsened; and 32% achieved only poor results. On the other hand, other investigators[7] found as high as 58% of patients achieving good to excellent results with demeclocycline. Mills et al[8] reported only 41% to achieve good to excellent results with demeclocycline, while 59% achieved only fair to poor response. The variation in response can be attributed in part to differences in dosage levels and length of studies. Nonetheless, there is almost universal agreement that a significant number of patients do poorly on antibiotic therapy. Clinicians handle this variable response to systemic antibiotics in different ways. Many choose to switch antibiotics when the therapeutic response falls short of what is routinely achieved in a similar length of time in a majority of their patients. They believe that the change is frequently rewarded by therapeutic success. Others maintain that, in such situations, all that is needed is patience and the patient will respond in time. There are no studies to date which attempt to systematically delineate the possible causes for antibiotic-resistant cases of acne.

Resistance of *P. acnes* to Antibiotics

A theroretical possibility for therapeutic failure is the development of resistance by *P. acnes* to whatever antibiotic the patient is using. If such a situation were to occur, then the switch to another antibiotic would be eminently rational and would explain the clinical observation that a change in antibiotic therapy often results in improvement in resistant cases. However, this author has failed to document such a situation to date, despite extensive searches conducted over the past 10 years. During that time, the author and collaborators processed cultures from over 1000 patients, and routinely searched for resistance of *P. acnes*. In addition to routine culture media, plates with 10μg/ml of demeclocycline, plates with 2μg/ml of erythromycin and, more recently, plates with 10μg/ml of clindamycin added were employed. No strain of either *P. acnes* or *Propionibacterium granulosum* which is resistant to these standard test doses has yet been detected.

In a comparative study of the susceptibility of anaerobic bacteria to various tetracyclines, Chow et al[9] commented that resistance was uncommon in *P. acnes*, in contrast to all other genera of anaerobic organisms. Similarly, in studies in which patients were treated with systemic tetracyclines, erythromycin, or clindamycin for 6 weeks or more, no strain of *P. acnes* developed a resistance to these antibiotics, even in those patients who showed a poor clinical response. Samples from patients taking tetracycline or erythromycin for as long as 3 years also failed to demonstrate resistant organisms.

Furthermore, attempts to induce resistance to erythromycin and tetracycline have failed. Exposing *P. acnes* or *P. granulosum* to concentrations well below the minimal inhibitory concentration of both tetracycline ($< 0.4 \mu g/ml$) and erythromycin ($< 0.2 \mu g/ml$) and then gradually increasing the concentration of the antibiotic did not result in resistant strains. Such a procedure frequently led to the selection or induction of resistant strains in other organisms, eg, *Escherichia coli* and *Staphylococcus aureus*. No resistant strains of *P. acnes* or of *P. granulosum* were found, despite numerous attempts to induce resistance. *P. acnes* and *P. granulosum* appear incapable of developing significant resistance to antibiotics. *E. coli* resistance to tetracyclines was shown to be due to a reduction in transport of the antibiotic across the cell wall.[10] The minimal inhibitory concentration of tetracyclines and erythromycins is so low that apparently more than enough of these antibiotics reach the intracellular areas of *P. acnes*.

The conclusions are clear. Resistant cases of acne are not due to resistance of the *P. acnes* and *P. granulosum*. While *P. acnes* does not develop resistance, the surface aerobic flora (coagulase-negative staphylococci, micrococci, and aerobic diphtheroids) rapidly develop resistance.[5] The development of resistance of the surface aerobic flora happened within 2 weeks in nearly all patients, and this in fact constitutes one of the pieces of evidence that the surface aerobic flora do not play a role in acne, for this resistance develops just as rapidly in those patients who show improvement as in those who fail to respond.

Failure of Patients to Comply

One important aspect frequently overlooked when evaluating patients who fail to improve on antibiotics is the possibility of deliberate or inadvertent failure to follow instructions. Two simple procedures which help in this diagnosis involve the use of the Wood light. With tetracyclines, a yellow-green fluorescence can be routinely seen in the mouth. Patients who have been taking their tetracycline faithfully will show a brilliant fluorescence on the buccal mucosa and tongue. In addition, large, deep, facial nodules will also frequently fluoresce in patients taking tetracycline. The second procedure, reported by Martin et al,[11] involved the examination of the nose and paranasal area under the Wood light to evaluate the intensity of follicular coral red fluorescence. This fluorescence is caused by a coproporphyrin secreted by *P. acnes*. After 3-4 weeks of antibiotic therapy (even at low doses such as 250 mg a day of tetracycline or erythromycin), follicular fluorescence will be markedly depressed. If, after such time, these areas show an intense fluorescence, the physician should consider that failure of patient compliance and the possibility of lack of intestinal absorption may be implicated.

Intestinal Absorption

The problem of intestinal absorption is well-recognized, particularly in the case of tetracycline, which can be significantly affected by milk and antacids. If a patient is doing poorly on antibiotics, and the Wood light examination shows a heavy follicular coral red fluorescence on the nose, then there are distinct possibilities that the antibiotic is not being fully absorbed and that concentrations insufficient to show a clinical improvement are reaching the follicular lumen.

A rather simple method of documenting such a situation involves measuring the resistance level of the surface aerobic flora. As mentioned above, the surface aerobic flora rapidly develop resistance during antibiotic therapy. The procedure used in the author's laboratory is to culture the skin surface and process the specimen on standard media and media to which either $2\mu g$ of erythromycin or $10\mu g$ of demeclocycline or clindamycin have been added. If the antibiotic reaches the surface, approximately 80% of the aerobic flora will be resistant, and there will be no significant difference in the growth seen on plates with and without added antibiotic. We employ techniques in our studies that permit precise quantification, but this is not absolutely essential. Rough, semi-quantitative estimates of the growth of aerobic surface organisms on media with and without antibiotic give valuable information. In continuing studies by the author and collaborators, it is found that, in the absence of a history suggestive of malabsorption (eg, a heavy ingestion of milk, antacids, or medications containing positive ions such as iron), malabsorption is an uncommon event. A careful history will detect most patients who are not absorbing sufficient amounts of the prescribed antibiotic.

Other Possible Causes of Antibiotic Resistance

If resistance of *P. acnes* to antibiotics, patient failure to comply with instructions, and malabsorption of antibiotics are relatively uncommon events, how then does one explain the significant number of patients who respond poorly to antibiotic therapy? Our evaluation of such patients is that the majority can be explained by one of the following mechanisms:

PERSISTENCE OF DEEP NODULAR LESIONS

Antibiotics do not produce involutions of existing inflammatory nodules. Such lesions are inflammatory reactions to extravasated material and their products, including keratinized cells, hair, lipids, and bacteria. The weight of existing evidence indicates that antibiotics work by suppressing the formation of new inflammatory lesions. Deep, large nodules can last up to 8 weeks, by which time the clinician may have decided that the antibiotic was not working, when in fact there was a significant decrease in new lesions which cannot be appreciated until the old lesions have involuted.

SINUS TRACT FORMATION

A small percentage of patients develop a type of lesion we will describe in detail elsewhere. In brief, dissecting sinus tracts form consisting of epithelialized, burrowing lesions which are constantly undergoing rupture and inciting marked inflammatory reactions. In a series of 20 patients observed by this author, 10 also had a history of evidence of pilonidal sinus tracts, and 4 had hidradenitis suppurativa. All 3 conditions display a similar pathology, ie, sinus tract formation. Sinus tracts rarely involute and often require surgical excision. Prolonged antibiotic therapy is at best temporarily effective.

ACNE MECHANICA

Mills and Kligman[12] emphasized the significant roles that friction or trauma can play in exacerbating inflammatory lesions (see Chapter 3). The habit of leaning and pressing on the face, or friction from football helmets, wrestling, *etc*, promotes rupture of the follicles and subsequent development of inflammatory lesions. A frequently overlooked source of excessive friction is the vigorous scrubbing practiced by some patients in attempts to "wash away" their acne. The use of brushes and other scrubbing techniques can induce significant inflammatory lesions despite antibiotic therapy. Elimination of the sources of excessive friction leads to rapid improvement of the aggravated condition.

EMOTIONAL OR PSYCHOLOGICAL INFLUENCES

There is little doubt in the author's mind that emotional or psychological factors significantly affect the acne process in some patients. In the author's experience, this occurs more commonly in women. A common clinical feature is a definite increase in seborrhea. This is most easily perceived on the scalp, and requires increased shampooing. The history of increasing seborrhea helps to evaluate the nature of the stress. All patients generally experience stress of some kind; a stress significant enough to aggravate acne will invariably be accompanied by noticeable seborrhea, possibly mediated through increased production of adrenal androgens.

HORMONAL ABNORMALITIES

A rare possibility, but one not to be overlooked, is that of a major endocrinological abnormality. Usually there will be signs sufficient to alert the physician to this possibility, such as a major change in menses or the development of hirsutism and acne simultaneously in a woman. Fortunately, such cases are extremely rare.

USE OF EXTERNAL COMEDOGENIC SUBSTANCES

Many cosmetics contain comedogenic substances. This author has observed patients who were using several products simultaneously which were capable of aggravating the acne process to the point that antibiotic therapy was ineffective.[13] Likewise, the prolonged use of topical corticosteroids will aggravate acne and even induce it in previously normal skin.[14] Evaluation of resistant cases of acne involves probing the patient in order to exact a full history of the materials applied.

AGGRAVATION BY SYSTEMIC MEDICATION

Anticonvulsive agents and systemic corticosteroids clearly aggravate the acne process (see Chapter 3, 9, 24, and 26).

Summary

For the patient who fails to respond to antibiotics, the author recommends the following: First, take a careful history. Look for the use of cosmetics, topical corticosteroids, anticonvulsive agents, and/or systemic corticosteroids. Inquire about marked increases in emotional or psychological stress accompanied by noticeable seborrhea. Probe the patient about habits of leaning on or squeezing acne areas. And, most importantly, inquire as to how often and in what manner the patient washes. In the physical examination, look for evidence of sinus tract formation, *ie*, extending, tunneling lesions with openings to the surface.

Use the Wood light to examine the density of follicular fluorescence in order to rule out malabsorption of an antibiotic; fluoresce the oral mucosa to rule out patient failure to comply to instructions when the antibiotic is a tetracycline. Culture the surface aerobic flora on routine media with and without the antibiotic in question to settle any question of malabsorption.

A systematic approach to these possibilities will usually uncover the factor or factors responsible for therapeutic failure. Clinical improvement promptly follows, once proper measures are initiated to neutralize the aggravating forces.

REFERENCES

1. Pochi PE, Strauss JS: Antibiotic resistance of *Corynebacterium acnes (Propionibacterium acnes)*. *J Invest Dermatol* 36:423, 1961.
2. Fulton JE, Farzad-Bakshandeh A, Bradley S: Studies on the mechanism of action of topical benzoyl peroxide and vitamin A acid in acne vulgaris. *J Cutan Pathol* 1:191, 1974.
3. Anderson AS, Galdys GJ, Green RC, et al: Improved reduction of cutaneous bacteria and free fatty acids with new benzoyl peroxide gel. *Cutis* 16:307, 1975.
4. Kligman AM, Mills OH, McGinley KJ, et al: Acne therapy with tretinoin in combination with antibiotics. *Acta Derm Venereol [Suppl] (Stockh)* 74:111, 1975.
5. Marples RR, Kligman AM: Ecological effects of oral antibiotics on the microflora of human skin. *Arch Dermatol* 103:148, 1971.
6. Plewig G, Petrozzi JW, Berendes U: Double-blind study of doxycycline in acne

vulgaris. *Arch Dermatol* 101:435, 1970.
7. Witkowski JA, Simons HM: Objective evaluation of demethylchlortetracycline hydrochloride in the treatment of acne. *JAMA* 196:397, 1966.
8. Mills OH, Marples RR, Kligman AM: Acne vulgaris. *Arch Dermatol* 106:200, 1972.
9. Chow A, Patten V, Guze L: Comparative susceptibility of anaerobic bacteria to minocycline, doxycycline, and tetracycline. *Antimicrob Agents Chemother* 1:46, 1975.
10. Zeew JR: Accumulation of tetracyclines by *Escherichia coli*. *J Bacteriol* 95:498, 1968.
11. Martin RJ, Kahn G, Gooding JW, et al: Cutaneous porphyrin fluorescence as an indicator of antibiotic absorption and effectiveness. *Cutis* 12:758, 1973.
12. Mills OH Jr, Kligman AM: Acne mechanica. *Arch Dermatol* 111:481, 1975.
13. Kligman AM, Mills OH Jr: "Acne cosmetica." *Arch Dermatol* 106:843, 1972.
14. Kligman AM, Leyden JJ: Adverse effects of fluorinated steroids applied to the face. *JAMA* 229:60, 1974.

Chapter 22

Treatment of Acne with Anovulatory Drugs
VINCENT P. BARRANCO, MD

It has been established that oral contraceptives are potentially beneficial in the treatment of acne[1-3] (see Chapter 12). Despite this, some patients taking oral contraceptives develop acne; some find that their conditions worsen; and still others experience no change.[4-6]

To better understand the effects of oral contraceptives on acne, it would be helpful to briefly discuss a few points regarding sex hormones and the sebaceous gland. At least one, if not the most important, factor in the pathogenesis of acne vulgaris is hypersecretion of the sebaceous glands. Androgens are the only known stimulus for direct sebaceous gland development and sebum secretion.[7] It has long been known that acne patients do not necessarily have higher plasma levels of androgen or higher daily androgen secretion rates.[8] To explain increased sebaceous output, the concept of "end-organ sensitivity" has been considered. This concept implies that the sebaceous glands in acne patients are more sensitive to the effects of androgen than are those in patients without acne. Recent evidence has shown that dihydrotestosterone is the cellularly active form of testosterone, and that acne-bearing skin converts higher rates of testosterone to dihydrotestosterone than does skin without acne.[9] The suggestion that the sebaceous glands in the acne-prone patient convert greater amounts of the cellularly active form of testosterone than do those in the patient without acne is the most plausible explanation of "end-organ sensitivity" to date.

Although they apparently have no direct effect on the sebaceous glands, estrogens are useful in the treatment of acne because of their ability to suppress sebum secretion. It is now generally believed that this effect occurs through the suppression of endogenous androgens, possibly of ovarian and/or adrenal origin.[3,10]

Oral contraceptives are composed of a synthetic estrogen and a synthetic progestogen. As expected, the estrogen component is responsible for the improvement seen in acne patients. When acne develops from the use of contraceptives, the progestogen must be the responsible agent.

The most commonly prescribed oral contraceptives in the United States combine one of five progestogens with one of two estrogens (Table I). Some of the newer "mini-dose" pills contain smaller doses of progestogens. Studies[11,12] on the biologic effects of these synthetic estrogens and progestogens shed some light on their effect on the sebaceous glands and acne. Although weakly androgenic, the three androgen-dominant progestogens also possess an anti-estrogenic effect. "Anti-estrogenicity" refers to the antagonistic effect of progestogens to estrogens when the two hormones are studied as a combination drug. In contrast, the progestogen, norethynodrel, is clearly nonandrogenic and possesses considerable estrogenicity with no anti-estrogenicity. The other estrogen-dominant progestogen, ethynodiol diacetate, is difficult to classify biologically, but evidence indicates that it has little or no androgenicity.

Androgen, as noted earlier, is the only known stimulus for direct sebaceous gland development and sebum production. Regarding the possible effect of oral contraceptives on the sebaceous glands in acne patients, oral contraceptives containing androgenic progestogens with significant anti-estrogenic effects are referred to as being "androgen-dominant," and those containing virtually nonandrogenic progestogens with greater estrogenicity and little or no anti-estrogenicity are referred to as being "estrogen-dominant."[13]

In 1974, two studies[13,14] were published that strongly support the theory that androgen-dominant oral contraceptives may cause or worsen acne. In one of these studies,[13] 13 of 19 women taking an androgen-dominant oral contraceptive either developed acne or experienced a worsening of their acne conditions. Moreover, 12 improved markedly when switched to an estrogen-dominant oral contraceptive. Most were switched to an estrogen-dominant oral contraceptive containing the same or lesser amounts of estrogen. This suggests that the improvement was due not to the change in the dose of estrogen, but to the change from an androgenic, more anti-estrogenic progestogen to a nonandrogenic, more estrogenic progestogen. The other study[14] was double-blind controlled, in which 10 women with acne were given one of two androgen-dominant oral contraceptives, while another group of 10 matched women with acne were given an estrogen-dominant oral contraceptive. Seven of the 10 receiving the androgen-dominant oral contraceptive experienced a worsening of their acne; 3 were unchanged; none improved.

Table I – Commonly Used Oval Contraceptives

Drug	Estrogen	mg/tab	Progestogen	mg/tab	Biologic Effect
Enovid-E®	mestranol	0.10	norethynodrel	2.5	estrogen-dominant
Enovid® 5	mestranol	0.075	norethynodrel	5.0	estrogen-dominant
Ovulen®	mestranol	0.10	ethynodiol diacetate	1.0	estrogen-dominant
Demulen®	ethinyl estradiol	0.05	ethynodiol diacetate	1.0	estrogen-dominant
Ovral®	ethinyl estradiol	0.05	norgestrel	0.5	androgen-dominant
Norinyl® 2 Ortho-Novum® 2	mestranol	0.10	norethindrone	2.0	androgen-dominant
Norinyl® 1+50 Ortho-Novum 1/50®	mestranol	0.05	norethindrone	1.0	androgen-dominant
Norinyl® 1+80 Ortho-Novum 1/80®	mestranol	0.08	norethindrone	1.0	androgen-dominant
Norlestrin® 1/50	ethinyl estradiol	0.05	norethindrone acetate	1.0	androgen-dominant
Norlestrin® 2.5/50	ethinyl estradiol	0.05	norethindrone acetate	2.5	androgen-dominant
——— Mini-Dose ———					
Lo/Ovral®	ethinyl estradiol	0.03	norgestrel	0.3	?
Modicon® Brevicon®	ethinyl estradiol	0.035	norethindrone	0.5	?
Loestrin® 1/20	ethinyl estradiol	0.02	norethindrone acetate	1.0	androgen-dominant
Loestrin® 1.5/30	ethinyl estradiol	0.03	norethindrone acetate	1.5	androgen-dominant
Zorane®	ethinyl estradiol	0.03	norethindrone acetate	1.5	androgen-dominant
Ovrette®	—	—	norgestrel	0.075	?
Micronor® Nor-Q.D.®	—	—	norethindrone	0.35	?

Eight of the 10 receiving the estrogen-dominant oral contraceptive experienced an improvement in their acne; and only one had her acne worsened. One of the androgen-dominant oral contraceptives in this study contained a lesser dose (Ovral®), and the other a greater dose (Ortho-Novum® 2) of the estrogen than did the estrogen-dominant oral contraceptive (Enovid®5). This observation further supports the concept that the acnegenic effect of androgen-dominant oral contraceptives is dependent on the progestogen rather than on the dose of estrogen.

Two other reports[15,16] support the concept that androgen-dominant oral contraceptives may stimulate acne. Both reports claimed that Ovral® precipitated acne in a total of 23 patients studied; one[16] speculated that the androgenic progestogen, norgestrel, was the causative agent.

There is no significant clinical data regarding acne and the effect of the newer "mini-dose" oral contraceptives. Experience with the full-dosage oral contraceptives should alert the physician whose patient's acne appears to be related to the use of oral contraceptives, especially those containing 1.0 mg or more of norethindrone acetate (Loestrin® and Zorane®).

The modern use of oral contraceptives emphasizes that these drugs should be tailored as closely as possible to the needs of the individual patient. Estrogen-dominant oral contraceptives containing 0.075 mg or more of estrogen (Enovid-E®, Enovid® 5, and Ovulen®) are the most beneficial in the acne-prone woman. In the author's experience, those estrogen-dominant oral contraceptives containing less than 0.075 mg of estrogen are less beneficial, but are nonacnegenic. It should be noted that the suppressive effect of estrogen-dominant oral contraceptives on sebaceous gland secretion may decrease after 14-24 months with a simultaneous exacerbation of acne.[3]

The most androgen-dominant oral contraceptives appear to be Ovral® and Norlestrin® 2.5/50. These contraceptives contain norgestrel or norethindrone acetate. Although those androgen-dominant oral contraceptives containing the norethindrone base are less of a problem, the greater the dose of norethindrone, the more likely is the oral contraceptive to be acnegenic. This author's experience with the new "mini-dose" oral contraceptives is considerably less than with the full-dosage drugs. The "mini-dose" oral contraceptives all contain a reduced amount of progestogen and appear to be less of a problem, with the possible exception of Loestrin® and Zorane®.

With increasing concern regarding estrogens and thromboembolic disease, it is questionable if estrogen-dominant oral contraceptives should be prescribed solely for acne. In the acne-prone woman who is already taking oral contraceptives, the switch to a more estrogen-dominant oral contraceptive (when not otherwise contraindicated), or to the newer "mini-dose" oral contraceptives containing minute doses of androgenic progestogen, may tip the scales in favor of an improvement in her acne. The discontinuing of the use of oral contraceptives appears to be occasionally associated with the development of adult-onset acne, or with the worsening of long-standing adolescent acne.[17,18] It would therefore seem prudent to consider this factor in the management of the acne-prone woman taking oral contraceptives.

REFERENCES

1. Palitz LL: Norethynodrel (Enovid®) in the control of acne in the female. *Arch Dermatol* 86:237, 1962.
2. Strauss JS, Pochi PE: Effect of Enovid® on sebum production in females. *Arch Dermatol* 86:366, 1963.

3. Strauss JS, Pochi PE: Effect of cyclic progestin-estrogen therapy on sebum and acne in women. *JAMA* 190:815, 1964.
4. Jelinek JE: Cutaneous side effects of oral contraceptives. *Arch Dermatol* 101:181, 1970.
5. Nelson JH: Clinical evaluation of side effects of current oral contraceptives. *J Reprod Med* 6:43, 1971.
6. Behrman SJ: Which pill to choose? *Hosp Pract* 4:34, 1969.
7. Strauss JS, Pochi PE: The human sebaceous gland: its regulation by steroidal hormones and its use as an end-organ for assaying androgenicity *in vivo*. *Recent Prog Horm Res* 19:384, 1963.
8. Pochi PE, Strauss JS, Rao GS, et al: Plasma testosterone and estrogen levels, urine testosterone excretion, and sebum production in males with acne vulgaris. *J Clin Endocrinol* 25:1660, 1965.
9. Sansone G, Reisner RM: Differential rates of conversion of testosterone to dihydrotestosterone in acne and in normal human skin—a possible pathologic factor in acne. *J Invest Dermatol* 55:366, 1971.
10. Montagna W: *The Structure and Function of Skin*, ed 2, pp 305-306. New York: Academic Press, 1962.
11. Drill VA: *Oral Contraceptives*, p 22. New York: McGraw-Hill, 1966.
12. Edgren RA, Jones RC, Clancy DP, et al: The biological effects of norgestrel alone and in combination with ethinyl estradiol. *J Reprod Fertil [Suppl]* 5:13, 1968.
13. Barranco VP, Jones DD: Effect of oral contraceptives on acne in the female. *South Med J* 67:703, 1974.
14. Barranco VP: Effect of androgen-dominant and estrogen-dominant oral contraceptives on acne. *Cutis* 14:384, 1974.
15. Gibbs WP: Acne and Ovral®. *Arch Dermatol* 109:912, 1974.
16. Woodward RK: Acne stimulation by Ovral®. *Arch Dermatol* 110:812, 1974.
17. Weigand DA, Olson RL: *Cutaneous Medicine Case Studies*, pp 60-61. New York: Medical Examination Pub, 1971.
18. Kligman AM: Pimples following the pill. *Arch Dermatol* 105:298, 1972.

Chapter 23

Physiotherapy
ERVIN EPSTEIN, MD

X-ray Therapy

One of the great unresolved medical conflicts of the last 20 years concerns the use of ionizing radiation in benign dermatoses, foremost of which is the psychic trauma-causing disease, acne vulgaris. Beliefs for or against dermatoradiotherapy have come to be little based on actual facts. The present philosophy is to use dermatoradiotherapy for the control of acne only in unusual cases, and then after other available therapies have been tried and found wanting. However, if x-radiation is safe and effective, its routine use should be encouraged. Furthermore, it should be considered as an adjunct to other therapeutic methods, rather than as an exclusive agent. It is not a question of whether antibiotics are safer and/or more effective than x-ray as used in the treatment of acne vulgaris; the two can and should be used together.

SAFETY OF X-RADIATION IN DERMATOLOGY

Ever since the atomic bomb was dropped over Japan, we have been deluged with propaganda regarding the hazards of radiation, a concern that was realized by 1897, one year after the discovery of this energy.[1] By 1940, it was well-recognized that ionizing radiation could lead to acute and chronic burns, leukemia, cancers of the skin and certain other viscera, fibrosis of many organs including the lungs, *etc.* However, it was clearly appreciated that these untoward problems resulted from overdosage. This latter realization was lost in the post-World War II hysteria, and soon we were told that any x-ray exposure was dangerous to us and to our progeny.[1] The linear hypothesis, or "no-threshold" theory, was born, has remained unproven, but is, nevertheless, embraced and nurtured by the x-ray abolitionists. Perhaps Brucer[2] put it most succinctly when he stated: "Animals can be killed in seconds by large amounts of radiation; but this does not make *radiation* dangerous—it makes *large amounts of radiation* dangerous." This author looks upon x-radiation as not being carcinogenic; only too much x-ray is capable of causing cancer. It is like water: a little may be beneficial and refreshing; too much can kill you.

In the postwar confusion, such concepts as quality of the rays and total body *vs* local x-ray exposure were lost. We soon saw scientists unable to appreciate the biologic difference between total dose given at one time and that administered in fractionation as employed by dermatologists. While the purpose of this Chapter is not to discuss the hazards of x-radiation as compared to its safety, it is necessary to touch upon these matters to show that this modality may be applied with reasonable safety if certain rules are followed.

It should be recognized, but unfortunately is not, that there is a very large safety range in x-radiation therapy. The usual dose of the Kienböck-Adamson epilation technique is 300 rads administered to 5 areas of the scalp during a single session. This author has seen the dose increased to 525 rads and even higher and administered to each area without complications.[1] Some 50 years ago, this author was given, because of a mistake in calibration, a total of 5400 rads to each of 3 areas of his face, one on his chest, and 3 on his back, and suffered no untoward side effects (12 weekly fractional treatments were given on 2 separate occasions, 2 years apart). Further, there is no explosive sensitivity to x-rays. Despite the "no-threshold" theory of x-ray damage, an individual receiving a single dose of 75 rads will not develop a radiodermatitis or a cancer. However, this author saw a patient die of thrombocytopenia after one aspirin tablet, and another, a physician, after 4 such pills. These two factors—the high level of therapeutic safety and the lack of explosive idiosyncracy—make x-radiation safe, in this author's opinion.

In most instances, if an individual develops a radiodermatitis, it is only a cosmetic defect. Also, it occurs only after extreme overdosage. Furthermore, the complications (*eg*, ulceration, keratoses, and cancer) occur only in the most severe examples of chronic radiodermatitis, and then in the most severely affected regions. If a malignancy supervenes, it is usually of comparatively low degree, and is cured easily. This author has seen one patient die of such a malignancy; however, death was due to a gross overdosage. The patient manifested both squamous cell carcinomas and sarcomas, and died of metastatic sarcoma.

While the aforementioned changes are predictable on the basis of overdosage, consider the unpredictable hazards of other systemic acne therapies. Aplastic anemia, colitis, thromboembolic phenomena, hypertension, ruptured peptic ulcers, spread of certain infections and malignancies, aggravation of diabetes, psychoses, *etc*, are all possible consequences which may result from the use of antibacterial and anovulatory agents, and corticosteroids. A radiodermatitis, in this author's opinion, is a risk preferable to any of these untoward side effects.

Furthermore, it should be remembered that there has never been a case of leukemia, genetic malformation, or skin cancer in a human being which was proven to be due to proper dermatoradiotherapy.

COMPLICATIONS

There are three potential complications involved in the use of x-radiation which have recently been brought to our attention, and which merit discussion.

Basal cell epitheliomas—Some physicians have been distressed at encountering basal cell epitheliomas in patients who had had x-radiation in the past without showing clinical evidence of cutaneous damage. These physicians should realize that basal cell epitheliomas are very common, that 30 years ago (or more), 25% of the patients who visited a dermatologist's office received x-ray therapy, and that it would be a miracle if none of these individuals manifested one or more of these tumors in later life. In fact, if these neoplasms did not appear in previously x-rayed individuals, the only reasonable assumption would then be that such therapy was of prophylactic value in the prevention of cutaneous cancers.

Thyroid cancer—It is well-established that x-ray therapy can cause cancer of the thyroid gland. However, this occurs principally in those who, in infancy, received comparatively deep x-ray treatments in large doses to the thymus or adenoids. This is not comparable to the treatment given to persons in late adolescence for the treatment of acne. Of course, some patients with thyroid cancer have received dermatoradiotherapy for acne, but the relationship is unproven and, in all probability, does not exist.

The danger of accepting such anecdotal evidence is well-illustrated by the experience of this author. Two of my classmates married and produced four children. The older two children had severe acne, and each received a full course of radiotherapy. The younger two had no acne, and therefore received no x-radiation. At the age of 18, the third sibling developed a thyroid cancer, and, upon reaching the same age, the youngest was found to have a benign nodule of the thyroid. If the situation had been reversed, *post hoc ergo propter hoc* reasoning could have involved this author in a probably indefensible malpractice action.

Breast cancer—Too much x-ray therapy can cause cancer in nearly any part of the body. Simon[3] recently reported 16 cases in which women with cancer of the breast had had x-ray therapy for acne or hirsutism. He sketchily described 5 cases only. Four of these individuals had chronic radiodermatitis; in other words, they had not received proper dermatologic radiotherapy. He had no idea of the dose, quality, fractionation, *etc*, which were involved. And again, we see the juxtaposition of two common events—breast cancer and x-ray therapy—20 or more years apart. At times, of course, the two do coexist; but what of the millions of women treated with x-radiation for acne who did not get breast cancer?

INDICATIONS AND CONTRAINDICATIONS

It is the contention of this author that x-ray therapy is safe. It should be used in combination with other therapeutic measures in the treatment of acne. Experience has shown that x-ray therapy should not be administered to an individual under the age of 18 because of the frequency of recurrences of the acne process in adolescents. Patients at the end of adolescence are less apt to suffer such a recrudescence once the acne is eliminated.

Of course, previous maximum x-ray therapy is a definite contraindication to dermatoradiotherapy. If the previous dosage cannot be determined, further therapy should not be administered. If the dose of radiation received previously is such that the amount which can be given safely is too small to produce the desired results, it is best to withhold these rays. A radiodermatitis would obviously be another reason for not employing x-ray therapy. X-ray therapy should not be administered during pregnancy. Therefore, we can say that x-ray therapy may be administered if the patient has acne; is older than 18 years; is not pregnant; and, has not had previous ionizing radiation to the involved areas.

On the other hand, most writings today insist that this modality should be reserved for very severe cases in which all other therapy has failed. For instance, in their new book, Braun-Falco et al[4] list the following criteria for the use of x-ray therapy in acne: *"1) Use only in extremely severe cases refractory to other types of therapy; 2) use only in patients over 17 years of age; 3) do not use in fair-skinned, blue-eyed, and red-haired patients; 4) do not use in drug-induced or occupational forms of acne; 5) insure protection of radiosensitive organs (eg, gonads, eyes, thyroid); and 6) never exceed the maximum permissible dose of 1000 rads per area and lifetime."* In this author's opinion, Number 1 and 3 are much too restrictive. Number 2, 4, 5, and 6 are reasonable and certainly should be followed.

TECHNIQUE OF THERAPY

The half-value layer (HVL) of aluminum of the x-ray beam that is suitable for the treatment of acne varies from 0.5-1.0 mm.[5] Since important structures lie under the skin of the face, neck, chest, and back, the least penetrating effective beam should be utilized. Traditionally, the usual HVL used is about 0.7 mm of aluminum. This is produced by a beam generated at 80 kilovolts, 5 milliamperes, 8-inch distance, with inherent filtration only.

Kilovoltages as low as 40-50 are recommended by some. This author uses 6- or 8-inch cones. Additional shielding is employed with lead rubber sheeting to cover areas such as the thyroid, neck, genitals, *etc.*

There are many different treatment schemes that range from 50-100 rads per treatment. The therapy is administered weekly for 3-4 months.

It was formerly the practice of this author to apply 75 rads every week for 6 weeks, and then the same amount every 2 weeks, for a total dose of 900 rads.[6] A study of 1051 patients receiving dermatoradiotherapy,[7] however, revealed that 50 rads administered weekly for 12 treatments for a total of 600 rads produced results as good as those achieved with the larger dose. A total of 600 rads is adequate if given over a long enough period. One advantage of the smaller dose is that more than 12 treatments can be administered if necessary. The 50 rads x 12 regimen produced results superior to a regimen in which 75 rads was given in 8 treatments. The number of treatments and the time over which they are given may be as important as the total dose. Sulzberger et al[8] demonstrated conclusively that a total dose of 1000 rads should not be exceeded if one wishes to avoid radiation sequelae, including that of cutaneous cancers.

The exact plan of therapy varies with the area being irradiated. On the face, treatments are given over the points of maximum involvement or over the zygomas. However, if there is marked involvement of the neck, the tube may be centered lower toward the chin. The distance must be measured from that part of the face closest to the tube. If there are severe manifestations of acne on the forehead, some clinicians apply a third treatment to this area. Although this author seldom administers a third treatment, those that do apparently experience no difficulty. As a rule, only one exposure is given over the sternum, but, in some patients, it may be necessary to administer 2 treatments to the upper lateral portions of the anterior trunk and to avoid the central area. The treatment of the upper back depends on the extent of the eruption. If only the mid-upper back is involved, one treatment is applied below the base of the neck. If the eruption is more extensive, therapy is given over the shoulders or scapulae as indicated. In more widespread eruptions, the dose may be applied also to the center of the lower back or to each side.

The patient must, of course, be protected from the back-scatter and bouncing rays. A lead sheet should be placed beneath the patient. In the author's installation, a lead rubber sheet is built into the table under the plastic upholstery. Lead eye shields are necessary if the face is being treated. The thyroid area, as well as the breast and gonads, must be protected with lead. This problem is solved by employing a lead rubber sheet which covers the entire body from the neck to the knees. If the anterior chest is being exposed, the sheet is temporarily moved up to the level of the diaphragm, shielding the face and neck. The female breasts should be covered. When the patient lies on his stomach, the lead rubber is placed over the low back, buttocks, and thighs. The head and posterior neck are covered with lead, too.

The danger is minimized and the therapeutic results are improved if the total dose is fractionated. Administering 75 rads weekly for 12 treatments is far more preferable therapeutically than giving the entire 900 rads at one time. The quality of the rays is as important as the quantity. For instance, the lethal dose of the hard radiation from an atomic bomb is said to be 300 rads of total body exposure. On the other hand, if one gives 7 treatments (3 to the face, one to the chest, 3 to the back) of 75 rads each at an HVL of 0.7 mm aluminum, the patient is exposed to 525 rads on the day of treatment without experiencing the slightest upset. If the patient receives 12 such treatments, his total exposure will be 6300 rads, and, to date, it has not been proven that this is a dangerous dose! With grenz rays, much larger amounts can be applied without any apparent harm or reaction.

As stated previously, radiation should be considered as an adjunct. To give the patient the best possible care, the physician should combine x-ray therapy with antibiotics, local applications, *etc.*

Irritating local remedies may produce erythema, which increases the biologic effect of ionizing radiation to a minor degree. It is therefore considered safer to avoid the use of such local therapies as vitamin A acid or benzoyl peroxide during the course of x-ray therapy. If the physician is not using x-rays in the treatment of acne, he is not giving his patients the advantage of every possible assistance in the management of their dermatosis.

RESULTS

The older literature is replete with articles extolling the therapeutic effectiveness of x-ray therapy in acne. In an attempt to secure a more realistic appraisal of the results of such therapy, 1051 patients treated with x-rays in the author's office over a 32-year period (1937-1969) were reviewed. This included 59.1% of the total number of those with acne encountered during that period. The two dosage schedules previously referred to were used. It was found that, although only about 14% cleared completely, 50% of the patients achieved results rated at 86-100%. Nearly 65% who received at least 6 treatments (half the recommended number) fell in the highly benefitted group.[7] To appreciate the results, one must consider the many parameters that had a bearing on the final outcome.

Patient cooperation—The 12 recommended treatments were completed by 50.5 of the 1051 patients, and 80% of the group received more than 6 treatments. Only 2.8% failed to return after the initial treatment. There was no decrease in these figures between 1946-1960, the years when so-called "patient resistance" was reputed to be the greatest. In fact, during those years, 62.6% accepted radiation therapy—more than the 59.1% average for the entire series.[7]

Age—The youngest group was the most cooperative, but achieved the poorest results, probably due to the activity of their physiologic processes.[7] Because of this observation, the author does not initiate treatment with x-radiation until the patient is 18 years of age.

Sex—Girls proved to be less cooperative than boys, but secured more benefit from the treatments.[7]

Location—Involvement of the face responded better than that of other areas.[7]

Duration of the disease—This variable had no effect on the therapeutic results.[7]

Severity—The effect of this factor is summarized thusly: the worse the eruption, the greater the cooperation; the greater the cooperation, the better the therapeutic results.[7]

Dosage—The results were better with increased number of treatments and, generally, when the full dose was given. However, as mentioned previously, the benefit obtained with a total dose of 600 rads given in 12 treatments was comparable to that resulting from 900 rads applied in 12 treatments.[7]

TRENDS IN X-RAY THERAPY

In 1971, the author sent a questionnaire to all the dermatologists in the United States, asking if they used x-ray therapy in acne. A total of 2871 (67.6%) responded. The results indicated that about 75% of the respondents had discontinued the use of this form of treatment for acne, and an additional 11% used it in less than 10% of their patients. Those queried were also asked why they had decreased or avoided the use of this modality. Many of them (37.3%) were impressed with the publicized hazards of this treatment. There were 30.4% who believed that better treatments were available. Nearly one-third did not want to contend with the public resistance to the use of these rays. It is probable that the real reason was lack of training, a factor mentioned by 13.6% of the respondents. The reluctance to use x-ray treatment was greatest (44.7%) among those who had not yet entered practice, and least (5.2%) in those who received their training 20 or more years earlier. Lack of equipment was given as a reason for nonuse by 11.5%, which dovetails with the "lack of training." Among all who answered, 11.9% considered x-ray therapy to be ineffective. It should be pointed out, on the other hand, that 240 practitioners (8.4%) had increased their use of this modality because: conviction of therapeutic efficacy (115); disappointment with other methods (73); safety (33); and other reasons (19).[9]

A questionnaire was sent to the members of the American Dermatologic Association, and it was found that, in 1950, these leaders in dermatology were administering x-ray treatments on 26.2% of the visits to their offices. By 1960, this had decreased by nearly one-half to 13.5%.[7]

In the past, more patients with acne than with any other dermatologic disease have been treated with x-radiation. The 1971 questionnaire was published under the title of "Dermatologic Radiotherapy—R.I.P."[9] The continued decline of the utilization of x-ray since that date makes the title of that communication prophetic. This author does not believe that this trend is warranted; nevertheless, it is a trend. But then, votes never established a scientific fact.

Grenz Ray Therapy

Grenz rays are a very soft form of ionizing radiation, the HVL being in the range of 0.020-0.040 mm of aluminum. This is produced by 10-20 kilovolts. Grenz ray therapy was originally introduced into the treatment of acne as a substitute for the "more hazardous" x-ray therapy. However, grenz ray therapy was soon discarded in this country. The problem concerned penetration: 99.5% of the beam is absorbed in the most superficial portion of the skin. Since biologic effect occurs only in the first millimeters, the grenz rays obviously do not penetrate sufficiently to affect the structures in the dermis that we recognize as being implicated in acne.

Surveys show that, at one time, 5% of the dermatologists employed this modality in the management of acne. Today it is used seldom for this dermatosis. The recommended dosage is high. Grenz rays can produce chronic radiodermatitis, but only in gross overdosage. Hyperpigmentation occurs commonly after grenz ray treatment, especially in dark-skinned individuals, although this cosmetic defect disappears, as a rule, with time. Most American dermatologists believe that grenz rays are not indicated for the treatment of acne; therefore, this discussion is most abbreviated.

Ultraviolet Light

Three types of ultraviolet light are available to the practitioner. At one time, the output was measured in ranges; today, however, the peak output is expressed as the measurement. For instance, the rays of the cold quartz (UVC) lamp are considered to have a single peak at 250 nm, thereby affecting the skin by producing erythema and burning while also possessing germicidal properties. Hot quartz (UVB) lamps give off rays that have many peaks ranging from 290-320 nm. The more important portion of its spectrum is concerned with longer rays, and the hot quartz lamp is said to exert its effect by "toning up" the skin in producing pigmentation, vitamin D, *etc*. The third type of ultraviolet, filtered ultraviolet light (UVA; the Wood light), is considered to peak at 360 nm.

Traditionally, ultraviolet light has been a mainstay of the attack against acne. Neither cold quartz- nor hot quartz-produced rays are as effective in this disease as natural solar irradiation. In fact, there is little evidence that ultraviolet radiation without photosensitizing agents is any more than a placebo.

In addition to destroying organisms, the cold quartz lamp produces desquamation, which might contribute to the therapy of this disease. However, certainly any form of ultraviolet therapy is very weak in anti-acne properties as compared to those of x-ray therapy, cryotherapy, certain local remedies, systemic antibiotics, *etc*. This therapeutic effect may be increased by the use of photosensitizing agents, especially systemically administered sulfonamides and psoralens. It is possible that the new, more intense PUVA as recommended for psoriasis and mycosis fungoides may prove to be valuable in the management of acne, although this has yet to be established. If, in the future, PUVA therapy is proven to be effective in the management of acne, it is probable that certain reactions to this procedure may limit its usefulness. The use of generalized ultraviolet light, such as that in a Zimmerman booth, may be more beneficial than localized treatment.

It should be remembered that ultraviolet light is carcinogenic, especially in fair-skinned blondes with blue eyes. Also, it can cause unsightly pigmentation, especially if used with a perfume-containing local remedy or cosmetic. This author knows of one patient who died from an ultraviolet light treatment. She had unrecognized congenital porphyria. Although ultraviolet light is one of the safest modalities available to the dermatologist, it is, unfortunately, also one of the least beneficial of the therapeutic agents used to control acne.

REFERENCES

1. Epstein E: Dermatologic radiotherapy 1965. *Arch Dermatol* 92:307, 1965.
2. Brucer M: Man must have developed in radioactivity: he has so much lead in his pants! (letter to the editor). *JAMA* 174:1651, 1960.
3. Simon N: Breast cancer induced by radiation: relation to mammography and treatment of acne. *JAMA* 237:789, 1977.
4. Braun-Falco O, Lukacs S, Goldschmidt H: *Dermatologic Radiotherapy*, p 132. New York: Springer-Verlag, 1976.
5. Cipollaro AC, Crossland PM: *X-rays and Radium in the Treatment of Diseases of the Skin*, ed 5, p 489. Philadelphia: Lea and Febiger, 1967.
6. Epstein E: Radiation therapy of benign dermatoses. *Dermatol Dig* 10:36, 1971.
7. Epstein E: X-ray therapy in acne: therapeutic response and patient cooperation. *Cutis* 8:321, 1971.
8. Sulzberger MB, Baer RL, Borota A: Do roentgen-ray treatments as given by skin specialists produce cancers or other sequelae? Follow-up study of dermatologic patients treated with low-voltage roengten rays. *Arch Dermatol Syphilol* 65:639, 1952.
9. Epstein E: Dermatologic radiotherapy—R.I.P. *Calif Med* 115:7, 1971.

Chapter 24

Other Therapies
JOSEPH A. WITKOWSKI, MD
LAWRENCE C. PARISH, MD

Internal Treatment

DIET

Is diet important in acne? Do certain foods ruin the complexion? Does chocolate really cause pimples? Can milk exacerbate acne? Physicians, parents, and patients are frequently at odds about this controversial aspect of acne therapy. Historically, dermatologists have recommended certain dietary restrictions for acne patients. Through the years, proponents of diet therapy have proscribed 4 food groups: 1) milk and milk products; 2) cacao bean derivatives; 3) fatty foods; and 4) halogenated foods (see Chapter 9 and 12).

Evidence—Is there any evidence for the role of diet in acne? Eskimos apparently were not plagued by acne vulgaris up until the time when so-called "junk foods," including chocolate, were introduced into their diet.[1] Curiously, these people had a diet already containing large amounts of fish and animal fat. When chocolate was tested in Americans, the results were different. Both a clinical[2] and an experimental[3] study failed to provide any evidence that chocolate made acne worse.

Although there are no good experimental data which conclude that dietary factors in general have an effect on acne, several reports[4-6] deserve mention. An acute form of papulopustular acne was found in a hospitalized patient undergoing prolonged intravenous hyperalimentation.[4] This was ascribed to the absence of several nonessential amino acids. In other patients, large quantities of milk, up to 2 gallons a day, were implicated as a cause of acne flares.[5] Yet some teenagers are able to consume huge quantities of dairy products and fatty foods without adverse effects. Finally, follicular wheals were observed in a patient within minutes after eating chocolate.[6] This was followed in 24 hours by an acne papule.

Major alterations in the diet can alter both the rate of sebum secretion and the composition of sebum. Although acne did not become worse in patients in the chocolate study,[3] careful examination of the data showed that, at the end of 2 weeks, the rate of sebum secretion was elevated in 60% of the patients, and all patients showed an increase in free fatty acids. A diet containing chocolate and skim milk altered sebum secretion activity within a minimum of 5 days.[7] On the other side of the spectrum, a decline in sebum secretion was noted after 1-4 weeks in patients on a starvation diet,[8] and changes in sebum composition were detected in as early as a few days.

Acne patients have been told that cola drinks are detrimental and that they should be avoided completely. There is no scientific evidence to support this restriction. Even a survey of the literature failed conclusively to condemn these beverages, contrary to folklore. However, support for this interdiction may be gleaned from the observation that children receiving cola syrups as an anti-emetic often develop an acneform eruption.

Iodides and bromides in pharmacologic doses can induce acneform eruptions. Clinicians have used this fact as a reason for restricting the intake of fish, shellfish, and even iodized salt. The amount of iodide in these foods and in other products (see Chapter 9 and 12) is insignificant as compared to the acne-inducing dose of these substances. Yet, worsening of acne following ingestion of these foods has been reported by patients.

Summary—Is there some reason for this discrepancy between scientific fact and clinical impression? Although acne is a disease in which multiple factors appear to be operative, retention hyperkeratosis is the common denominator in its pathogenesis. This is the stage upon which all agents must act. Without blocked follicular orifices, dietary products may have no influence on inducing acne lesions.

Several factors need to be considered. Acne is characterized by wide, natural fluctuations in activity. The cause-and-effect relationship may not be as immediate as it is in acute urticaria. An exacerbation of acne may not become evident for several days after a dietary indiscretion, making it even more difficult to implicate a particular food. The time of ingestion of aggravating foods may be the essential determinant. Cola and chocolate had no effect on acne when taken immediately after meals, but did aggravate acne when ingested as a between-meal snack.[9]

Finally, individual susceptibility may be the overriding determinant which governs responses to a variety of agents. It is conceivable that there are trigger mechanisms in the sebaceous gland system that vary widely from patient to patient.

The clinician should be prepared to give dietary advice, even though he may not offer it. Patients and their parents or spouses have been geared to believe that diet is an important part of acne therapy, if not the entire cause of the condition. Thus, they ask for views on the importance of diet in acne. The clinician should point out that acne may be aggravated by certain foods, but that this is probably an individual matter.

This is a good opportunity to offer sound, nutritional advice. Although the concept of a well-balanced diet is somewhat nebulous, the patient should be encouraged to eat a varied diet and to avoid overconsumption of "junk foods." Suspect foods should be eliminated for at least 2 weeks; if the acne improves, then, obviously, that food should be avoided. Nevertheless, it is important to remember that even the strictest diet has never cured acne, and severe dietary restrictions just do not make sense.

SYSTEMIC CORTICOSTEROIDS

Adrenal corticosteroids are helpful in suppressing the inflammatory component of acne. Two modes of therapy have been found useful: short courses of full therapeutic doses, and long-term, low-dosage therapy (see Chapter 12).

Full therapeutic doses should be reserved for the treatment of patients with severe nodular acne unresponsive to other forms of therapy (eg, acne fulminans [acute febrile ulcerative acne]),[10] to help control acute exacerbations and to ameliorate severe acne until more conventional treatment becomes effective. Short courses are recommended. Prednisone or its equivalent is administered in doses of 20-40 mg, once every morning, for 1-2 weeks, followed by reduced dosage and then withdrawal, preferably within 2 weeks. There is no justification for routine long-term use of full therapeutic doses of corticosteroids in patients. Prolonged use of high-dosage therapy will result in the appearance of new lesions on the shoulders and face (ie, corticosteroid acne) after 1-2 months.

Low-dosage maintenance treatment with prednisone, 5-10 mg, once a day, has been effective in controlling cases of women with severe nodular acne unresponsive to conventional modes of therapy. Hirsutism is often an associated finding. An adrenocortical hydroxylase deficiency after 24-hour adrenocorticotropic hormone (ACTH) infusion was demonstrated in many of these women.[11] Mild acne which may occur in women taking estrogenic progestogen-containing oral contraceptives can also be controlled by low-dosage adrenocorticosteroid therapy.

ZINC SULFATE

Zinc Sulfate, 220 mg, 3 times a day, has been reported as being useful in the treatment of inflammatory acne. A double-blind study[12] demonstrated a statistically significant reduction of comedones and inflammatory lesions in as early as 4 weeks after initiation of therapy. Opinion is divided as to the effectiveness of zinc in the treatment of acne. Although the exact mode of action is not known, possible roles played by zinc sulfate in the metabolism of vitamin A as well as in enzyme activity were postulated.[12] The importance of zinc in the correction of defective white blood cell chemotaxis was also recently described.[13]

Patients receiving zinc sulfate should avoid the concomitant use of tetracycline. Zinc-tetracycline complexes are probably formed, thus preventing absorption.

DIURETICS

Exacerbation of acne during the 7-10 days prior to menstruation is not uncommon. Women so affected often complain of weight gain during this stage of the menstrual cycle. Premenstrual fluid retention with dermal hydration and, possibly, keratin swelling are thought responsible for this phenomenon. Support for this clinical impression was recently demonstrated.[14] Direct measurement of the pilosebaceous orifice showed[14] that the duct is smallest between the 15th-20th days of the cycle. This reduction in size could cause significant resistance to sebum outflow and subsequent induction of inflammatory lesions. Although a recent double-blind study[15] in which hydrochlorothiazide was administered to women premenstrually failed to show a significant effect in the control of premenstrual acne exacerbations, this is not in keeping with the clinical experience of some observers. Orally administered diuretics seem to be of greatest benefit in the treatment of women who had had moderately severe acne in adolescence, but who are now plagued by a 1-6 papule premenstrual flare (see Chapter 12).

INTRALESIONAL CORTICOSTEROIDS

Baer and Witten[6] described the use of intralesional corticosteroids in 1959. They injected suspensions of hydrocortisone acetate, prednisolone, and triamcinolone diacetate into cystic lesions. The intralesional use of triamcinolone acetonide was reported by Rebello[16] in 1962. In 1965, Leeming[17] described the use of the Dermajet® apparatus in delivering the corticosteroid to the skin. The efficacy of this form of treatment has since been substantiated by the authors[18] in a controlled study in 1967.

Inflammatory nodules, indurated plaques, and abscesses are the primary indications for the use of intralesional corticosteroids. Without such treatment, these lesions invariably heal with scar formation. Either triamcinolone diacetate (25 mg/cc) or triamcinolone acetonide (10 mg/cc) is diluted with water, saline, or 1% lidocaine to a concentration of 2.5-5.0 mg/cc. Betamethasone sodium phosphate-acetate (6 mg/cc) is diluted to a final concentration of 0.3-0.6 mg/cc. One-tenth to 0.5 ml is injected directly into the lesion through a #25-27 gauge needle. The volume of the injected material is determined by the size of the lesion. Slight distension of the lesion is the desired result. Well-liquified abscesses can be drained through a small stab incision. Infiltration of open lesions is best accomplished with the Dermajet®, as this allows more uniform dispersion of the corticosteroid throughout the lesions with less leakage. If an abscess is incised but does not drain freely, excessive manipulation is to be avoided. The lesion should be infiltrated with the Dermajet®; this will often help to liquify the contents, after which the lesion may be drained.

Treated lesions usually flatten within 2-3 days, and completely resolve within 7-10 days. A slight depression in the skin at the treated site is occasionally seen after treating large lesions. This depression in the skin surface usually becomes imperceptible after a few months. Recurrences, although rare, may be retreated 2-3 times at no more than 2-3 week intervals (see Chapter 25).

Another indication for the use of intralesional corticosteroids is in the treatment of hypertrophic and keloidal acne scars. Several injections at 2-4 week intervals are usually necessary to soften and flatten hypertrophic scars. Keloids, however, usually require protracted treatment with full-strength corticosteroids before they will respond.

Intravascular injection must be avoided. Every attempt to distribute the corticosteroid evenly throughout the lesion should be made in order to prevent deposition of too high a concentration at any one point in the skin. Finally, the total dose of injected corticosteroid should be kept well below 20 mg per treatment. Adrenal suppression was described[19] when 20 mg or more of triamcinolone acetonide was administered during a single treatment.

Physical Irritants

Since the beginning of time, physicians have used a variety of methods to make the skin red and cause it to peel. In the 1920's, Giraudeau[20,21] introduced into the treatment of acne the use of a slush consisting of a mixture of solid carbon dioxide, acetone, and sulfur. Over the years, dermatologists have employed numerous variations of the Giraudeau technique (see Chapter 25).

CRYOSLUSH

Method—A 50-pound tank of carbon dioxide with a siphon is a convenient source of carbon dioxide. The soft snow can be collected in a chamois or towel held over the end of a "pig-tail adapter" which is screwed on the tank nozzle. Slush can be prepared and applied in several ways. The ball of carbon dioxide can be mixed with acetone in a porcelain mortar and ground until a slush is obtained. The slush is then applied to the skin with a gauze-covered tongue blade. Some add sulfur to the slurry. The ball can instead be wrapped in small sack of gauze and dipped in acetone; it is then pressed against or slowly drawn across the skin. Or, a gauze-covered tongue blade moistened with acetone can be rubbed across a ball of carbon dioxide snow held in a chamois. The carbon dioxide-laden tongue blade or carbon dioxide ball is then applied to the skin with a short, stroking motion. Greater pressure can be applied when a deeper freeze is required. Each operator develops his own timing technique, depending on the pressure he exerts.

Results—Application of slush causes superficial freezing of the skin. The effect appears to be the greatest on closed comedones and inflammatory papules; impaired heat diffusion allows these lesions to freeze more easily than the surrounding skin. Even the lightest application will cause momentary freezing to the lesions. Within minutes after treatment, the skin resumes its usual color or becomes slightly red. The more deeply frozen lesions become edematous within an hour. The edema persists for several hours, and is followed by blistering and crusting after 1-2 days. The more superficially frozen areas begin to peel within 2-3 days. The peeling is complete in 5-7 days. The resulting desquamation appears to help convert closed comedones into open lesions, aids in the removal of more superficial open comedones, and decapitates pustules. The deeper freezing aids in the involution of papules and seems to help prevent scarring. It is quite likely that the increased blood flow potentiates the effect of systemically administered antibiotics, although no studies have yet been done to substantiate this thinking.

Most patients experience a stinging or burning sensation during application of the carbon dioxide slush. While tolerated by the majority of patients, there are some who find this form of therapy unacceptable. Too vigorous application over bony prominences can cause a burn. This often results in postinflammatory pigmentation. Occasionally, dark-skinned patients experience hypopigmentation.

SOLID CARBON DIOXIDE

Method—Individual lesions may be treated with solid carbon dioxide. A pencil of carbon dioxide can be fashioned from a block of carbon dioxide. This can also be made by pushing soft carbon dioxide snow into a narrow plastic cylinder. The Kidde® Apparatus is a convenient method of forming a carbon dioxide pencil. The pencil is applied with pressure to individual papules and nodules. It is pressed against the lesion for periods of up to one minute, depending on the pressure used.

Results—The lesions freeze upon application of solid carbon dioxide. They subsequently undergo involution within 7-10 days.

LIQUID NITROGEN

Liquid nitrogen has been used for nearly 30 years in treating skin disease. Allington[22] first used liquid nitrogen for cryotherapy in 1950 by applying the refrigerant to the skin with a cotton-tipped applicator. Eleven years later, Cooper[23] utilized a closed liquid nitrogen system, and in 1970, Torre[24] treated milia by channeling liquid nitrogen through a doorknob. Although liquid nitrogen has been used in treating acne and acne scars for many years, Graham's recent work[25] has re-emphasized its use.

Equipment—The refrigerant effect of liquid nitrogen may be delivered to the skin in several ways: spray, probe, or cotton-tipped applicators. Commercially available units include the Kryospray®, the TT-32®, the Zacarian C-21™, and the CE-8®. The last two units may be used with either spray or probe attachments. The CE-8® has the advantage of holding 31 liters of liquid nitrogen. Depending on the frequency of usage, refilling may not be necessary for 2-4 weeks, as the liquid nitrogen has an evaporation rate of 0.33 liters per day.

A variety of spray tips are available from the manufacturers. These include point tips with apertures of 2 mm or less in diameter, and an acne spray tip 19 mm wide. Other spray tips fashioned from disposable hypodermic syringes and angiocatheters may be attached to the probe handle with a Luer-lok® Adapter. In addition, probes of various sizes and shapes are also available with the CE-8® unit.

Technique—Application of liquid nitrogen is useful when employed as an adjunct to conventional acne therapies. It can replace incision and drainage of acne lesions, ultraviolet light (UVL) therapy, and, in some instances, intralesional corticosteroid treatment. Open comedones will still require expression. Treatments with liquid nitrogen may be repeated every 2-4 weeks until the acne is controlled.

In general, factors determining the size of the area to be frozen are the aperture diameter, the tip-to-skin distances, and the rate of flow of liquid nitrogen. When treating small superficial lesions, a tip with a 1 mm aperture is best. The tip is held 2-10 mm from the skin surface, and the individual lesions are frozen for 3-5 seconds. Larger lesions require a larger aperture spray tip and are frozen for 15-20 seconds.

Diffuse superficial peeling of the skin may be accomplished by spraying with a 2-3 mm pointed tip or with the acne spray tip. The tip is held 3-5 cm from the skin surface, and is moved back and forth over the skin surface until momentary blanching occurs. This technique may also be used to treat acne scars. For this purpose, however, atrophic, convoluted scars are maintained in the frozen state for 15-30 seconds by repeated sprayings. Hypertrophic or keloidal scars should be frozen for 30-60 seconds and occasionally longer, depending on the size of the lesion. Retreatment every 4-6 weeks seems optimal for resolution of these lesions.

Probes may also be used to treat papules and nodules. The probe is placed directly on the lesion without pressure. Contact is maintained for 3-20 seconds, depending on the size and depth of the lesion. Larger lesions may require several applications before they will freeze entirely. Applying the probe with pressure results in faster and deeper freezing. Probes have the advantage of greater precision of application and less lateral spread of freezing.

Cotton-tipped applicators saturated with liquid nitrogen are useful for freezing inflammatory lesions (2-5 seconds) and thick scars (10-15 seconds).

Results—Complexion modifies the overall response to freezing. Fair-skinned patients will require less freezing than brunettes. Most patients describe a stinging sensation at the moment of freezing. This usually subsides within minutes for small lesions, and rarely persists for more than 45 minutes for larger lesions. Should this be unacceptable, cold compresses will alleviate the discomfort.

Erythema of the frozen site appears almost immediately after thawing of the lesions. This is evanescent for lightly frozen lesions; more deeply frozen lesions become edematous within minutes. This may be followed during any time between 15 minutes and 3 days by blister formation. If not ruptured, this vesicle or bulla collapses and crusts over within 1-2 days. In most instances, the crust separates within 5-10 days. The residual erythema may persist for 1-4 weeks.

Papules resolve within 2-5 days. Closed comedones are unroofed during that time. Nodules become crusted in 3-4 days, and heal within a week.

Advantages—The application of liquid nitrogen is a noninvasive technique which helps to reduce scarring, the usual sequela of papular and nodular acne. Lesions treated with liquid nitrogen rarely recur. Reactive vasodilation resulting in increased blood flow, release of hydrolytic enzymes causing liquefaction of tissue components, and increased fibrinolysis have all been postulated as possible mechanisms of action of cryotherapy.[26] The response could also be immunologic by enhancing delayed hypersensitivity to *Propionibacterium acnes*.

Chemical Irritants

At the turn of the century, precipitated sulfur and salicylic acid in petrolatum was very much in vogue for use in the treatment of acne.[27] This causes peeling and induces dryness and erythema, much as other chemicals that have been used since. Although these agents have no effect on the rate of sebum production or output, they appear to cause a decrease in oiliness by virtue of their defatting effect on the outermost layer of the skin. Their irritant properties may cause increased shedding of the stratum corneum, both on the surface of the skin and possibly in the follicular canal. This effect may help decapitate pustules and superficial papules, permitting drainage of these lesions. Although perhaps not influencing the evolution of lesions, it certainly shortens their life span.

More frequent application of exfoliants, or the concomitant use of several agents having similar properties, seems to have an additive effect on the skin. Additional peeling and even more erythema will result. Interestingly, the erythema due to enhanced blood flow may help to resolve deeper inflammatory lesions. Although erythema may further the therapeutic effect, it will often be unacceptable to the patient unless he is previously alerted.

In view of these circumstances, familiarity with a few preparations is essential. The clinician should learn what each one will do individually or in combination, keeping in mind that any agent will have an exaggerated effect on patients with drier skins. It is generally best to begin with a relatively mild preparation and then gradually increase the effect.

Two additional factors should be considered concerning the use of topically applied medications. The skin will eventually become tolerant to any irritant; consequently, either more frequent applications or higher concentrations of the agent are necessary to achieve the desired effect. Secondly, changes in humidity and in exposure to wind may further modify the effect of locally applied medications. For this reason, winter often potentiates the effect of irritants, with patients requiring less frequent applications or lower concentrations.

VARIETIES

Topical medications used in the treatment of acne contain varying combinations of elemental sulfur, sulfur compounds, resorcin, salicylic acid, alcohol, and acetone. These compounds are found in lotions, creams, solutions, gels, compresses, and cleansing preparations in varying concentrations. Lotions are prescribed in both clear and tinted vehicles. Tinted vehicles are useful in camouflaging individual lesions while they undergo involution.

A note of caution regarding elemental sulfur is warranted. Although precipitated sulfur is a time-honored constituent of many acne preparations, there is reason to suspect that its prolonged use may perpetuate the acne process while seeming to alleviate it. Although no clinical confirmation is yet available, both human and animal assays have shown that sulfur is comedogenic. Thus, by inducing the formation of new comedones, sulfur may be promoting the development of new acne lesions. Sulfur compounds, however, are free of this comedogenic effect.[28]

Despite the media commercials which imply that clean skin is clear skin, there is no conclusive evidence that acne is the result of a cleansing failure. "Medicated" soaps should be looked upon as just another method of cleansing the skin. If properly rinsed, very little of the incorporated chemicals remain on the skin after washing. Scrubbing the skin should be proscribed. In the authors' view, abrasives generally have no place in the treatment of acne.

Some of the commercially available lotions contain small amounts of hydrocortisone. The prime indication for the use of these medications is the presence of pruritus and underlying seborrheic dermatitis, eczematization, or very dry facial skin. The authors do not recommend the topical application of fluorinated corticosteroids, either alone or in combination with conventional acne therapy. Although these preparations initially have a suppressive effect on the inflammatory component of acne, their continued use will result in an explosive exacerbation of the disease[29] (see Chapter 3).

Vleminckx's solution is a most useful preparation for the treatment of severe inflammatory acne. Applied as a hot compress, usually at bedtime, it helps resolve inflammatory lesions. Except for the disagreeable odor of Vleminckx's solution and its ability to possibly tarnish metals, no serious side effects are known.

REFERENCES

1. Shaefer O: Nutrition Today, Nov/Dec. 15, 1971.
2. Grant JD, Anderson PC: Chocolate as a cause of acne: a dissenting view. *Missouri Med* 62:459, 1965.
3. Fulton JE Jr, Plewig G, Kligman AM: Effect of chocolate on acne vulgaris. *JAMA* 210:2071, 1969.
4. Schlappner OL, Shelley WB, Ruberg RL, et al: Acute papulopustular acne associated with prolonged intravenous hyperalimentation. *JAMA* 219:877, 1972.
5. Shelley WB: *Consultations in Dermatology,* p 155. Philadelphia: WB Saunders, 1972.
6. Baer RL, Witten VH (Eds): "Acne Vulgaris: Remarks on Recent Advances in Knowledge and Management," in *The Year Book of Dermatology, 1959-60*, pp 7-32. Chicago: Year Book Medical Pub, 1960.
7. MacDonald I: Effects of skim milk and chocolate diet on serum and skin lipids. *J Sci Food Agric* 19:270, 1968.
8. Pochi PE, Downing DT, Strauss JS: Sebaceous gland response in man to prolonged total caloric deprivation. *J Invest Dermatol* 55:303, 1970.
9. Mullins JF, Naylor D: Glucose and the acne diathesis: an hypothesis and review of pertinent literature. *Tex Rep Biol Med* 20:161, 1962.
10. Goldschmidt H, Leyden JJ, Stein KH: Acne fulminans. *Arch Dermatol* 113:444, 1977.
11. Rose LI, Newmark SR, Strauss JS, et al: Adrenocortical hydroxylase deficiency in acne vulgaris. *J Invest Dermatol* 66:324, 1976.
12. Michaelsson G, Juhlin L, Vahlquist A: Effects of oral zinc and vitamin A in acne. *Arch Dermatol* 113:31, 1977.
13. Weston WL, Huff JC, Humbert JR, et al: Zinc correction of defective chemotaxis in acrodermatitis enteropathica. *Arch Dermatol* 113:422, 1977.
14. Williams M, Cunliffe WJ: Explanation for premenstrual acne. *Lancet* 2:1055, 1973.
15. Jelinek JE: Hydrochlorothiazide and the control of premenstrual exacerbation of acne. *Arch Dermatol* 105:79, 1972.
16. Rebello DJ: Intralesional triamcinolone acetonide in skin diseases other than psoriasis. *Br J Dermatol* 74:358, 1962.
17. Leeming JA: Intradermal triamcinolone in the treatment of cystic acne. *S Afr Med J* 39:567, 1965.
18. Parish LC, Witkowski JA: The enigma of acne therapy: the acne abscess. *Am J Med* 254:769, 1967.
19. Potter RA: Intradermal triamcinolone and adrenal suppression in acne vulgaris. *J Invest Dermatol* 57:364, 1971.
20. Giraudeau R: Cryotherapie directe a l'aide d'un melange de la neige carbonique et de acetone. *Bull Soc Fr Dermatol Syphiligr* 35:463, 1928.
21. Giraudeau R: La cure d'exfoliation par le melange de la neige carbonique acetone, soufres dans l'acne. *Bull Soc Fr Dermatol Syphiligr* 36:654, 1929.
22. Allington HV: Liquid nitrogen in the treatment of skin diseases. *Calif Med* 12:153, 1950.
23. Cooper IS, Lee AS: Cryostatic congelation: a system for producing a limited,

      controlled region of cooling or freezing of biologic tissues. *J Nerv Ment Dis* 133:259, 1961.
24. Torre D: "Cryosurgery in Dermatology" in Von Leyden H, Cahan WF (Eds): *Cryogenics in Surgery*. New York: Medical Examiners Pub, 1971.
25. Graham GF: Cryosurgical treatment of acne. *Cutis* 16:506, 1975.
26. Leyden JJ, Mills OH, Kligman AM: Cryoprobe treatment of acne conglobata. *Br J Dermatol* 90:335, 1974.
27. Grindon J: *Diseases of the Skin*, p 344. Philadelphia: Lea Brothers, 1902.
28. Mills OH Jr, Kligman AM: Is sulfur helpful or harmful in acne vulgaris? *Br J Dermatol* 86:620, 1972.
29. Kaidbey KH, Kligman AM: The pathogenesis of topical steroid acne. *J Invest Dermatol* 62:31, 1974.

Chapter 25

Surgery for Acne: Preventive, Therapeutic, and Rehabilitative

NORMAN ORENTREICH, MD
NANCY P. DURR

Optimal improvement for most acne patients requires some degree of surgery. In mild cases, the surgery consists simply of the expression of open and closed comedones. In more severe cases, it includes intralesional injections of anti-inflammatory corticosteroids and/or incision and drainage of pustules and cysts. Ultimately the scars are treated with reconstructive procedures (Figure 1): intralesional corticosteroids, excision, punch elevation, punch excision with full-thickness grafting, silicone-induced collagen augmentation, and dermabrasion. Judicious acne surgery is both prophylactic and therapeutic for comedonal, pustular, and cystic acne.

Procedures for Active Acne

EXPRESSION OF OPEN AND CLOSED COMEDONES

Both open and closed comedones can become inflamed and pustular. Open comedones sometimes persist for many months before becoming inflamed. Generally, the longer a comedo persists, the larger it will become. Thus it follows that the larger the comedo, the longer the period of inflammation (average—13 days) of the ensuing pustule or cyst.[1] Expression of open and closed comedones reduces the chances of their evolving into papules, pustules, and cysts, with consequent dermal destruction (see Chapter 12).

Skillful comedo expression should be done with a minimum of trauma to the patient. Care should be taken that the comedo contents are not forced into the dermis. The instrument selected should be the one that best affords manual dexterity and efficacy during the procedure.

The skin is cleansed with ethanol to allow visualization of the lesions. Open comedones are usually obvious, while closed comedones may require stretching of the skin. A sharp, sterile #11 blade is used to open the orifice or to loosen the top of the comedo. The rim of the comedo extractor is placed around the ostium of the comedo. Proper force and direction with appropriate eccentric manipulation of the instrument will express the contents of the closed comedo.

CHEMOEXFOLIATION

A light application of 20% trichloracetic acid may be desirable for therapeutic exfoliation in patients with either active acne or mild acne-associated hyperpigmentation.

CRYOSURGERY AND CRYOEXFOLIATION

Ethyl chloride, Freon®, solid carbon dioxide, and liquid nitrogen (see Chapter 24) are cryotherapeutic modalities used to speed the resolution of inflammatory lesions and/or to produce beneficial cryoexfoliation of acne and postacne hyperpigmentation.

CUTANEOUS CORTICOSTEROID INJECTION THERAPY

The treatment of acne was facilitated by the development of intralesional corticosteroid injections.[2] Corticosteroids, intralesionally injected, hasten the resolution of inflamed lesions and thus inhibit scarring. The morbidostatic corticosteroids are vasoconstricting, antimitotic, anti-inflammatory, and antipruritic (see Chapter 12 and 24).

The effect of a specific corticosteroid is directly related to the number of milligrams deposited in the skin. Papules and cysts respond to 0.05-0.1 ml of triamcinolone acetonide, administered in a suspension containing 2.5-5 mg/ml. While 5 mg/ml is employed for most lesions of the body, 2.5 mg/ml is used for facial lesions. Temporary atrophy, least acceptable on the face, is minimized with the use of the lower concentration.

Only aqueous corticosteroid suspensions are used for cutaneous injection. The administration of reproducible doses of a suspension requires a uniform distribution of the corticosteroid particles. The corticosteroid sediment in the multidose vial should be thoroughly agitated within the container for even resuspension before it is withdrawn through a large-bore needle. The material should then be used before it settles in the syringe. Should the particles settle, they may be resuspended by drawing air into the syringe and inverting the syringe several times. The air bubble is then expelled.

The use of a 1.0 ml syringe and a #30-gauge needle provides for a controlled, efficient and relatively painless injection. The tattooing technique, by either multi-jet or hand jet hypospray-type administration, allows material to be wasted, and can be more painful and more traumatic to tissues. This technique does not afford accurate control of dosage at the site of administration, and may produce superficial atrophy.

Dilution of commercially available corticosteroids is usually necessary in order to avoid atrophy. Corticosteroid suspensions should be diluted with isotonic saline (0.9% sodium chloride with 0.9% benzyl alcohol as a preservative). Lidocaine is not an optimal diluent; it is more painful upon injection and may produce local vasospasm.[3] Diluents containing phenol or parabens may cause flocculation of the corticosteroid suspension. Suspensions containing crystals of 50μ or larger (as seen on microscopic examination) should be discarded, unless the crystals are reduced to less than 10μ by sonification. Early use of a diluted suspension avoids crystal growth. Large crystals, when injected into the face or scalp, can cause amaurosis.[4]

INCISION AND DRAINAGE

Incision and drainage of pustular and cystic lesions is the cornerstone of acne surgery. Lesions resolve more rapidly and with less scar formation when this procedure is properly performed (see Chapter 24). A small stab-incision (1-3 mm) at the summit of the lesion is made with a #11 blade. The contents are gently expressed. Corticosteroids may then be injected into the lesion. When done skillfully, incision and drainage is well-tolerated. Prior refrigeration with ethyl chloride or Freon® of the area to be treated lessens the discomfort. The application of solid carbon dioxide helps resolve the lesion and provides anesthesia for incision and drainage.

FREQUENCY OF ACNE SURGERY

Acne surgery can be painful and can cause temporary irritation and erythema. Weekly to monthly execution of the appropriate surgical procedure prevents the patient from performing inept acne surgery on himself, thereby possibly rupturing the wall of the lesion and releasing material into the dermis. Self-induced scarring in the form of neurotic excoriations is a problem frequently observed in acne patients. Sometimes it is preferable to only use corticosteroid injection therapy instead of incision and drainage when the latter causes undue scarring.

Procedures for Acne Scars

DERMABRASION

Improvement of acne scarring with dermabrasion depends upon the type and depth of the defects, the number and level of dermabrasions, and the healing capabilities of the individual. A single dermabrasion effectively improves most imperfections in the upper third of the dermis. A defect which

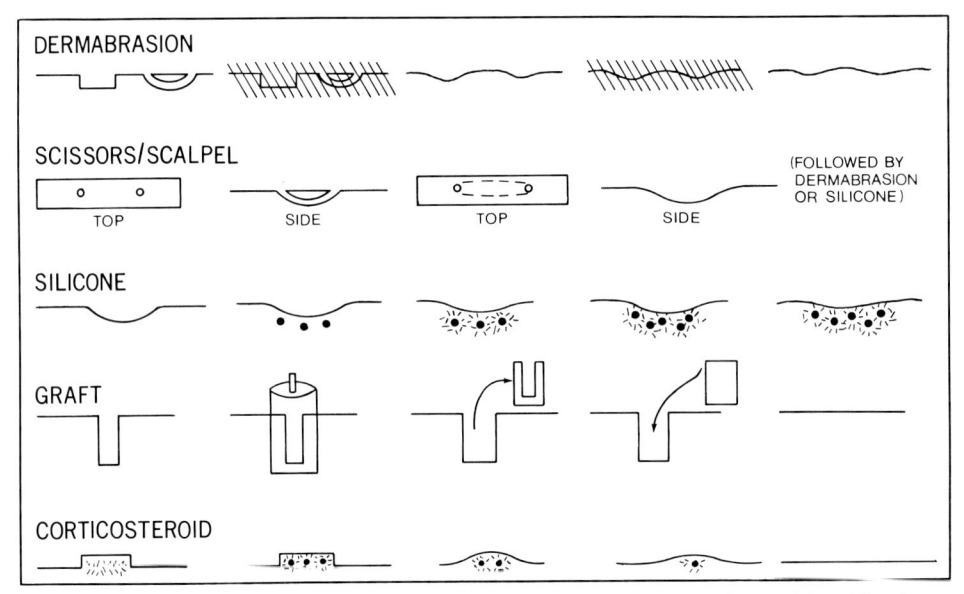

Figure 1. Treatments for Acne Scars. Acne scarring is multiform, and a variety of treatments may be required for optimal improvement. Dermabrasion smoothes sharp-edged scars and breaks up their fibrotic bases. Either dermabrasion or excision unroofs epithelialized tunnels. Silicone droplets at dermal-subcutaneous interface stimulate collagen augmentation of depressed scars. Free full-thickness earlobe skin grafts replace deep scars. True intralesional injections of corticosteroids atrophy hypertrophic/keloidal scars.

extends into the deeper dermis usually requires more than one dermabrasion, or other procedures, to produce satisfactory improvement.

Acne scarring is multiform, consisting of scars which may be narrow, deep, pitted, "ice pick"-like, crater-like, hypotrophic, diffusely depressed, hypertrophic, or keloidal (Figure 1) (see Chapter 11). Skin resurfacing by dermabrasion may remove superficial scars and minimize deeper ones. Scarring need not be totally corrected to see an improvement in the general appearance of the skin. For example, acne scars with sharp edges will cast distinct shadows and give the skin surface a "moonscape" appearance. Dermabrasion bevels the sharp edges of scars, reducing these shadows. Dermabrasion also breaks up the bases of depressed scars, allowing them to heal with less indentation. Scars which rise above the skin's surface are planed down.

Dermabrasion is not optimal, however, for certain types of scars. For example, in the deep "ice pick" scars (ie, patulons, infundibular, epithelial tracts), bands of collagen often extend down to the subcutaneous layers, keeping the epithelial invagination stable. These scars are better treated by punch excision, with or without graft replacement. Areas of atrophy or depression are better treated by silicone-induced collagen augmentation. Generally, the scars which improve on manual stretching of the skin at the

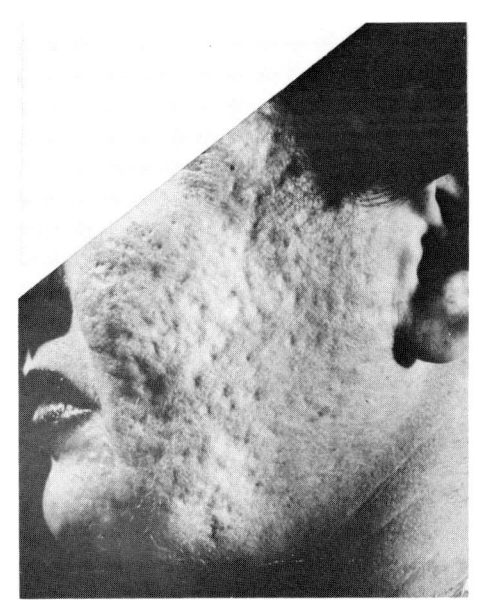

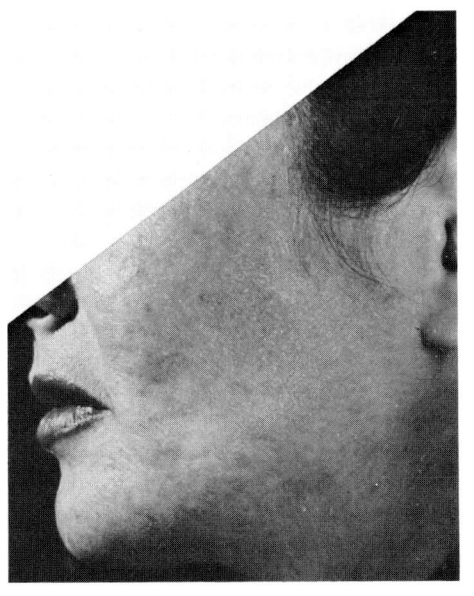

Figure 2. Three dermabrasions provided excellent improvement. Had other scar treatment methods been performed, 2 dermabrasions would have sufficed.

time of examination are those which improve from 50-75% with a single dermabrasion. Additional dermabrasions can further improve the condition of the skin (Figure 2).

Although dermabrasion is usually performed for the cosmetic improvement of certain skin defects, it can be therapeutic and prophylactic for active acne. Dermabrasion removes cysts and epithelialized sinuses, drains infected lesions, and alters the orifices of sebaceous glands. Before the advent of corticosteroids and antibiotics, dermabrasion was frequently used to ameliorate severe acne. Although dermabrasion is rarely used as a primary treatment for acne, certainly the patient with active but controlled acne need not postpone dermabrasion treatment of scarring.

The Black patient with acne scarring fares extremely well with dermabrasion. Although there is a period of very obvious hypopigmentation after surgery, the eventual return of pigment and its blending with untreated areas is good. Contrary to expectations, there is no increased incidence of hypertrophic scarring or keloid formation following dermabrasion or facial grafting in the Black patient. The pigment of Asiatics, however, is more volatile; hyperpigmentation following surgery can take months to normalize, even with treatment.

Dermabrasion requires manual training and dexterity. If dermabrasion is too superficial, the degree of improvement may be disappointing. If dermabrasion is too deep, unnecessary hypopigmentation and scarring can occur. Expertise in the technical aspects of the procedure and a thorough understanding of the indications, postoperative care, sequelae, and psychological factors involved are essential for optimal results.

Contraindications—Dermabrasion removes the entire epidermis and the upper part of the skin adnexa. Re-epithelialization and repigmentation take place in the residual portion of the hair follicles, and in the sebaceous glands and sweat ducts. If these adnexa are diminished or absent (*eg*, due to radiation damage), postdermabrasion healing may be poor (*eg*, healing may be delayed, hypotrophic, or hypertrophic). Acne scarring in conjunction with radiodermatitis requires a very light dermabrasion.

Although dermabrasion has been successfully performed on patients with active herpes simplex, delaying the procedure minimizes the possibility that the virus will disseminate to the abraded areas, causing an eruption similar to that of Kaposi's varicelliform eruption.

Dermabrasion is usually limited to the face and neck for the management of acne scars. Dermabrasion of the back or chest is rarely performed, because the adnexa in these areas are less dense, and thus healing is less optimal. There is also greater potential for keloid formation and for cosmetically unacceptable pigment contrast between abraded and nonabraded areas. Other methods, described below, are more suitable for the treatment of scars on the back or chest.

Preoperative Instructions—Loose, comfortable clothing that does not have to be removed over the head is suggested. Long hair should be tied back or braided; short hair should be brushed back off the face. The areas to be abraded should be shaved prior to the operation. Hair washing should be done the night before, since it is not advisable to shampoo until 4-5 days after undergoing surgery. A light breakfast is suggested on the morning of the operation.

Photographs are taken in the office, after the area to be abraded has been washed with soap and water.

Anesthesia—Dermabrasion is an office procedure not requiring general anesthesia. Fifty to 75 mg of meperidine hydrochloride is usually given intramuscularly, one half hour prior to surgery. Immediately before or else during dermabrasion, key facial nerves may be injected with 1% or 2% lidocaine with a #30-gauge needle to produce block anesthesia of the forehead, cheeks, nose, chin, or upper lip. Deep injection avoids tissue distortion.

Refrigeration of the skin produces anesthesia, rigidity of tissues, and avascularity. Ethyl chloride, Freon®, or mixtures used with a blower to enhance evaporation will easily freeze a 2 x 2-inch area to -30°C in 15-20 seconds. The skin remains frozen for 15-30 seconds, which is ample time for the physician to abrade the area. With proper planning and the aid of a trained assistant, a full-face dermabrasion can be completed within 20 minutes. A room fan and adequate ventilation reduce the unpleasant fumes of the refrigerant. Excessive freezing may prolong healing time and cause a protracted erythema, and is thus to be avoided. Abraded areas are overlapped by 1-2 cm to prevent demarcation.

As each area is finished, it may be covered with gauze saturated with a 2% lidocaine-saline solution. This reduces the burning sensation that occurs with thawing. Tolerance for pain varies. Most patients experience discomfort during only the first 10 seconds of freezing.

Method—While a dermabrasion can be performed by an unassisted physician, the operation is facilitated by the presence of two surgical assistants. Each wears a protective plastic gown and a clear, hard, plastic face shield. The primary assistant wears cotton gloves covered by rubber gloves for insulation against the freezing by the anesthetic. This assistant places gauze pads on the skin to demarcate the 2 x 2-inch areas to be frozen; gauze pads are also used to protect the patient's eyes, ears, and nose. The other assistant helps with the refrigeration anesthesia. Four fine-spray bottles of ethyl chloride are used simultaneously with a blower to accomplish adequate freezing: 2 are directed by the surgeon and 2 by the assistant. Adequate freezing can be accomplished with only 2 cans of Freon®.

For a full-face dermabrasion, the face is usually divided into 17 areas: 4 on each cheek; 2 on the chin; 2 on the nose; 2 on the upper lip; and 3 on the forehead. Spraying and abrading one area at a time, the physician usually moves from the outermost and dependent areas towards the central and upper areas of the face.

Wire brushes, $3/4$ inches in diameter and $3/16$ inches wide, are preferred over the diamond fraise, as they are more abrasive. The brushes are available in "soft," "regular," and "coarse" grades. After being used several times, the brushes become less abrasive as the wire bristles are bent backwards. In a new brush, all the bristles are positioned in the direction of rotation to maximize the abrasive effect. The surgeon should inspect the brushes for abrasiveness.

The selection of the appropriately abrasive instrument depends on the thickness of the skin and the depth of the scarring to be abraded. A narrow wire brush disc permits point contact at its perimeter on rigidly frozen skin. Removal of defects can be precisely controlled. The brush is held by its mandrel in a chuck attached to a flexible cable from a $1/10$ hp motor, producing 23,000 rpm. The speed of the motor is controlled by a foot pedal connected to a rheostat.

The rotating wire brush is moved by the surgeon over the frozen skin with firm, steady, back-and-forth strokes. Greater pressure is applied to areas of deeper scarring. Whenever possible, the abrasion ends at a natural fold, at a line of demarcation, or at a relatively hidden site (*eg*, at the nasolabial fold, at the hairline, or under the jawline).

The forehead is abraded from the hairline into the eyebrow. Abrasion of the chin and upper lip is carried on to the vermilion border. Immediately after the dermabrasion, a light chemical exfoliating agent (*eg*, 20-30% aqueous trichloracetic acid) is applied to the surrounding, unabraded areas for additional pigment blending.

In patients with severe scarring, a second dermabrasion is usually required. The second operation may be performed as early as 6 weeks after the first. Usually, only the deeply scarred areas require this second procedure. To avoid obvious lines of demarcation, a "feathering" stroke is used at the edges of the abraded areas. Occasionally, 3 or more dermabrasions are needed.

Postoperative Office Care—After the operation, the lidocaine-soaked gauze pads which were applied to each abraded area, now blood-soaked, are removed. The areas are again sprayed with 2% lidocaine solution and fresh, sterile gauze pads are applied. The bleeding that follows dermabrasion lasts only a few minutes. Cotton strips coated with antibiotic ointment are applied to the abraded surface. Over these are placed thick, absorbent pads, and the entire face is wrapped with gauze.

It is recommended that the patient be accompanied home because of the effects of preoperative medications and bandage-restricted vision.

Postoperative Home Care—The patient initially can do little else but rest and take the prescribed medications. Swelling is inevitable, especially during the first 48 hours after surgery. It is not unusual for the eyelids to become swollen, even though abrasion is not performed on these areas. With time and gravity, the neck becomes edematous. To speed this drainage, the patient should sit up, and walk about. During sleep, the head should be elevated on several pillows. Oral corticosteroids may be given to reduce inflammation and edema.

Most patients do not complain of discomfort, but describe a sensation similar to that of a warm sunburn. Some experience a slight throbbing sensation. Mild analgesics are prescribed; however, they are rarely needed after the first 3 days. When insomnia is a problem, a medication for sleep is prescribed.

Twenty-four hours after surgery, all the bandages are removed. At this time, or as soon as the serum ooze has begun to gel, the patient applies an antibiotic ointment frequently. The ointment can be applied directly to the area with a sterile tongue blade, sterile gauze, a cotton swab, or a clean finger. This ointment facilitates healing by preventing any dessication. At no time should the abraded area be allowed to become dry; it should always remain flexible and soft. Because the serum and ointment may drip, a cotton bib may be draped around the neck. The ointment and serum may be wiped from nonabraded areas; the abraded area, however, should not be cleansed for 5 days. A stretchable headband will help keep hair off the face. Large, white, plastic bags may be taped over the pillows to avoid soiling and to prevent the healing skin from adhering to the pillow case.

On the fifth day after surgery, warm water soaks are applied to the abraded areas for 15-minute periods. A clean washcloth is dipped in warm water, held to the face, removed, dipped again, and reapplied. With each soaking, a considerable amount of the caramel-colored gel of serum and ointment is removed. These soaks are done 2-3 times a day until the gel is gone (usually 7-10 days). If hard crusts inadvertently form, they should not be forcibly removed; rather, ointment should be reapplied to soften them, and soaking continued.

When re-epithelialization occurs, cool compresses of equal parts of water and milk may be applied by the patient 3 times a day for 5-minute periods to reduce erythema and to relieve pruritus that may accompany the final stages of healing. Between and after compresses, a light layer of 2% hydrocortisone cream is applied to taut, dry, or irritated areas.

Until healing is complete, patients should avoid extreme exercise; straining, lifting, and bending; excessive heat, cold, and wind; direct sunlight; and all nonprescribed skin preparations. Within 10 days, men can usually shave, and women can apply a nonmedicated makeup.

The time required for re-epithelialization increases with the age of the patient and the depth of dermabrasion. Re-epithelialization usually occurs within 7-10 days. Initial repigmentation usually takes 4-6 weeks, while more complete restoration of pigmentation takes several months.

Postoperative Sequelae—Erythema occurs in all patients and can last for 2 weeks to 2 months. Topical, intralesional, and systemic corticosteroids may relieve the condition.

Milia formation occurs in one-third of the patients. It is best treated by pinpoint electrodesiccation, or by removal with a #11 blade and a comedo extractor.

Eczematization occurs in one-tenth of the patients, and usually responds to topical anti-inflammatory corticosteroids. Occasionally, intralesional and/or systemic corticosteroids are used.

Pigmentary alteration occurs in all patients for several weeks. Initially, there is hypopigmentation with erythema. The skin pigmentation returns in about 6 weeks. Postinflammatory hyperpigmentation is seen in 10% of the patients. It is usually temporary, and will disappear within a few weeks. Occasionally it will require topical treatment (eg, 20% aqueous trichloracetic acid, salicylic acid, hydroquinone, ammoniated mercury, retinoic acid, and/or corticosteroids). Dermabrasion can produce persistent hypopigmentation in a few patients. Loss of pigment occurs more frequently in radiodermatitis-affected skin.

The incidence of hypertrophic reactions varies with the underlying problem: acne scars, 1%; wrinkles, 5%; radiodermatitis, 25%; tattoos, 75%. These reactions may subside with time, but resolve more quickly with intralesional corticosteroid injections.

CHEMOSURGERY

In the opinion of the authors as well as others who have performed chemosurgery with phenol or trichloracetic acid preparations, chemosurgery is relatively ineffective for the treatment of acne scarring, and has been displaced by dermabrasion.

PUNCH ELEVATION

A depressed scar may be improved by punch elevation.[5] The plug containing the depressed scar is raised to a level flush with the surrounding skin; it may be necessary to desiccate the edges after healing. An elliptically shaped defect can be conformed to the circle of a punch by stretching the defect across its short axis.

PUNCH EXCISION WITH FULL-THICKNESS GRAFT REPLACEMENT

Punch excision surgery, either with or without graft replacement, is suited for patients with either a few discrete acne scars or scars not suitable for dermabrasion or silicone augmentation. The ideal scar for punch removal is the "ice pick" scar.

Although punch elevation is helpful in treating some acne scars, punch excision followed by full-thickness, normal skin graft replacement usually gives better results. The donor and recipient sites are anesthetized with lidocaine. The scar is excised by punch (typically 2-3 mm), and is discarded. The graft of normal tissue is excised from the posterior earlobe usually with a slightly larger punch. Trimming of fat or suturing is rarely needed. Antibiotic ointment and a small Band-Aid® or Clearon® are applied.

For an optimal cosmetic result, the fully-healed graft edges can be blended by electrodesiccation several weeks later. If the graft heals lower than the surrounding skin, it may be treated with silicone augmentation, or re-excised and elevated or replaced with a larger punch graft.

If the patient has extensive and multiform acne scarring, dermabrasion is usually done after grafting, since the dermabrasion will smooth previous grafts. Dermabrasion, however, may uncover epithelialized sinus defects which might require subsequent grafts.

EXCISION OF EPITHELIALIZED SINUSES

Acne may be associated with an inflammatory, necrotic reaction to keratin, sebum, and bacteria trapped beneath the surface of the skin in epithelialized tunnels and sinuses (see Chapter 11 and 21). These epithelialized sinuses or tunnel scars may either be large enough to thread with a scissors, or small enough to thread with a needle. Dermabrasion unroofs these sinuses, but they can also be effectively unroofed with a scissors or scalpel.

COLLAGEN AUGMENTATION

When a minute amount of liquid polydimethylsiloxane (silicone) is introduced into the dermal-subcutaneous interface, it is surrounded by fibrocytes which form collagen[5] (Figure 1 and 3). It is this formation of new collagen which corrects the defect, and not the small volume of silicone

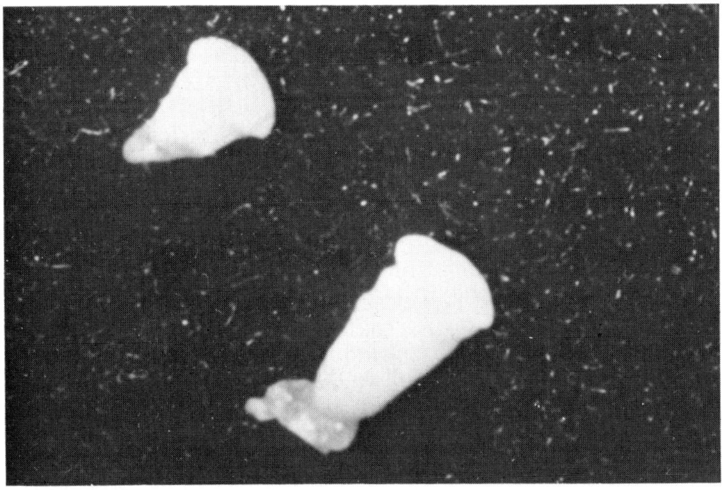

Figure 3. A site on the medial aspect of an arm was injected with 0.2 ml of pure medical-grade silicone. One year later, this site (right plug) and untreated adjacent site (left plug) were punch-biopsied. Augmentation of treated site is obvious. Reproduced with permission from Selmanowitz VJ, Orentreich N: Medical-grade fluid silicone: a monographic review. *J Dermatol Surg Oncol* 3:597, 1977. Copyright © 1977, The Journal of Dermatologic Surgery and Oncology, Inc, New York.

injected. Since collagen deposition is not immediate, the full effect of injected silicone is not evident for 1-3 months. The number of injections required for correction of an individual scar depends on the degree of collagen response. Since collagen deposition is the purpose of these injections, the droplet size is kept to a minimum to provide the greatest surface area-to-volume ratio. Each droplet should be administered as a separate injection, so that there is no pooling of the material.

Dermabrasion does not eradicate the benefits of previous silicone treatments, and, during his 25 years of experience in combining silicone injections and dermabrasion, regardless of sequence, one of the authors (NO) has found them to be fully compatible procedures.

The silicone used is 100% pure, medical-grade, polydimethylsiloxane. It has a viscosity of 360^{cs}, and is filtered through diatomaceous earth. It is handled and stored in glass-stoppered or other nonreactive bottles, and is autoclaved. The viscous fluid is administered with a special hydraulically designed ¼ ml, long-barrel, narrow-bore syringe with a Luer-lok® Adapter and a #30-gauge needle.

COLLAGEN REDUCTION

Whereas collagen formation is induced by silicone, it is reduced by corticosteroids. Intralesional injections of triamcinolone acetonide, ranging in concentration from 2.5-10 mg/ml, are useful in the treatment of hypertrophic or keloidal scars. The dosage is 1 mg per cubic centimeter of hypertrophic tissue. Several injections, at least one month apart, may be required to produce the desired degree of atrophy in the hypertrophic site.

Solid carbon dioxide also reduces hypertrophic or keloidal scars when applied with sufficient pressure to compress and refrigerate the scar in depth (see Chapter 24).

REFERENCES

1. Orentreich N, Durr NP: The natural evolution of comedones into inflammatory papules and pustules. *J Invest Dermatol* 62:316, 1974.
2. Orentreich N: "Cutaneous Corticosteroid Injection Therapy," in Maibach HI (Ed): *Dermatopharmacology*. St. Louis: CV Mosby (to be published).
3. Epstein E: Herpes zoster and post-zoster neuralgia: intralesional triamcinolone therapy. *Cutis* 12:898, 1973.
4. Selmanowitz VJ, Orentreich N: Cutaneous corticosteroid injection and amaurosis: analysis for cause and prevention. *Arch Dermatol* 110:729, 1974.
5. Selmanowitz VJ, Orentreich N: Medical-grade fluid silicone: a monographic review. *J Dermatol Surg Oncol* 3:597, 1977.

Chapter 26

Summing Up

SAMUEL B. FRANK, MD

Despite intensive research over the past 20 years, many questions as to the pathogenesis of acne remain unanswered. Sulzberger presented many of the problems that yet require solutions (see Chapter 1). We do not know why one individual has just a few comedones and another has a nodulocystic acne that scars him for life. We have no understanding as to what initiates the process in the follicular canal that produces the changes which finally result in an acne lesion. The recent observations of Knutson,[1] derived from his studies utilizing the electron microscope, have resulted in new observations as to what occurs in the follicular canal. One can well realize that Knutson had to examine many follicles to find the various states of development which lead to the comedo, since, at any given time, there are only a finite number of sebaceous follicles that are developing comedones.

    The clinician is frequently asked by the patient as to why lesions are more numerous in one area of the skin than in another, and absent in still others, and, when a comedo does form, why one becomes inflamed while another does not. The unmanipulated open comedo rarely produces the inflammatory lesions of acne. The closed comedo has been regarded as the precursor of inflammatory acne. It appears, however, that microcomedones, lesions that cannot be seen or felt, are more important than the visible comedones in the pathogenesis of acne lesions. What contributes to the process? What stops it? What is the role of heredity? What part does the psyche play?

    We can only conjecture as tc what precipitates acne. Much investigation has been done in regard to hormones. The chemistry of sebum has also received a good deal of attention. The proliferation of bacteria, the activity of the sebaceous glands, and the alterations of sebum have aroused much productive study.[2] But we still have many more questions than answers.

Various theories have been suggested to explain why acne resolves in most patients at the end of their teens. Sulzberger hypothesized that the pilosebaceous follicles involved in acne are hardened or destroyed during the acne-bearing years. He believed that these changes explain why, in adult patients with tropical acne, lesions appear in areas not previously involved during adolescence. Perhaps the pilosebaceous unit's exquisite sensitivity to hormones is lost in adulthood. An additional possibility suggested[3] for the spontaneous involution of acne is that the lining of the follicle might accommodate to the bacterial products and become immune to them. Here, too, the riddles are unanswered.

The existing lack of knowledge must be pushed aside and replaced by what we do know about acne. And we do know a great deal. The successes of the past few years are most exciting. The chapters in this book have presented the accomplishments of both laboratory and clinical investigators. When reviewing the history of acne (see Chapter 2), it is reassuring to note how much progress has been made in recent years.

Pathogenesis

SEBUM

There is general agreement that sebum output is usually higher in individuals with acne than in those without, and that it is particularly high in patients with severe acne. These observations are not always consistent; high sebum levels are found in individuals who do not have acne, and the reverse is also true. Plewig and Kligman pointed out that sebum continuously escapes from the follicular channel which contains a comedo (see Chapter 11). They described the extrusion of horny material from open comedones as occurring in a "glacier-like" fashion.

The sebaceous follicle, a special type of follicular unit containing large sebaceous glands and rudimentary hairs, has been implicated as the site where acne begins.[4] The sebaceous follicles are more numerous in individuals with acne than in those without. These sebaceous glands have cells that are almost twice the size of those seen in normal sebaceous glands[5]—cells that appear to have a genetic explanation. Knutson[1] observed lipid engorgement in the lining of the infrainfundibular portion of the follicular channel (see Chapter 10). These fat droplets are not of sebaceous gland origin. Knutson also noted in the infrainfundibular cells a decrease in the lamellar granules, structures that contain hydrolytic enzymes, the presence of which are considered to be necessary to produce the normal separation of the cornified layer cells. This may explain the presence in the follicular lining of the conglomeration of cells which ultimately form the comedo. The ready separation normally seen of the cells which line the follicle does not occur in the acne follicle, where the cells adhere to each other.

Attention has centered on the lipolysis that occurs in sebum. Bacterial lipases, particularly those from *Propionibacterium acnes*, have been shown to act on the triglycerides to produce free fatty acids and glycerol. Although the involvement of free fatty acids has aroused interest, no role has been attributed to the glycerol thus far. Since it was shown by Strauss and Pochi[6] that free fatty acids are irritants when injected intradermally, it appeared logical to explain inflammatory acne as due to the release of free fatty acids. The free fatty acids with chain lengths between C_8 and C_{12} appear to be the most irritating components of sebum.[7] The free fatty acid hypothesis was further substantiated by the findings[8] that tetracycline produced a decrease in free fatty acids on the skin surface and also diminished bacterial growth. Puhvel and Sakamoto[9] showed, however, that free fatty acids in the follicular canal do not exist in amounts capable of inducing anything more than a mild inflammation. Investigating the inflammatory role of *P. acnes*, Puhvel and Sakamoto[10] observed that physiologic quantities of the components of skin lipids (including free fatty acids) were less inflammatory than physiologic amounts of *P. acnes*, when intradermally injected in humans.

Voss[3] pointed out that sebum contains components other than lipases which may be implicated in the pathogenesis of acne. Bacterial enzymes such as proteases, neuraminidase, hyaluronidase, and lecithinase may also contribute to the acne process. Bacterial antigens and toxins could well serve as inducers of inflammation. Puhvel and Reisner[11] showed that the concentration of tetracycline able to suppress lipases *in vitro* is several times that which exists in the acne follicle. Fulton,[12] as well as Weeks et al,[13] further cast doubt on the role of free fatty acids in acne with the observation that a pyridyl phosphate (fospirate) that specifically inhibits lipases and reduces free fatty acids did not have any clinical effect on the course of acne (see Chapter 8).

The chemical composition of the sebum in acne patients is not distinctively different from that observed in acne-free individuals. Recent work indicated that the fatty acid, octadeca-5,8-dienoic acid, was increased in acne patients, but subsequent study failed to establish the significance of these findings.[14,15] The suggestion that acne may be a product of increased sebum viscosity[16] has neither been substantiated.[17] Cunliffe et al[18] suggested that a blocking of the follicular orifice occurs due to hydration after polythene occlusion. Wheatley suggested that, in addition to the possible environmental factor referred to by Cunliffe et al, hormonal effects may contribute to the creation of the milieu which incites comedo formation (see Chapter 4).

BACTERIA

The predominant organism in the follicular canal is the anaerobic diphtheroid, *Propionibacterium*. It is divided into two groups, *P. acnes* (group I) and *P. granulosum* (group II).[19] Anaerobic diphtheroids grow luxuriantly in comedones, particularly in the closed ones.[20] Leyden et al[21] reported that *Propionibacterium* is more numerous in acne patients during adolescence than in control individuals of the same age. Kligman[22] emphasized that the inflammatory lesions of acne are dependent on the products of *P. acnes*, and that the rupture of the comedo is determined by this organism. Besides the *Propionibacterium*, *Staphylococcus epidermidis* is found in acne lesions. The role which this microorganism plays in acne is small, if any. *Pityrosporon* organisms are also present on the skin, but their role is still not clarified.

A gamut of other organisms is found in acne pustules, including *Staphylococcus aureus*, coliform organisms, *Proteus*, and *Klebsiella-Aerobacter*. They are either secondary invaders or else appear because ecological changes have been produced by antibiotic or bacteriostatic therapy.[23-25]

Puhvel demonstrated, by agglutination, complement-fixation, precipitation, and immunodiffusion tests to *P. acnes*, high levels of circulating antibodies in the blood serum of acne patients (see Chapter 6). Individuals who do not have acne do not have these high levels, despite the presence of diphtheroids in their follicles. Skin sensitivity to *P. acnes* is greater in patients with acne than in acne-free individuals. This immediate skin hypersensitivity is even greater in patients with the more severe forms of acne.[26] In contrast, cell-mediated immunity appears to be reduced or absent in conglobate acne. Further work is needed to interpret these observations, and immunology studies are now being conducted in research centers throughout the world.

Corynebacterium parvum and *P. acnes* were recently identified serologically and biochemically as being the same organism. *C. parvum* has been shown to have immunologic-stimulating and antitumor qualities. Thus, the diphtheroid of acne, if it is truly identical with *C. parvum*, can be considered as possibly playing a role in immunologic competence (see Chapter 6). This observation suggests the need for studies on the incidence of tumor growths in individuals who have had active acne. It may be fanciful thinking, but it is conceivable that the acne sufferer may be more immunocompetent than an acne-free individual, and therefore less prone to malignancies, although the opposite has been found to be true in the case of leukemia (see Chapter 6).

Puhvel suggested that the repeated eruptions of acne which are associated with massive *P. acnes* infections may, perhaps, have the same effect on the host's reticuloendothelial system as multiple injections of a *P. acnes* vaccine (see Chapter 6). Recently, Goldman et al[27] revived interest in vaccine therapy. They used the predominant acne organism, *P. acnes*, as the basis for a vaccine. They found that 16 of 27 patients undergoing vaccine therapy experienced improvement of their acne within 6-8 weeks.

HORMONES

It is well-recognized that an association exists between acne and hormonal changes. Over 40 years ago, Hamilton et al[28-30] observed the development of acne in castrates and eunuchoid individuals which was due to the administration of androgens. There is no doubt that the sebaceous gland is sensitive to male hormone. And yet it has not been demonstrated that elevated androgen levels occur consistently in the plasma and urine of acne patients.[31,32] On the other hand, elevated levels of serum androgen were recently found[33] in about half of female patients with acne. The higher readings, however, could not be correlated with the types or severity of acne.

It was shown that exogenous androgen does not stimulate the sebaceous glands in adult men, probably because the sebaceous glands are already maximally stimulated.[34] This phenomenon does not occur in the normal female, however. It was shown that 5α-dihydrotestosterone is increased in acne-bearing skin of both sexes;[35] this observation suggests that acne patients have a greater end-organ activity, and certainly warrants further investigation.

Androgens are derived from the testes, ovaries, and adrenals. There is no doubt that the testis is the major source of androgen in the male, but there is uncertainty as to how important a source for androgens is the ovary in the female. Nor has the role of the adrenals in both sexes been fully evaluated.

It is unlikely that androgens are the only hormonal factor in the acne process. It has been shown in the experimental animal that the products of the pituitary (eg, growth hormone and melanocyte-stimulating hormone) have a permissive or synergistic action when they are combined with androgenic hormones. Thyrotropic hormone is also able to increase sebum output when combined with testosterone.[36] This effect may, however, be due to the increased thyroid hormone itself. Acromegalics have increased sebum output associated with severe acne,[37] while patients with hypopituitarism have diminished sebum production.[38] Several years ago, Lasher et al[39] suggested a product of the pituitary gland exists that has a sebum-stimulating activity; they termed this product "sebotropin." The role of sebotropin has not gained full acceptance, and is still considered uncertain.[40] Thody and Shuster[38,41] demonstrated that a melanocyte-stimulating hormone is sebotropic in animals.

Progesterone has been thought to be responsible for increased sebaceous gland activity.[42] The premenstrual flare of acne is attributed to this hormone, but it is difficult to clinically define the exact timing of this flare and to coordinate exacerbations of acne in the female with increased progesterone levels. Burton et al[43] observed that the lowest level of sebum production occurred in the mid-cycle, and that levels increased during the luteal phase of the cycle. However, they found a definite but unexplained drop in sebum production during the premenstrual phase, and were therefore unable to correlate acne activity with the endocrine variations of the menstrual cycle. Strauss and Kligman[44] also were unable to demonstrate changes in sebum production during the cycle to explain the premenstrual flare of acne.

The hormones from other glands of internal secretion were studied by many investigators, but the findings to date have not led to an accepted, distinctive role in acne for any of them.

OTHER FACTORS

Diet—In the past, certain foods were held responsible for aggravating acne. This is a subject that has generated much heated discussion among practitioners. Up until a few years ago, almost all physicians agreed that chocolate had acnegenic qualities. The work of several investigators[45-47] has denied chocolate's ability to flare acne. Mackie and Mackie[48] questioned the experimental format used by some of the investigators. Similarly, foods containing iodidies and bromides were considered capable of influencing the severity of acne.[49] It is conceivable that extraordinary amounts of iodides and bromides, if ingested, may be acnegenic, but many clinicians have questioned whether the amount of these halides in the usual diet is able to exacerbate acne. It is the experience of this author that the emphasis on diet in acne has diminished since more effective agents have become available for the management of the disease. I believe that, as acne therapy further improves, diet restrictions in the treatment of acne will be dropped entirely, except in the most unusual situations. Certainly, as Reisner pointed out, the present evidence does not justify the adding of dietary restrictions to the problems that the young must already face (see Chapter 9, 12, and 24).

Drugs—The list of drugs that are capable of aggravating or inducing acne is a long one (Table 1[50])(see Chapter 12 and 24). Corticosteroids or corticotropin, given in high, nonphysiologic doses, will produce enlargement of the sebaceous glands in prepuberal boys and in postpuberal girls.[40,51] The acneform lesions associated with corticosteroid administration is attributed to a type of follicular hyperkeratinization which is different from that which occurs in acne (see Chapter 3).

Heredity—Most observers accept the concept that genetics play some part in acne. This author has observed many instances of the same manifestations of acne in several members of the same family. Similar acne conditions are usually seen in identical twins.[52] Attention has been called to the form of nodulocystic acne seen in individuals with the XYY genetic pattern.[53] In spite of much study to date,[54,55] the role of heredity in acne has not been defined.

Psyche—The relationship between the psyche and acne also requires clarification. Although numerous studies have been conducted as to the psychological factors which may contribute to the pathogenesis of acne, there is no general agreement regarding the role of the psyche in acne.[56] Cunliffe[57] even questioned the degree to which the psyche is affected by the presence of acne or its sequelae. Tranquilizing medications appear to be justified only for the treatment of pyoderma faciale (see Chapter 3).

Cosmetics—Kligman and Mills[58] have called attention to what they

Table I—Drugs Capable of Inducing or Aggravating Acne

Barbiturates
Chloral hydrate
Cod liver oil
Diphenylhydantoin
Disulfiram
Halides
   bromides
   chlorine hydrocarbon compounds
   halothane anesthesia
   iodides
Hormones
   adrenocorticotropic hormone (ACTH)
   corticosteroids (topical and systemic)
   "mini" pill
   progestogens
   testosterone
   thyroid hormone

Isonicotinic acid hydrazide
   (isoniazid)
Lithium
Lysergic acid diethylamide (LSD)
Methamphetamine
MK-672
Paramethadione
Quinine
Salicylates
Tetracycline (and other anti-
   biotics that produce
   an ecologic shift)
Tetraethylthiuram
Thiouracil
Thiourea
Trimethadione
Vitamin B_{12}

---

termed "acne cosmetica." They attributed the acne seen in adult women to the use of cosmetics, especially moisturizers. In some women, this type of acne may first appear after their teenage years. In others, acne had been present in adolescence. Acne cosmetica usually appears on the chin and is characterized by small, closed, grain-like comedones and persistent papules. Using the rabbit ear as a model, Kligman and Mills[58] identified certain ingredients, usually components of facial creams, which they believed to be responsible for acne cosmetica. Leyden[59] regarded the aggravating factor of cosmetics as being chemical rather than mechanical.

    Soap—Mills and Kligman[60] emphasized that the frequent use of soap and water (6-10 times a day) on acne-bearing areas further aggravates acne; they termed this form of acne "acne detergens." From our present knowledge of the comedo and how deeply it is entrenched in the follicle, it is overoptimistic to believe that washing with soap and water will dislodge or alter the comedo.[59] Consequently, little is to be gained by recommending the use of soap and water as having therapeutic value.

    Trauma—Mills and Kligman[61] identified an acne aggravated by trauma as "acne mechanica." This manifestation of acne was recognized previously by other observers.[62,63] Such mechanical acts as friction, pressure, stretching, rubbing, or pulling of the skin, produced by such postures as cupping the chin in the hands, or by contact with such external agents as the violin chin-rest, football shoulder pads, and similar sources of trauma, can aggravate acne. Even turtleneck garments were found able to aggravate acne.[64] Leyden[59] believed that the clinician may mistakenly think the therapy the patient is receiving inadequate in situations where friction may actually be responsible for the continued exacerbation of acne.

    Sun—Several years ago this author[56] recognized that, following sun exposure, some patients developed an acne-like eruption consisting of pointed or dome-shaped, uniform, keratinous cysts of 2-3 mm in size. I called this eruption "miliary acne." Since then, Hjorth,[65] and later, Mills and Kligman,[66] described this manifestation of acne as "acne aestivalis," or "Mallorca acne." This condition can appear in patients who may or may not have active acne. It is refractory to treatment, but slowly involutes spontaneously.

Other considerations—Thirty or 40 years ago, the clinician emphasized that the acne patient should correct any poor sleeping or hygienic habits. Queries were made as to bowel habits, and constipation was treated. A regimen of 6 glasses of water a day was recommended. Today, little, if any, attention is paid by the clinician to any of these considerations.

Classification of Acne Types and Their Management

In recent years, 7 therapeutic measures[67] have stood out as being significantly valuable for use in the treatment of acne. These treatment methods include oral and topical antibiotics, retinoic acid (tretinoin, vitamin A acid), benzoyl peroxide gel, intralesional and oral corticosteroids, and cryotherapy. These treatments are used individually, but are more frequently employed in combination, in the management of acne. Successful management for the vast majority of patients can be accomplished with these measures. Although the treatment of acne is still demanding, it is now much less difficult than it was only a few years ago.

In order to use the aforementioned measures more effectively, this author has found it useful to distinguish 7 types of acne (Table II).[67]

1) NONINFLAMMATORY COMEDONAL ACNE

In this type of acne, both open and closed noninflamed comedones are seen. Plewig and Kligman pointed out that the comedo is the result of the sticking together of the intrafollicular horny cells (see Chapter 11). One of the best therapeutic agents presently available to counteract this phenomenon is tretinoin. Various strengths of vitamin A acid are available in lotion, cream, and gel vehicles. The one chosen is dependent not only on the number and character of the comedones, but also on the willingness of the patient to accept the irritating effect that some experience from the particular tretinoin preparation. The 0.25% gel and the 0.1% retinoic acid lotion produce the most rapid results, but frequently at the expense of much reaction on the skin. On the other extreme, the 0.1% and 0.05% creams are not as irritating, but their use requires almost twice as long as that of the lotion or gel to accomplish elimination of the comedones, and, in some patients, they may not be adequately effective. Papa presented rules to aid the physician in selecting the proper tretinoin preparation for the patient (see Chapter 13). Since improvement requires at least 8-12 weeks of use of the strong lotion, the choice of concentration used takes on real importance.

Table II – The 7 Types of Acne and their Therapeutic Measures[67]

#	Type	Therapy
1	Noninflammatory comedonal acne	Tretinoin
2	Inflammatory comedonal acne	Tretinoin; Antibiotic lotion (tetracycline, erythromycin, clindamycin)
3	Mild papular acne of early adolescents	Antibiotic lotion; tretinoin
4	Papulopustular acne of women	Antibiotic lotion; Benzoyl peroxide gel (5%); Tretinoin
5	Moderately severe acne of adolescents	Tretinoin and Benzoyl peroxide gel (5% or 10%) combined treatment; Oral antibiotics; Antibiotic lotion
6	Severe acne of adolescents	Tretinoin (cream or gel) and Benzoyl peroxide gel (5% or 10%) combined treatment; Oral antibiotics; Antibiotic lotion; Intralesional corticosteroid solution; Liquid nitrogen
7	Nodulocystic/conglobate acne	Same regimen as for Type 6, and oral corticosteroids

Applications of tretinoin, on an alternate-night basis for the initial 1-2 weeks of therapy, and on 2 of every 3 nights thereafter, will produce enough "hardening" of the skin in 3-4 weeks so that most patients will afterwards be able to use the tretinoin preparation nightly with little or no irritation. Hydration of the skin, produced by washing with soap and water, appears to accentuate irritation and drying. The patient should therefore be advised to apply tretinoin at least 30 minutes after washing. The vitamin A acid should be applied several minutes before bedtime in order that the possible tingling and flushing which some patients experience is kept from affecting sleep. The patient should be prepared to see, after a few applications, a possible redness appearing around the comedones. Papa believed this to be due to the increased permeability of the follicular wall which thus allows the follicular contents to be exposed to irritation (see Chapter 13 and 14). Papa emphasized that tretinoin therapy should be continued despite the occurrence of this erythema, because this phenomenon is short-lived. The patients are advised to apply tretinoin at night to avoid the "shiny" look that may be seen during the day. The expression of comedones is also helpful.

It is recognized by some that the action of vitamin A acid is not dependent on irritation. The mode of action of tretinoin lies in this agent's ability to prevent the horny cells of the follicle from adhering to each other.[68]

2) INFLAMMATORY COMEDONAL ACNE

This form of acne is usually seen in the younger adolescents. Both inflamed and noninflamed comedones are present, most often on the fore-

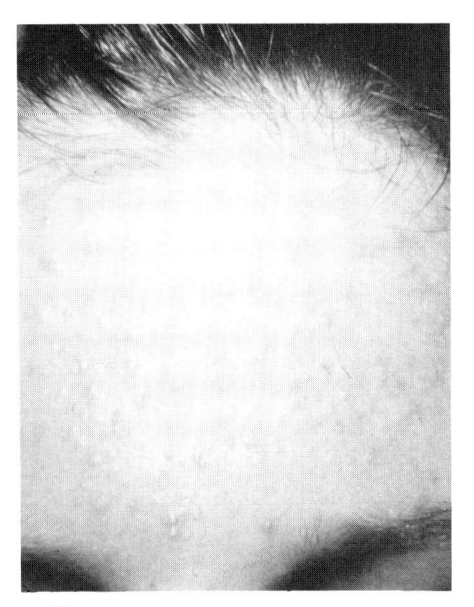

Figure 1. Inflammatory comedonal acne. Reproduced with permission from Frank SB: An update on acne vulgaris. *Int J Dermatol* 16:409, 1977. Copyright © 1977, JB Lippincott, Philadelphia.

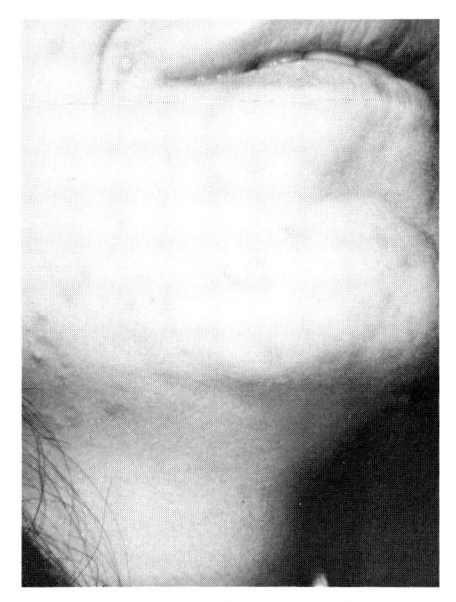

Figure 2. Papulopustular acne of women. Photograph courtesy W. Minkin, MD.

head, although the cheeks and chin may also be involved (Figure 1). Minute, pitted scars develop in some of the patients. Applications of a topical antibiotic (formulations appear further on in this Chapter), in the morning and afternoon, and retinoic acid, at bedtime, are useful in this type of acne. Comedo removal hastens progress.

3) MILD PAPULAR ACNE OF EARLY ADOLESCENTS

This type of acne is characterized by the presence of only a few papules and pustules, some of which may be acuminate and small, with only a few mature comedones. An antibiotic lotion is, at times, dramatically effective. The comedones can usually be eliminated by expression. If removal is not effective, a mild tretinoin preparation should be prescribed.

4) PAPULOPUSTULAR ACNE OF WOMEN

The lesions of this form of acne usually occur on the chins of women who are between 20-30 years of age (Figure 2). For this reason, it has been designated as "chin acne."[56] Kligman and Mills[58] attributed this form of acne to the use of cosmetics. Although there are usually only a few papules and pustules present at any one time, their duration can be quite prolonged, and their presence can be most annoying to the patient. Only a few comedones are seen.

An antibiotic lotion is particularly effective for the management of this type of acne and is the only therapy needed for many women. Benzoyl peroxide gel (5%) can also be used to hasten the resolution of the inflamed papules and pustules, if they are numerous. This author recommends that the gel initially be applied to the lesions on alternate nights, at bedtime. In 1-2 weeks, it is applied to the entire acne-bearing area, at first on an alternate-night basis. When the benzoyl peroxide gel begins to lose its desquamative quality, it is applied more frequently until, ultimately, it is used once a day. Most patients can achieve daily use in 3-4 weeks. For those unable to tolerate daily application, the use of benzoyl peroxide gel on an every-other-day basis can usually be maintained. A burning sensation may occur when benzoyl peroxide gel is applied. However, Montes[69] observed that the benzoyl peroxide acetone gel does not produce this reaction. Fulton suggested applying benzoyl peroxide once a day for 3-4 hours duration at the onset (see Chapter 15), instead of on alternate nights as this author advised. He recommended increasing the time of application until the gel is used for several hours and the level needed to maintain control is achieved. Comedo expression and, in some patients, the application of retinoic acid on alternate nights may be needed. When benzoyl peroxide gel is used together with tretinoin, alternate-night applications usually suffice.

It is usually possible to discontinue the use of both benzoyl peroxide and tretinoin when the condition is controlled. Papa pointed out that tretinoin also produces a decrease in the number of papules and pustules as well as comedones (see Chapter 13). When resolution occurs, the antibiotic lotion must be continued to maintain control. To eliminate the perpetuating effect of comedogenic cosmetics, the patient is advised to use oil-free cosmetics, preferably water-base makeup preparations.

5) MODERATELY SEVERE ACNE (GRADE II[70])

This form of acne is characterized by the presence of a moderate number of comedones, papules, and pustules. The combined use of retinoic acid and benzoyl peroxide gel (5% or 10%, depending on the severity) is particularly effective for the treatment of this condition. It is the practice of this author to initiate treatment with one or the other, depending on whether comedones are the predominant lesion type (in which case tretinoin is used), or whether inflammatory lesions are the more prominent (in which case benzoyl peroxide is used). Benzoyl peroxide gel is applied in the morning, on alternate days, first to the lesions and ultimately to the entire acne-bearing area. Retinoic acid is applied at night, in the same fashion and on the same schedule as outlined above. When daily use is achieved with the former agent, then the latter is applied on a daily basis as well. A few patients are unable to achieve daily use of both therapies. These patients are usually able to apply each one on alternate nights.

Fulton recommended that the vitamin A acid be applied and allowed to dry for 10-15 minutes, after which the benzoyl peroxide preparation is applied (see Chapter 15). This author has avoided applying the two agents at the same time, thinking they would chemically affect each other, but apparently this reaction has not been Fulton's experience. Hurwitz stated that, at the very outset of treatment, he used the benzoyl peroxide gel and the tretinoin, one applied in the morning and the other at bedtime, without starting first one and then the other, as this author has done. In fact, it has been Hurwitz's experience that the combined use of these agents reduced irritation (see Chapter 16).

If the combined tretinoin-benzoyl peroxide treatment is not adequately effective, oral antibiotics are prescribed in tapering doses (see Chapter 20). Akers and Maibach presented the present-day thinking as to the indications and contraindications for the use of oral antibiotics. The choice of antibiotic, the dosage, the frequency of follow-up visits, and the required precautions were included in their discussion (see Chapter 20). Tetracycline and its analogues or erythromycin are the antibiotics of choice. Akers and Maibach discussed the relatively uncommon side effects and adverse reactions produced by these two antibiotics, and they made a good case for the long-term employment, when needed, of antibiotics in the treatment of acne. This author suggests that topical antibiotic therapy should also be employed as an adjunct, with applications made at noon and in the early evening. It is not necessary to use the same antibiotic in the topical preparation as the one that is taken orally. It is this author's impression that the combined use of a topical and an oral antibiotic in the treatment of acne makes it possible to more rapidly reduce the dosage of the systemic agent, as well as to reduce the duration of use of oral antibiotics.

6) SEVERE ACNE (GRADE III[70])

A few cystic and indurated lesions, besides a greater number of the kinds of lesions described in Type 5, may be present in this type of acne. In addition to the therapies outlined for moderately severe acne, an intralesional corticosteroid is injected into the cysts which appear in severe acne (see Chapter 24 and 25). Equal parts of intralesional corticosteroid solution and saline are injected into the pocket of the cyst. This author believes that the incidence of atrophy is reduced if the material is injected into the cyst cavity rather than into the infiltrated area surrounding the cyst. For this reason, the corticosteroid should be injected only into those lesions where a space exists. The Dermajet® is useful in this procedure as suggested by Witkowski and Parish (see Chapter 24). This author also applies a liquid nitrogen-saturated, cotton-tipped applicator stick directly to the nodular, indurated lesions for a period of 5 seconds.

7) NODULOCYSTIC/CONGLOBATE ACNE (GRADE IV[70])

The management of this type of acne requires all of the measures listed

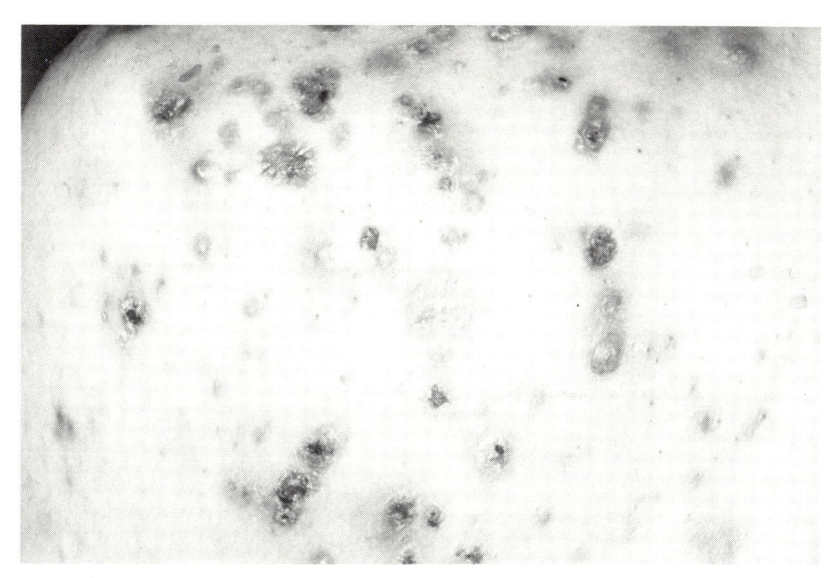

Figure 3. Acne fulminans. Photograph courtesy H. Goldschmidt, MD.

in Type 6. In addition, oral corticosteroids may be required. Initially, prednisone is taken in dosages of either 40 mg, every other day (once in the early morning), or 20 mg, every day (5 mg, 4 times a day). Then the dose is gradually reduced to 5 mg, taken either every day or every other day. Treatment should be discontinued as soon as possible, but 1-2 months of this treatment may be required (see Chapter 24).

The use of oral corticosteroids is rarely needed in an active acne practice, but, when indicated, can be very effective in the treatment of nodulocystic or conglobate acne. Fortunately, adolescent acne patients, if they require such therapy, rarely have any concomitant condition that contraindicates the use of oral corticosteroids.

Baer et al[71] reported prescribing high daily doses of tetracycline, starting with an average of 2000 mg, to 31 patients who had this type of acne which was also resistant to other treatments. They reduced the dose in the usual manner as improvement occurred. Fourteen of the 31 experienced clearing of their acne. Urinalysis, complete blood counts, selected blood, liver, and kidney function tests were performed at the outset and at 3-6 month intervals. Only 3 of the patients had to discontinue treatment because of severe side effects.

The combined use of oral corticosteroid therapy (starting with 30 mg a day of prednisone, and reducing gradually) and full-dosage oral antibiotic therapy (tetracycline, 500 mg, 3 times a day; demeclocycline hydrochloride, 300 mg, 2 times a day; or cephalexin monohydrate, 500 mg, 3 times a day) was recommended by Goldschmidt et al[72] for the treatment of acne fulminans (Figure 3). This author has found that therapy of similar magnitude may be needed for the other extremely severe acnes described by Kligman and Plewig (see Chapter 3).

DISCUSSION

With the 7 therapeutic measures described above, this author rarely finds it necessary to prescribe preparations that contain elemental sulfur, resorcin, or salicylic acid. Mills and Kligman[73] demonstrated, with the rabbit ear model, that sulfur is comedogenic. Fulton, however, did not agree (see Chapter 15). Even so, most observers have found that sulfur does help resolve individual inflammatory acne lesions. A resorcin-sulfur lotion appears to be helpful in the very mild acne of the pre-adolescent. The occurrence of allergic contact sensitivity to elemental sulfur is practically nil (see Chapter 15).

Fulton pointed out that the incidence of allergic reactions to benzoyl peroxide occurs in about 1-2% of patients, and suggested a 6-item patch test kit (see Chapter 15). Sensitivity to tretinoin rarely occurs (see Chapter 13).

There does not appear to be any substantiation for the claims made of the effectivity of various surface antibacterials that are incorporated in some soaps, even though these agents have their adherents. It has been this author's experience that an ordinary, nonmedicated soap is all that is needed in the aforementioned regimens. Abrasive soaps are also unnecessary and might possibly accentuate the irritation which is produced, in some patients, by the use of benzoyl peroxide and tretinoin. Many clinicians have discontinued recommending such soaps.

Acne is not cured: it either involutes spontaneously or is controlled. As improvement from treatment appears, the clinician has to interpret the reason for the improvement. If the patient is in his late teens or early twenties, a decision must be made about the continuation of treatment. Most therapists titer down both oral and topical therapy. Antibiotics are prescribed in decreasing levels to the equivalent of 250 mg of tetracycline a day or every other day, and finally ceased. If activity manifests itself, the oral antibiotic is resumed. The same tapering-off method is used with topical agents. Benzoyl peroxide or tretinoin are used on alternate days, then one is stopped and ultimately the other is discontinued. The applications of antibiotic lotions are reduced to once a day until finally their use is ended.

In adult patients, the frequency of applications and doses is reduced to the lowest level. At times, one or more measures may be stopped, but it is not usual that all treatment can be discontinued in adult acne.

Other Therapies

X-RAY THERAPY

The relationship between the rate of sebum excretion and severity of acne has lead to utilizing such measures as x-ray and estrogens to reduce sebum output. The use of x-radiation in the treatment of acne was presented by Epstein (see Chapter 23). Much debate has developed regarding the use of x-ray treatments. Epstein believed that x-ray therapy should be employed as an adjunct in the treatment of acne, and should be used in the treatment of most patients who have active acne. Others strongly believe that this treatment should only be used for extremely severe manifestations of acne unresponsive to other therapies, and a third group believes, just as adamantly, that x-radiation should not be used at all. This author finds this form of radiation to be only temporarily effective; its benefit does not last long enough (only a few months, at most) to warrant its use. Only those individuals who have reached the end of their acne-prone years will achieve lasting benefit from this type of treatment. The one exception I make to the avoidance of this treatment is in the rare situation where improvement of a short duration is helpful, *eg*, when a psychiatrist indicates that a few months of relief would aid in the management of a seriously disturbed patient. It is strongly recommended that, if x-ray therapy is to be used, it should be entrusted only to the therapist who is familiar with the capabilities of this modality and who knows how to handle it technically (see Chapter 12).

PUVA THERAPY

When the combined use of psoralen and ultraviolet A energy was introduced, some were encouraged to believe that this form of photosensitization would be useful for the treatment of acne. However, PUVA was found to have no effect on the course of acne.[74]

REHABILITATIVE SURGERY

Orentreich and Durr stated that they do not depend on dermabrasion alone to help correct the scarring of acne (see Chapter 25). This author fully agrees that the physician must be able to use, as required, the other surgical procedures that are available.

Two types of calcium deposits associated with long-term inflammation in acne were described: calcification with and without bone formation.[75] There is no effective treatment for these calcifications other than physical removal with a pointed implement (see Chapter 11).

HORMONE THERAPY

It is well-established that estrogens, in adequate dosage, can produce improvement in acne. The feminizing effects produced in the male by the use of estrogens, however, limits its usefulness to the female. Estrogens produce a lowering of sebum, but to accomplish this decrease usually requires a daily intake of approximately 60-75 μg of ethinyl estradiol or mestranol. The "mini" anovulatory drugs usually have 50 μg or less of estrogen, a dosage level too low to be consistently effective in most women for the control of acne.[76,77] Some women, however, do respond to lower doses. Pochi and

Strauss[78] observed some suppression of sebum with doses of estrogen just above 20 μg, and a large decrease of output with 250 μg. The amount of decrease varied from patient to patient.

When estrogens are prescribed for the female in doses high enough to reduce sebum output, changes will occur in the menstrual flow, and the menstrual cycle as a whole will be altered. The use of anovulatory combinations was welcomed by the acne therapist because a monthly flow was maintained. The "mini" pill which was subsequently favored by the gynecologist for its reduced estrogen content has resulted in inconsistent effectiveness as employed in the treatment of acne. The effect of the androgen-dominant progestogens has further limited the use of some of anovulatory preparations available (see Chapter 22).

Other steroids besides estrogens inhibit sebaceous activity (see Chapter 7). A norprogesterone, 17α-methyl-B-nortestosterone, antagonizes the action of androgens at their target sites. In this sense, these compounds are anti-androgenic. Experimentally, anti-androgens have been shown able to reduce sebaceous output, but, because of their undesirable effects, none of the anti-androgens are considered useful for acne therapy.

ORAL AND TOPICAL ANTIBIOTIC THERAPY

The role played by *P. acnes* and its lipase enzyme has been offered as an explanation for the effectiveness of antibiotics in the treatment of acne, but doubt has recently been cast on this hypothesis. Exactly how antibiotics work in acne is still unclear. Sensitivity tests to both *P. acnes* and *S. epidermidis* do not parallel the effectiveness of the antibiotics that are usually successful in the treatment of acne, nor are the tests a means of determining which antibiotic will be clinically beneficial in the treatment of a particular patient. It has been shown that both the anaerobic diphtheroids and staphylococci are sensitive to penicillin, yet this antibiotic is ineffective in treating acne. It is fortunate that the diphtheroids do not develop resistance to the antibiotics that are usually effective in acne therapy (see Chapter 21).

Clinical improvement can be achieved by the use of antibiotics in doses well below those usually required to treat bacterial diseases.[56] Reductions in the bacterial population cannot always be correlated with clinical improvement. Resh and Stoughton[79] found no diminution of *P. acnes* in comedones following the application of an erythromycin or a tetracycline lotion; yet both of these antibiotics are clinically effective topically. Mills et al[80] stated that bacterial decrease does not always accompany improvement.

The reduction of free fatty acids on the skin surface was used as a criterion of effectiveness by Fulton and Pablo[81] when they first studied which antibiotics would be effective for the topical therapy of acne. Anderson et al,[82] however, did not observe a reduction in free fatty acids on the skin of acne patients, despite successful treatment with topical tetracycline. These observations indicate that bacterial counts as well as free fatty acid findings are not necessarily determinants of the effectiveness of an antibiotic.

Leyden pointed out that antibiotics do not cause the resolution of nodular lesions and sinuses (see Chapter 21). Antibiotics do have an effect, however, in reducing the formation of new lesions. It is difficult to explain why both oral and topical antibiotics reduce the number of comedones in some patients. This observation was documented by many observers.[56,83,84] Despite the conflicting observations noted above, the effectiveness of antibiotics in acne therapy is well-established, even though their mode of action has not been fully explained.

Attention has centered on the follicular canal as the place where acne begins. Knutson's[1] studies of the early ultramicroscopic changes in the follicular canal as seen in comedo formation generated an avid interest in this area. Hyperkeratinization of the follicle had been observed for many years, but the clinician could only reach the follicular area consistently by systemic therapy or x-radiation. It was always hoped that the topical desquamative agents could produce changes in the follicular canal as well as on the skin, but there were always those who doubted whether the topical desquamative formulations used were able to reach the follicular channel. In the past several years, topical agents have become available in vehicles which contain penetrant ingredients. The high alcohol-containing lotions that are combined with water or propylene glycol, as well as the gel vehicles, have proved to be effective in bringing antibacterial agents into the follicular canal. Penetrants such as n-decyl methyl sulfoxide or methyl pyrrolidone have also been used successfully in vehicles for topical antibiotics.

Esterly et al[85] demonstrated that, in concentrations comparable to or below therapeutic level, tetracycline, erythromycin, and clindamycin produced a definite inhibitory effect on leukocyte chemotaxis. These findings may help to explain the effectiveness of antibiotics in the treatment of inflammatory acne. Further studies in this direction are awaited.

Fulton and Pablo[81] and Mills et al[80] reported that erythromycin, when incorporated in a proper vehicle, was effective in the treatment of acne. Soon after, topical tetracycline[84] and clindamycin[86] were also reported as being beneficial in the treatment of acne.

The use of topical antibiotics for treatment of acne was explored as early as 1957,[87] but this method of treatment never became popular, probably because of a concern that the local application of an antibiotic might sensitize those undergoing such therapy, and thus the usefulness of important systemic antibiotics would be diminished. It is now realized that skin sensitization produced by erythromycin,[88,89] tetracycline, and clindamycin is extremely low. In addition, it should be emphasized that topical antibiotics do not produce the undesirable side effects that systemic antibiotics are known to produce. Many clinicians hesitate to prescribe oral antibiotics because of the long periods of use required to treat acne. They not only want to avoid side effects, but are equally concerned about the possibility of altering the skin and internal bacterial ecology. The use of topical antibiotics makes it possible to avoid systemic therapy (and its possible adverse effects) in acne treatment.

In addition, antibiotic lotions have great patient acceptance. When used alone, the patient is pleased not to experience the drying and desquamation often produced by the use of most other topical anti-acne preparations. The clinician should be aware, however, of the types of acne that can be treated with topical antibiotics alone and those that require additional forms of treatment. This author has found that, by identifying the several types of acne as previously discussed, it is easier to determine those situations in which topical antibiotics would be useful.

There is no doubt that, for an antibiotic lotion to be effective, it must have a vehicle that carries the active agent into the follicular canal. Much of the evidence of penetration is inferential, and is demonstrated by the clinical benefit received. Stoughton and Resh[86] measured the amount of penetration accomplished by various antibiotics in their pyrrolidone vehicle by using an *in vitro* bioassay method. They found that clindamycin and erythromycin demonstrated definite penetration into the corium. They also observed that tetracycline had an ability to penetrate, but one less active than that of clindamycin or erythromycin. In addition, Blaney and Cook[90] showed by fluorescence, light microscopy, and radiographs that tetracycline penetrates the follicular channel.

The effect of aging on topical antibiotics has not yet been completely studied. Chalker et al[91] evaluated the clinical effect of the constituted tetracycline lotion after aging for 6 and 11 weeks at room temperature, and for 9 weeks at 32.2°C (calculated to be equivalent to 24 weeks of aging at 21.1°C). Each group experienced significant clinical effectiveness for at least 8 weeks.

Wechsler et al[92] noted that the tetracycline lotion was not effective in patients in whom the predominant lesions were cystic or comedonal. Fulton and Bradley[93] found, as did this author,[94] that topical erythromycin is particularly beneficial in treatment of the acne of the adult woman.

Much discussion has developed as to which of the three topical antibiotics is the most effective. There are proponents for each agent among clinicians who have used all of them. To adequately determine which antibiotic is the best, controlled studies will have to be performed.

Topical Antibiotic Formulations

Tetracycline[84]

Tetracycline hydrochloride	*0.22%*
4-epitetracycline hydrochloride	*0.28%*
N-decyl methyl sulfoxide	*0.125%*
Sucrose esters	*0.125%*
Sodium bisulfite	*0.1%*
Ethyl alcohol	*40 parts*
Water	*60 parts*

The preceding is the formulation for Topicycline®. It is the only topical antibiotic approved at this time by the Food and Drug Administration. This lotion was well-studied (see Chapter 17), and was found to be stable and to have an effectiveness comparable to that of oral tetracycline. A small percentage of patients experience slight stinging and yellow discoloration of the skin, but these reactions are transitory and, in the patients studied, did not cause the use of the lotion to be discontinued.

Erythromycin

Erythromycin gluceptate injectable	*500.0 mg*
Ethyl alcohol (95%)	*12.5 ml*
Propylene glycol	*12.5 ml*
Water, distilled	*2.5 ml*

This author has found the above formulation to be admirably effective. The water is needed to remove the erythromycin gluceptate from its ampule. The preparation is dispensed in an amber bottle to protect it from light. The patient is advised to keep the lotion in the refrigerator in order to reduce evaporation and prevent deterioration. The lotion is applied with the fingers rather than with absorbent cotton to reduce wastage.

When the pharmacist attempts to make a lotion using erythromycin base or stearate tablets with either the above vehicle or variations of it, he finds it necessary to grind, triturate, or crush the commercial tablet. This leaves particulate matter floating in the liquid. If filtered, some of the active erythromycin is lost. Consequently, the more expensive gluceptate or lactobionate has been used by some clinicians. Two vehicles are now available in which the commercial tablet can be dissolved (E-Solve® Lotion and Vehicle/N®). Berman[95] recommended the E-Solve®, as did Hurwitz (see Chapter 16) and Fisher.[89] Vehicle/N® provides a filtering applicator head.

This author believes that erythromycin estolate should be avoided because, if internal absorption should occur, a possible hepatotoxic effect could result. This is, admittedly, a remote possibility; even so, since other analogues are available, the estolate does not have to be used.

Clindamycin

Clindamycin phosphate	*1%*
Ethyl alcohol (95%) } *Water, distilled* }	*equal parts*

Stoughton and Resh[86] recommended the use of the above formulation. Others use the following, or similar preparations[67] (see Chapter 19):

Clindamycin phosphate injectable or clindamycin HCl hydrate	*600.0 mg*
Propylene glycol	*3.0 ml*
Water, distilled	*27.0 ml*
Isopropyl or ethyl alcohol (95%)	*30.0 ml*

To be effective, any topical antibiotic must penetrate into the follicular channel. Although only a few milligrams of the antibiotic is applied each day, the possibility that some minute amount can be absorbed is a very real one. It is not known how much clindamycin would have to be absorbed to produce a diarrhea or, worse, the pseudomembranous colitis. Most clinicians do not believe enough of the antibiotic penetrates the skin to produce a deleterious effect. Stoughton has known of only a very few instances of diarrhea that could possibly be attributed to the topical clindamycin treatment of acne (see Chapter 19). Voron[96] reported, however, that some systemic absorption of clindamycin does occur. Clindamycin was recovered in the urine of 4 of 9 patients who had undergone topical clindamycin therapy for 1-7 weeks. Voron also reported that a protoscopy revealed a marked inflammation of the mucosa in one patient who developed diarrhea while using topical clindamycin for acne. Patients who receive topical clindamycin therapy should, therefore, be advised to discontinue use of the topical clindamycin if diarrhea develops; such patients should also be observed for any severe reaction.

ORAL RETINOID THERAPY

Peck[97] reported that an oral retinoid, 13-*cis*-retinoic acid, proved to be most effective for the treatment of cystic and conglobate acne. Twelve of 14 patients (16-48 years of age) were successfully cleared of these most intractable forms of acne after 4 months of therapy employing an average dose of 140 mg a day (80-240 mg a day) of this retinoid. Of the remaining 2 patients, one had an 82% response, and the other, a 75% response. What is most exciting is that, after this retinoid therapy was discontinued, the patients held their improvement, some for as long as 20 months (at the time this book went to press). Only 2 of the 14 developed an occasional cyst; none of the rest experienced renewed acne activity (G. Peck, personal communication, November 1978).

Strauss et al[98,99] observed an inhibition of the sebaceous glands during administration of the retinoid. A change occurred from adult characteristics to those seen in prepuberty in sebum lipid composition (cholesterol plus cholesterol esters increased, whereas wax esters and squalene decreased). The evidence of the possibility that this retinoid is able to alter sebaceous gland activity is impressive.

The retinoid's effect on the sebaceous gland suggests the possibility of a new therapeutic tool for the management of acne. Peck[97] described a long list of dose-dependent side effects (*eg*, cheilitis, facial dermatitis, xerosis, nosebleeds, and other minor reactions), but he found that each could be controlled; none were major in consequence. This work merits close attention.

REFERENCES

1. Knutson DD: Ultrastructural observations in acne vulgaris: the normal sebaceous

follicle and acne lesions. *J Invest Dermatol* 62:288, 1974.
2. Wheatley VR: Sebum, lipogenesis, lipolysis and acne. *Cutis* 17:475, 1976.
3. Voss JG: A microbial etiology of acne. *Cutis* 17:488, 1976.
4. Strauss JS, Kligman AM: The pathologic dynamics of acne vulgaris. *Arch Dermatol* 82:779, 1960.
5. Tosti A: A comparison of the histodynamics of sebaceous glands and epidermis in man: a microanatomic and morphometric study. *J Invest Dermatol* 62:147, 1974.
6. Strauss JS, Pochi PE: Intracutaneous injection of sebum and comedones: histologic observations. *Arch Dermatol* 92:443, 1965.
7. Ray T, Kellum RE: Acne vulgaris: studies in pathogenesis: free fatty acid irritancy in patients with and without acne. *J Invest Dermatol* 57:6, 1971.
8. Freinkel RK, Strauss JS, Yip SY, et al: Effect of tetracycline on the composition of sebum in acne vulgaris. *N Engl J Med* 273:850, 1965.
9. Puhvel SM, Sakamoto M: A reevaluation of fatty acids as inflammatory agents in acne. *J Invest Dermatol* 68:93, 1977.
10. Puhvel SM, Sakamoto M: An *in vivo* evaluation of the inflammatory effect of purified comedonal components in human skin. *J Invest Dermatol* 69:401, 1977.
11. Puhvel SM, Reisner RM: Effect of antibiotics on the lipases of *Corynebacterium acnes in vitro*. *Arch Dermatol* 106:45, 1972.
12. Fulton JE Jr: Lipases: their questionable role in acne vulgaris. *Int J Dermatol* 15:732, 1976.
13. Weeks JG, McCarty L, Black T, et al: The inability of a bacterial lipase inhibitor to control acne vulgaris. *J Invest Dermatol* 69:236, 1977.
14. Morello AM, Downing DT, Strauss JS: Octadecadienoic acid in human skin surface lipid. *J Invest Dermatol* 64:207, 1975.
15. Morello AM, Downing DT, Strauss JS: Octadecadienoic acids in the skin surface lipids of acne patients and normal controls. *J Invest Dermatol* 66:319, 1976.
16. Cunliffe WJ, Shuster S: Pathogenesis of acne. *Lancet* 1:685, 1969.
17. Burton JL: The physical properties of sebum in acne vulgaris. *Clin Sci* 39:757, 1970.
18. Cunliffe WJ, Perera WD, Tan SG, et al: Pilo-sebaceous duct physiology. 2. The effect of keratin hydration on sebum excretion rate. *Br J Dermatol* 94:431, 1976.
19. Whiteside JA, Voss JG: Incidence and lipolytic activity of *Propionibacterium acnes* (*Corynebacterium acnes* group I) and *P. granulosum* (*C. acnes* group II) in acne and in normal skin. *J Invest Dermatol* 60:94, 1973.
20. Izumi AK, Marples RR, Kligman AM: Bacteriology of acne comedones. *Arch Dermatol* 102:397, 1970.
21. Leyden JJ, McGinley KJ, Mills OH, et al: *Propionibacterium* levels in patients with and without acne vulgaris. *J Invest Dermatol* 65:382, 1975.
22. Kligman AM: An overview of acne. *J Invest Dermatol* 62:268, 1974.
23. Fulton JE Jr, McGinley K, Leyden J, et al: Gram-negative folliculitis in acne vulgaris. *Arch Dermatol* 98:349, 1968.
24. Leyden JJ, Marples RR: Ecologic principles and antibiotic therapy in chronic dermatoses. *Arch Dermatol* 107:208, 1973.
25. Leyden JJ, Marples RR, Mills OH Jr, et al: Gram-negative folliculitis—a complication of antibiotic therapy in acne vulgaris. *Br J Dermatol* 88:533, 1973.
26. Puhvel SM, Hoffman IK, Reisner RM, et al: Dermal hypersensitivity of patients with acne vulgaris to *Corynebacterium acnes*. *J Invest Dermatol* 49:154, 1967.
27. Goldman L, Michael JG, Riebel S: The immunology of acne: a polyvalent propionibacteria vaccine. *Cutis* 23:181, 1979.
28. Hamilton JB: Treatment of sexual underdevelopment with synthetic male hormone substance. *Endocrinology* 21:649, 1937.
29. Hamilton JB: Male hormone substance: a prime factor in acne. *J Clin Endocrinol* 1:570, 1941.

30. Hamilton JB, Mestler GE: Effect of orchiectomy and oöphorectomy upon existent and potential acne. *J Invest Dermatol* 41:249, 1963.
31. Pochi PE, Strauss JS, Rao GS, et al: Plasma testosterone and estrogen levels, urine testosterone excretion, and sebum production in males with acne vulgaris. *J Clin Endocrinol* 25:1660, 1965.
32. Pochi PE: "Hormonal and Microbial Influences on the Sebaceous Follicles in Acne," in Jadassohn W, Schirren CG (Eds): *XIII International Congress of Dermatology*, pp 762-763. New York: Springer-Verlag, 1968.
33. Förström L, Mustakallio KK, Dessypris A, et al: Plasma testosterone levels and acne. *Acta Derm Venereol (Stockh)* 54:369, 1974.
34. Strauss JS, Kligman AM, Pochi PE: The effect of androgens and estrogens on human sebaceous glands. *J Invest Dermatol* 39:139, 1962.
35. Sansone G, Reisner RM: Differential rates of conversion of testosterone to dihydrotestosterone in acne and in normal skin—a possible pathogenic factor in acne. *J Invest Dermatol* 56:366, 1971.
36. Ebling FJ, Ebling E, Skinner J: The effects of thyrotrophic hormone and of thyroxine on the response of the sebaceous glands of the rat to testosterone. *J Endocrinol* 48:83, 1970.
37. Burton JL, Libman LJ, Cunliffe WJ, et al: Sebum excretion in acromegaly. *Br Med J* 1:406, 1972.
38. Shuster S, Thody AJ: The control and measurement of sebum secretion. *J Invest Dermatol* 62:172, 1974.
39. Lasher N, Lorincz AL, Rothman S: Hormonal effects on sebaceous glands in the white rat. III. Evidence for the presence of a pituitary sebaceous gland tropic factor. *J Invest Dermatol* 24:499, 1955.
40. Strauss JS, Pochi PE: The human sebaceous gland: its regulation by steroidal hormones and its use as an end-organ for assaying androgenicity *in vivo*. *Recent Prog Horm Res* 19:385, 1963.
41. Thody AJ, Shuster S: Sebum secretion after drugs which affect melanocyte-stimulating hormone secretion. *J Endocrinol* 72:413, 1977.
42. Smith JG Jr: The aged human sebaceous gland: the effects of hormone administration and a comparison with adolescent gland function. *Arch Dermatol* 80:663, 1959.
43. Burton JL, Cartlidge M, Shuster S: Variations in sebum excretion during the menstrual cycle. *Acta Derm Venereol (Stockh)* 53:81, 1973.
44. Strauss JS, Kligman AM: Effect of progesterone and progesterone-like compounds on the human sebaceous gland. *J Invest Dermatol* 36:309, 1961.
45. van Scott EJ: "Significance of Changes in Pilosebaceous Units in Acne and Other Diseases," in Rothman S (Ed): *The Human Integument, Normal and Abnormal*, pp 113-126. Washington: American Association for the Advancement of Science, 1959.
46. Grant JD, Anderson PC: Chocolate as a cause of acne: a dissenting view. *Mo Med* 62:459, 1965.
47. Fulton JE Jr, Plewig G, Kligman AM: Effect of chocolate on acne vulgaris. *JAMA* 210:2071, 1969.
48. Mackie BS, Mackie LE: Chocolate and acne. *Aust J Dermatol* 15:103, 1974.
49. Hitch JM, Greenberg BG: Adolescent acne and dietary iodine. *Arch Dermatol* 84:898, 1961.
50. Frank SB: Uncommon aspects of common acne. *Cutis* 14:817, 1974.
51. Strauss JS, Kligman AM: The effect of ACTH and hydrocortisone on the human sebaceous gland. *J Invest Dermatol* 33:9, 1959.
52. Niermann H: Bericht über 230 Zwillinge mit Hautkrankheiten. *Z Menschl Vererb Konstitutionsl* 34:483, 1958.

53. Voorhees JJ, Hayes E, Wilkins J, et al: XYY chromosomal complement and nodulocystic acne. *Ann Int Med* 73:271, 1970.
54. Damon A: Constitutional factors in acne vulgaris. *Arch Dermatol* 76:172, 1957.
55. Hecht H: Hereditary trends in acne vulgaris: prevention of acne. *Dermatologica* 121:297, 1960.
56. Frank SB: *Acne Vulgaris.* Springfield: Charles C Thomas, 1971.
57. Cunliffe WJ, Cotterill JA: *The Acnes,* pp 277-278. Philadelphia: WB Saunders, 1975.
58. Kligman AM, Mills OH Jr: "Acne cosmetica." *Arch Dermatol* 106:843, 1972.
59. Leyden JJ: Pathogenesis of acne vulgaris. *Int J Dermatol* 15:490, 1976.
60. Mills OH Jr, Kligman AM: Acne detergens. *Arch Dermatol* 111:65, 1975.
61. Mills OH Jr, Kligman AM: Acne mechanica. *Arch Dermatol* 111:481, 1975.
62. Gaul LE: Habitual manipulations in acne vulgaris. *J Indiana State Med Assoc* 49:1192, 1956.
63. Yaffee HS: The role of trauma and other thoughts about acne. *Cutis* 12:579, 1973.
64. Goldman L: Turtleneck shirt and sweater acne (letter to the editor). *Arch Dermatol* 113:109, 1977.
65. Hjorth N, Sjølin KE, Sylvest B, et al: Acne aestivalis—Mallorca acne. *Acta Derm Venereol (Stockh)* 52:61, 1972.
66. Mills OH Jr, Kligman AM: Acne aestivalis. *Arch Dermatol* 111:891, 1975.
67. Frank SB: An update on acne vulgaris. *Int J Dermatol* 16:409, 1977.
68. Kligman AM, Fulton JE Jr, Plewig G: Topical vitamin A acid in acne vulgaris. *Arch Dermatol* 99:469, 1969.
69. Montes LF: Acne vulgaris: treatment with topical benzoyl peroxide acetone gel. *Cutis* 19:681, 1977.
70. Pillsbury DM, Shelley WB, Kligman AM: *Dermatology,* p 810. Philadelphia: WB Saunders, 1956.
71. Baer RL, Leshaw SM, Shalita AR: High-dose tetracycline therapy in severe acne. *Arch Dermatol* 112:479, 1976.
72. Goldschmidt H, Leyden JJ, Stein KH: Acne fulminans: investigation of acute febrile ulcerative acne. *Arch Dermatol* 113:444, 1977.
73. Mills OH Jr, Kligman AM: Is sulfur helpful or harmful in acne vulgaris? *Br J Dermatol* 86:620, 1972.
74. Mills OH, Kligman AM: Ultraviolet phototherapy and photochemotherapy of acne vulgaris. *Arch Dermatol* 114:221, 1978.
75. Basler RSW, Watters JH, Taylor WB: Calcifying acne lesions. *Int J Dermatol* 16:755, 1977.
76. Pochi PE, Strauss JS: Treatment of acne. *Mod Treat* 2:847, 1965.
77. Strauss JS, Pochi PE: "Acne Vulgaris," in Yaffee HS (Ed): *Newer Views of Skin Diseases,* pp 191-201. Boston: Little & Brown, 1966.
78. Pochi PE, Strauss JS: Sebaceous gland suppression with ethinyl estradiol and diethylstilbesterol. *Arch Dermatol* 108:210, 1973.
79. Resh W, Stoughton RB: Topically applied antibiotics in acne vulgaris: clinical response and suppression of *Corynebacterium acnes* in open comedones. *Arch Dermatol* 112:182, 1976.
80. Mills OH Jr, Kligman AM, Stewart R: The clinical effectiveness of topical erythromycin in acne vulgaris. *Cutis* 15:93, 1975.
81. Fulton JE Jr, Pablo G: Topical antibacterial therapy for acne: study of the family of erythromycins. *Arch Dermatol* 110:83, 1974.
82. Anderson RL, Cook CH, Smith DE: The effect of oral and topical tetracycline on acne severity and on surface lipid composition. *J Invest Dermatol* 66:172, 1976.
83. Christian GL, Krueger GG: Clindamycin *vs* placebo as adjunctive therapy in moderately severe acne. *Arch Dermatol* 111:997, 1975.
84. Frank SB: Topical treatment of acne with a tetracycline preparation: results of a

multi-group study. *Cutis* 17:539, 1976.
85. Esterly NB, Furey NL, Flanagan LE: The effect of antimicrobial agents on leukocyte chemotaxis. *J Invest Dermatol* 70:51, 1978.
86. Stoughton RB, Resh W: Topical clindamycin in the control of acne vulgaris. *Cutis* 17:551, 1976.
87. Hollander L, Shelton JM, Hardy SM: Achromycin lotion: an adjunct in treating acne vulgaris. *Am Pract Dig Treat* 8:1602, 1957.
88. Fisher AA: Erythromycin as a nonsensitizing topical antibiotic for acne (answer to question). *JAMA* 236:2798, 1976.
89. Fisher AA: Erythromycin "free base"—a nonsensitizing topical antibiotic for infected dermatoses and acne vulgaris. *Cutis* 20:17, 1977.
90. Blaney DJ, Cook CH: Topical use of tetracycline in the treatment of acne: a double-blind study comparing topical and oral tetracycline therapy and placebo. *Arch Dermatol* 112:971, 1976.
91. Chalker DK, Smith JG Jr, Wehr R: The effect of storage or aging upon the efficacy of topical tetracycline in treating acne vulgaris. Presented at the Southern Medical Association, Section on Dermatology, November 1975.
92. Wechsler HL, Kirk J, Slone J: Acne treated with a topical tetracycline preparation for a period of one year: results of a multi-group study. *Int J Dermatol* 17:237, 1978.
93. Fulton JE Jr, Bradley S: The choice of vitamin A acid, erythromycin or benzoyl peroxide for the topical treatment of acne. *Cutis* 17:560, 1976.
94. Frank SB: Treatment of acne with topical antibiotics. *Postgrad Med* 61:92, 1977.
95. Berman L: A practical, inexpensive method of preparing stable antibiotic lotions for acne therapy. *Dermatol Dig* 16:27, 1977.
96. Voron DA: Systemic absorption of topical clindamycin. *Arch Dermatol* 114:798, 1978.
97. Peck GL: Synthetic retinoid used in dermatopathies. *JAMA* 240:610, 1978.
98. Strauss JS, Peck GL, Olson TG, et al: Alteration of skin lipid composition by oral 13-*cis*-retinoic acid: comparison of pretreatment and treatment values. *J Invest Dermatol* 70:223, 1978.
99. Strauss JS, Peck GL, Olsen TG, et al: Sebum composition during oral 13-*cis*-retinoic acid administration. *J Invest Dermatol* 70:228, 1978.

Index

Illustrative material, eg, charts, graphs, and photographs, have been indexed and are indicated by "illus." Chapter titles have also been indexed.

Accommodation
  hardening, 3
  to benzoyl peroxide, 253
Acne
  acromegalics, incidence in, 59, 60
  adolescent, *see* Adolescents
  aestivalis, *see* Acne aestivalis
  androgen levels, 54
  antibiotic-resistant, "Choice of Antibiotics: Management of Antibiotic-resistant Acne," 198-205
  associated with growth hormones, 59, 60
  cell-mediated immunity, 70, 71
  classification, "Classification of Acne and Its Variants," 13-26
    morphologic criteria, 13
    species, 13
    summary, 250-256; illus, 251
  conglobata, *see* Acne conglobata
  cosmetica, *see* Acne cosmetica
  decreased therapy, 256
  definition, 81
  detergens, *see* Acne detergens
  development, "Hormones," 53-60
  due to physical agents, *see* Physical irritants
  enigmas, "Enigmas and Hypotheses," 1-6
  etiology, microbial, 36-43
  facial, treatment, illus, 48
  follicular, "Noninflammatory and Inflammatory Acne," 91-113
  Fox's "proper use of term . . ." (1879), 7, 8
  fulminans, *see* Acne fulminans
  genetic susceptibility, 6
  history, "History of Acne," 7-12
  hypotheses, "Enigmas and Hypotheses," 1-6
  illus, *Portfolio of Dermochromes*, 11
  immunology, "Immunology," 47-52
  in immunotherapy of cancer, 49, 50
  inflammatory, 117-120
    "Noninflammatory and Inflammatory Acne," 91-113
    successful treatment with antibiotics, 199
    treatment, 250-256
  involution, spontaneous, 244
  lesions, *see* Acne lesions
  management, *see* Acne treatment
  mechanica, *see* Acne mechanica
  medications, 74-78
  neonatorum, *see* Acne neonatorum
  noninflammatory,
    "Noninflammatory and Inflammatory Acne," 91-113
    treatment, 116, 117
  occupational, *see* Occupational acne
  pathogenesis, *see* Acne pathogenesis
  related miscellaneous factors, 74-80
  remission after adolescence, 2-5, 244
  scars, *see* Acne scars
  textbooks, first, 9
  therapy, *see* Acne treatment
  treatment, *see* Acne treatment
  tropical, *see* Tropical acne
  true, species, 13
  venenata, *see* Acne venenata
  vulgaris, *see* Acne vulgaris
Acne aestivales
  "miliary acne," 250
  see also Mallorca acne
Acne conglobata
  and suppressed cellular immune response, 51
  bacterial agglutination titers, 49
  description, 19
  effective oral retinoid therapy, 262
  hemorrhagic nodules, 106; illus, 107
Acne cosmetica
  acnegenic agents, 20, 21
  character, 249
  discussion, 19-21
  illus, 20
  (passim), 248, 249
  prevalence, 19
Acne detergens, 249
Acne fulminans
  description, treatment, 16
  illus, 109, 255
  ulcerative lesions, 109
Acne lesions
  bacteria of, 186
  characteristic of acne fulminans, 109
  development, factors,

"Bacteriology," 35-43
draining sinuses, see Draining sinuses
affected by antibiotics, 202, 203
formed by free fatty acids, 187
from comedones, 149
hemorrhagic nodule, see
   Hemorrhagic nodule
hidradenitis suppurativa-like, see
   Hidradenitis suppurativa-like
   lesions
inflammatory, 102-109; reduced by
   erythromycin, 169
microorganic constituents, 38
nodules, see Nodules
papules, see Papules
pustules, see Pustules
treated with benzoyl peroxide, 142, 143

Acne management
see Acne treatment

Acne mechanica
illus, 18
traumatic factors, 17-19, 203; summary, 249

Acne neonatorum
incidence, significance, 17

Acne, occupational
see Occupational acne

Acne pathogenesis
factors, 148, 149
   anti-androgen treatment, 62, 64
   bacteria (summary), 245, 246
   general (summary), 248-250
   hormones (summary), 246-248
   sebum (summary), 244, 245
"Free Fatty Acid Hypothesis: Summarized," 67-73
"Hormones," 53-66
myths and theories, 67
"Other Pathogenic Factors," 74-80
theoretical mechanisms, 40-42
   and *Propionibacterium acnes*, 47-51
   and sebaceous gland, 29-33
unanswered questions, 243, 244; summary, 244-250

Acne scars
and oral antibiotic treatment, 180
atrophic scars, see Atrophic scars
complex, 110; illus, 111
crateriform, see Crateriform scars
dermabrasion, see Dermabrasion
keloidal, see Keloidal scars
surgery, rehabilitative, 257

therapy, recommended, using
   intralesional corticosteroids, 224
   physical irritants, 224-227

Acne surgery
in acne management, 117, 257
"Surgery for Acne," 231-242
see also individual techniques

Acne treatment
adverse drug reactions, 189-193
"An Overview of Acne Treatment," 114-120
antibiotic, 149; summary, 258-262
   "Choice of Antibiotics . . . ," 198-205
   "Oral Antibiotics," 179-197
      complications, illus, 189
      efficacy, 187, 188
      rationale, 186, 187
      safety, 188, 189
benzoyl peroxide, 150
   "Benzoyl Peroxide Topical Therapy," 141-147
   and tretinoin, 151-156
chemotherapeutic agents, 117
comedo removal, 116
corticosteroids, 117, 118
cosmetics, 119
diet, 119
diuretics, 118
drying and exfoliating agents, 149
effective, 149
estrogen therapy, 118
goal, 149
hindered by etiological concepts, 148
miscellaneous, 119, 120
"Other Therapies," 220-230
peeling agents, 116
radiation, "Physiotherapy," 211-219
related to etiology, 35
sulfones, 119
summary, 250-256
"Surgery for Acne . . . ," 231-242
therapeutic measures, illus, 251
topical
   "Combined Vitamin A Acid and Benzoyl Peroxide Topical Therapy," 148-158
   "Topical Clindamycin Therapy," 171-178
   "Topical Erythromycin Therapy," 168-170
   "Topical Tetracycline Therapy," 159-167

INDEX

"Vitamin A Acid Topical Therapy," 121-135
"Vitamin A Acid Topical Therapy: Ultrastructural Effects," 136-140
tretinoin, 129-131, 150-157; illus, 129, 130
vaccines, 50, 119, 246
x-ray therapy, 119, 211-217
Acne venenata, 19-22
see also individual types
Acneform eruptions
  distinguished from acne vulgaris, 13, 14
  due to drugs, 23-25
  miscellaneous factors, "Other Pathogenic Factors," 74-80
Acromegaly
  incidence of acne in, 59, 60
  sebum production in patients, 59
ACTH
  inducing adrenocortical hydroxylase deficiency, 222
Adolescent(s)
  "burned out" theory, 3, 4
  counselling need, in acne therapy, 115
Adrenocorticotropic hormone
  see ACTH
Aerobic flora
  resistance to antibiotics, 201, 202
Allergy
  rare effect of antibiotic therapy, 193
American Academy of Dermatology surveyed, "Oral Antibiotics," 179-197
American Dermatologic Association member usage of x-radiation, 217
Anaerobic diphtheroids
  growth suppression, due to clindamycin, 161
  in acne lesions, 38
  in skin flora, 38
  sensitive to penicillin, 258
  see also individual names
Androgen production
  excessive, in masculinizing syndromes, 16
Androgenic hormones
  "Hormones," 53-66
  in acne pathogenesis, 68, 71; summary, 246-248
  see also Androgens and individual names
Androgenic steroids

and pituitary hormone, synergistic action, 56-59
Androgen(s)
  activity, effect on sebaceous glands, 31, 54-59, 247
  metabolism in skin, pathways, illus, 61
  producing true acne, 75
  sources, 247
  stimulus for sebaceous gland development, 206
  see also Androgenic hormones
Anesthesia
  in dermabrasion, 236, 237
Anovulatory drugs
  hazards, 209, 213
  "mini," low-estrogen content, 257, 258
  "Treatment of Acne with Anovulatory Drugs," 206-210
  see also Oral contraceptives
Anterior pituitary
  in the onset of puberty, 2
Anti-androgens
  in acne vulgaris treatment, 62-64
  "reversed two-phase therapy," 63
  unsuitable for acne therapy, 258
Antibacterial agents
  in acne therapy, 42; selected hazards, 213
  in soaps, therapeutic agent, 256
Antibiotics
  absorption, hazards of, 262
  American Academy of Dermatology Survey, 179-197
  "Choice of Antibiotics . . .," 198-205
  decreased, in decreased therapy, 256
  effect on acne lesions, 202, 203
  in acne therapy, 117, 149 (*passim*), 251-256
  summary, 258-262
  lotions, patient acceptance, 260
  oral, in acne therapy
    concomitant therapy, 183
    contraindications, 180, 181
    dosage, 183
    drug reactions, 189-194
    efficacy, 187-188
    erythromycin prescription formulas, 184
    indications, 180, 181
    laboratory tests, initial and follow-up, 181, 182

"Oral Antibiotics," 179-197
  prescription refills, frequency, 182
  rationale, 186, 187
  safety, 168, 169
  therapy cessation, 182, 183
penetration vehicle, 260
P. acnes' resistance to, 200, 201
systemic, in acne therapy, 199
therapy, no uniform success, 200
topical, in acne therapy
  effect of aging, 260
  effect on *P. acnes*, 172; illus, 172, 174
  primary goal, 171
  usage survey, 174; illus, 176-178
  vs systemic, 259, 260
see also individual antibiotics
Antibodies
  anti-*P. acnes*, titration methods, 49
  circulating, levels, in acne conglobata, 48, 49
  in acne pathogenesis, 40, 41
  see also individual antibodies
Anticonvulsants
  in acneform eruptions, 75
Atrophic scars, 112; illus, 112
Bacille Calmette Guérin, *see BCG*
Bacitracin
  effect on *P. acnes in vitro*, illus, 172
Bacteria
  "Bacteriology," 35-46
  decreased, in improved acne, 258
  follicular, in acnegenesis, 69, 71
  in acnegenesis, summary, 245, 246
  in comedones, illus, 99
  see also individual names
Bacterial enzymes
  in acne process, 245
Bacterial lipase inhibitors
  in free fatty acid suppression, 70
Bacterial vaccines, 50
Basal cell epitheliomas
  in x-radiated patients, 213
Bateman, Thomas (1778-1821)
  acne classification ("tubercles"), 8
BCG (bacille Calmette Guérin)
  in immunotherapy of malignancies, 49
Benzoyl peroxide
  acetone, in papulopustular acne, 253
  allergic reactions, 146, 147
  and tretinoin, 142, 143, 145, 151-156
    "Combined Vitamin A Acid and Benzoyl Peroxide Topical Therapy," 149-158
    illus, 151, 153-155, 157
  "Benzoyl Peroxide Topical Therapy," 141-147
  bioassay, illus, 173
  catalytic cleavage, 142
  chemistry, 141
  clinical response, 143-145
  commercial preparations
    efficacy, 144
    patient use, 144, 145
  dermatologic use, 142
  effect on free fatty acids, 160
  efficacy and stability, 143
  FDA-approved, 198
  in acne vulgaris therapy, 150
  in *P. acnes* reduction, 198, 199
  industrial use, 142
  incidence of allergic reactions, 256
  moderately severe acne, therapy, 253, 254
  obstructive acne management, 116 *(passim)*, 256
  topical forms, 150
  traditional role in skin disease therapy, 10
  use in sycosis barbae, 150
Betamethasone sodium phosphate-acetate
  intralesional, in acne therapy, 223, 224
"Blackhead" (open comedo), 149
Blacks
  and pomade acne, 21
  successful treatment with dermabrasion, 235
Blood
  affected by antibiotic therapy, 191
Breast cancer
  and x-ray therapy, 213, 214
Bromides
  in acne form eruptions, *see Iodides and bromides*
  in acnegenesis, 221
Bulkley, L. Duncan (1845-1928)
  on acne instrumentation, 10
  on acne treatment, 9
Bullous drug eruption
  effect of antibiotic therapy, 192
Calcium deposits
  in inflamed acne *(passim)*, 257
Cancer

breast, *see* Breast cancer
immunotherapy, and *P. acnes*, 49, 50
thyroid, *see* Thyroid
see also Malignancy
Carbon dioxide
  effect on scars, 242
  slush, in acne therapy, 224, 225
  solid, in acne therapy, 225, 233
Cell(s)
  sebaceous, *see* Sebaceous cell
Chemical irritants
  in acne therapy, 227, 228
Chemoexfoliation
  in acne therapy, 232
Chemosurgery
  in acne therapy, 239, 240
Chemotherapeutic agents
  see under Antibiotics and *individual names*
"Chin acne"
  as acne mechanica, 17
  as papulopustular acne, 252
  attributed to cosmetic use, 252
Chlorinated hydrocarbons
  inducing occupational acne, 21, 22
Chloroxine
  effect on *P. acnes in vitro*, illus, 172
Chlortetracycline
  effective in acne therapy, 187
Chocolate
  in acnegenesis, 78, 119-221, 248
Climate
  factor in acne pathogenesis, 77
  see also Heat and humidity
Clindamycin
  and *P. acnes* resistance, 200, 201
  bioassay, illus, 173
  effect on *P. acnes*, 172; illus, 172, 174
  effective antibiotic agent, 259-262
  formulation, 261
  in reduction of follicular fluorescence, 39
  judged effective in treating acne vulgaris, 187
  phosphate, lotion, in comedo sterilization, 172
  stability, in hydroalcoholic preparations, 176, 177
  therapy, *vs* oral tetracycline, illus, 175
  topical
    absorption hazard, 262
    agent, in acne therapy, 159, 199

"Topical Clindamycin Therapy," 171-178
  varying prescriptions (survey), 185
  vehicle effectiveness, 173, 174; illus, 175
Cola drinks, in acnegenesis, 221
Colitis
  effect of antibiotic therapy, 193
Collagen
  augmentation, 240, 241
  reduction, 241, 242
Comedo(nes)
  affected by tretinoin, "Vitamin A Acid Topical Therapy: Ultrastructural Effects," 136-140
  age, and hair count, 93
  bacteria in, illus, 99
  beginning, description, 81-90
  closed, described, 95-100; illus, 97
  core and wall in tretinoin therapy, 137
  described, 69
  disintegrated, after tretinoin therapy, illus, 139
  epithelial changes with tretinoin therapy, 136-140
  evolution, 95-101
  expression, 231-233
  expulsion, with tretinoin therapy, 122, 123; illus, 125
  faulty keratinization, 149
  follicular portion, illus, 124
  formation
    abnormal keratinization, 69, 70
    "Comedo Formation: Ultrastructure," 81-90
    horny cells, illus, 89
    illus, 86, 87
    mature, closed, illus, 88
  hairs, illus, 101
  horny framework after tretinoin therapy, illus, 138
  in acne pathogenesis, 243
  lipid content, 31
  microcomedo, 95; illus, 96
  microflora, microorganic constituents, 38
  open, 149; illus, 98, 123
    description, 100
    sterilization and *P. acnes*, illus, 175
  P. acnes affected by antibiotics, 173
  polyporous, 100, 112, 113; illus, 104
  potential inflammation, 231

removal, in acne therapy, 116
rupture, 100
secondary, 100, 101; illus, 102
types, 95
Comedonal acne
  described, 19
  inflammatory, management, 251, 252; illus, 252
  noninflammatory, and tretinoin, 250, 251
  surgery as therapy, 231, 232
Constipation
  acne aggravator, 77
Contact acne
  see Acne venenata
Contraceptives
  see Oral contraceptives; Anovulatory drugs
"Cork" concept
  (comedo-retained sebum), 93
Corticosteroid(s)
  cutaneous, injection therapy, 232, 233
  factor in collagen formation reduction, 241, 242
  fluorinated, nonrecommended in acne therapy, 228
  in acneform eruptions, 23-25
    characteristic features, 25
    illus, 24
  in acne treatment, 117, 118, 222
    hazards, 213, 222
  in cystic acne, use, 50
  intralesional, indications and use, 223, 224, 232, 233, 254
  oral, in conglobate acne therapy, 255
  producing enlarged sebaceous glands, 248
  topical, prolonged use aggravating acne, 204
Corynebacterium acnes
  in acne process, 39-40
  see also Propionibacterium acnes *and* Propionibacterium granulosum
Cornynebacterium parvum
  identified with *P. acnes*, 246
  in immunotherapy of malignancies, 49
Cosmetics
  "acne cosmetica," *see* Acne cosmetica
  aggravating acne process, 203, 204
  in acne management, 119

in acne pathogenesis, 19-21;
  description and treatment, 76, 77
Crateriform scars
  "ice-pick," 110; illus, 110
Cryoslush
  method and results, 224, 225
Cushing's syndrome
  cortisol-induced, features, 16
Cyproterone acetate
  and sebaceous gland activity, 62
  and sebum secretion, illus, 62, 63
Cryotherapeutic modalities
  in treating inflammatory lesions, 232
Cysts
  acne scars, 112, 113
  cystic acne
    oral retinoid therapy, 262
    surgery indicated, 231
    unimproved, with tetracycline, 165
  illus, 103
  secondary comedonal, 100
Demeclocycline
  in acne treatment, prescriptions (survey), 184; *(passim)*, 199, 200
Demodex, see Follicular mites
Dermabrasion
  in acne therapy, 233-239; illus, 234, 235
  contraindications, 236
  in treating crateriform scars, 110
  method, 237, 238
  postoperative care and sequelae, 238, 239
  preoperative considerations, 236, 237
  prophylactic for active acne, 235
Dermatologic instruments
  early use, 9, 10
Dermatoradiotherapy, *see* X-ray therapy
Diabetes insipidus syndrome
  effect of antibiotic therapy, 190, 191
Diacyl peroxide
  industrial use, 142
  see also individual names
Diarrhea
  effect of clindamycin therapy, 262
Diet
  in acne management, 119, 220-222
  in acne pathogenesis, 78, 79;
    summary, 248
  "junk" foods, 220
  see also Food(s) *and individual foods*
Dihydrotestosterone

converted from testosterone, 32, 68, 206, 247
  in acne patients, 68
  by sebaceous gland, 31, 32
Diuretic(s)
  in acne management, 118, 119
  in acne therapy, 223
Doxycycline
  in acne therapy, 185, 186; dosages, 186
  questionable efficacy, 187
Draining sinuses
  as acne lesion, 106-108
  illus, 108
Drug reaction, adverse, 189-193
Drug(s)
  acne inducing or aggravating, illus, 249
  common, in acnegenesis, 74, 75
  factor in acneform eruptions, 23-25 illus, 249
  miscellaneous, significance in acnegenesis, 75
  see also Anovulatory drugs and individual drugs
Duhring, Louis (1845–1913)
  recommendations for acne therapy, 9
Emotional stress
  in acne pathogenesis, 77, 78, 203
"End-organ sensitivity"
  in increased sebaceous activity, 207
Epithelioma, basal cell
  see Basal cell epithelioma
Erythema
  occurrence with tretinoin, 251
Erythromycin
  and P. acnes resistance, 200, 201
  anti-inflammatory agent, 169
  bioassay, illus, 173
  effect on P. acnes, 172; illus, 172, 174
  effect on sebum free fatty acids, 160
  effective antibiotic agent (passim), 258-261
  estolate, suggested avoidance, 261
  formulation, 261
  in management of moderately severe acne, 254
  judged effective in acne therapy, 187
  penetration ability, 260
  topical
    agent in acne therapy, 159, 199
    "Topical Erythromycin Therapy," 168-170; illus, 170

stability in "homemade" formulations, 170
  varying prescriptions (survey), 184
  with tretinoin in acne therapy, 133
Estradiol
  effect on sebaceous gland activity, 62
  in acne management, 118
  intake required for sebum reduction, 257
  treatment and sebum secretion, illus, 62, 63
Estrogens
  affecting menstruation, 258
  effect on sebaceous gland activity, 60-62
  in acne management, 118, 207, 257, 258
Exercise, and acne aggravation, 77
Exfoliating agents
  additive effect on skin, 227, 228
  traditional, in acne therapy
  see also Peeling agents and individual techniques
External contactants
  in acne pathogenesis, 76, 77
Fatty acids
  and comedogenesis, 149
  hypothesis challenged, 70, 71; and acne therapy, 71
  in acne
    factors and proposals, 68
    inflammatory (summary), 245
    lesion formation, 187
    pathogenesis, "Free Fatty Acid Hypothesis: Summarized," 67-73
  in sebum, affected by tetracycline, 160, 161, 187, 245
  irritant, in acne, 68, 69, 245; in sebum, 187, 245
  reduction, effectiveness, 161
  suppression with bacterial lipase inhibitors, 70
  surface, in acnegenesis, 29, 30, 36, 40
Favre-Racouchot
  see Senile (solar) comedones
5α-reductase
  testosterone-converting enzyme, 68
Follicular canal
  site of acne pathogenesis, 243
Follicular epithelium
  affected by tretinoin, 125-127
Follicular mites
  in sebaceous follicles, 93

274 INDEX

Food(s)
  proscribed (traditionally) in acne therapy, 220
  types, factor in acne pathogenesis, 78, 79
  see also Diet and *individual foods*
Fox, George Henry (1846–1937)
  "on the proper use of the term 'acne'," 7, 8
Fox, Howard (1873–1954)
  therapeutic effects of phototherapy, 10
Free fatty acids
  see Fatty acids
Gamma globulin(s)
  elevated levels in acne conglobata, 49
Gastrointestinal upset
  effect of antibiotic therapy, 189, 190
Gram-negative folliculitis
  type I and II, effect of antibiotic therapy, 19, 192
Grenz ray therapy, 218
Halides (halogens)
  in acne pathogenesis, 74, 75
  illus, 249
Hardening, 3
  to benzoyl peroxide, 253
Heat and humidity
  acne aggravators, 3, 77, 119
Hemorrhagic nodule
  acne lesions, 106; illus, 107
Hepatic toxicity
  side effect of antibiotics, 190, 191
Heredity
  genetic susceptibility in acne, 6
  undefined rule in acnegenesis, 248
Hidradenitis suppurativa-like lesions, 108, 109
Hirsutism
  finding with prednisone therapy, 222
  treatment with anti-androgens, 62-64
Hormones
  acnegenic
    in acneform eruptions, 75
    in tropical acne, 3
  androgenic, *see Androgenic hormones*
  "Hormones," 53-66
  in acnegenesis (summary), 246-248
  pituitary, *see Pituitary hormones*
  sex, *see Sex hormones*
  steroid, mechanism of action, 31
  therapy (summary), 257, 258

  see also Androgens and *individual hormones*
Hydrocortisone
  topical use, indications, 228
Hygiene
  and acne pathogenesis, 77
Hypothalamus
  onset of puberty, 2
"Ice-pick" scars
  see Crateriform scars
Immunity
  cell-mediated, in acnegenesis, 70, 71
Immunology, "Immunology," 47-52
Incision and drainage, 233
Infection(s)
  effect of antibiotic therapy, 191, 192
Infrainfundibulum, 136
Interfollicular stratum corneum
  after tretinoin therapy, illus, 128, 132
  illus, 126
Intestinal absorption
  abnormal, in unsuccessful antibiotic therapy, 202
Intravenous hyperalimentation
  prolonged, causing acne, 220
Iodides
  in acnegenesis, 74, 75; summary, 248
  see also Iodides and bromides
Iodides and bromides
  in acnegenesis, 221; summary, 248
  precipitating acneform eruptions, 23
Isoniazid
  see Isonicotinic acid hydrazide
Isonicotinic acid hydrazide
  in acne pathogenesis, 75
  in acneform eruptions, 23
Keloidal scars
  described, 110-112; illus, 111
Keratinization
  follicular, and retinoic acid, 199
  in acroinfundibulum, 136
  in comedo formation, 69, 70, 82-90
  in infrainfundibulum, 136
  process, faulty, in acne vulgaris, 148, 149
Kidney failure
  and antibiotic therapy, 190
Kienböck-Adamson
  epilation technique, dosage, 212
Laboratory tests
  in antibiotic therapy (survey)
    routine, 181

follow-up, 181, 182
Lincomycin
　effect on *P. acnes in vitro*, illus, 172
　effective agent, 187, 199
　varying prescriptions (survey), 185
Lipid(s)
　comedonal, 30, 31
　epidermal, secretion rate and determination, 28
　skin surface
　　composition, 30
　　sources, 28
　　triglyceride presence, 40
　see also individual lipids
Lipogenesis
　in sebaceous glands, 31, 32
　"Sebum: Lipogenesis," 27-34
Malignancy
　immunocompetence among acne sufferers, 246
　result of radiation overdose in acne therapy, 212
　see also Cancer
Mallorca acne, 123
　"miliary acne," 250
Masculinizing syndromes, 16, 17
Menstruation
　affected by estrogen therapy, 258
　exacerbation of acne during, 223
　premenstrual acne due to progesterone, 247
Mestranol, 118, 257
Microorganisms
　growth in sebaceous follicle, 36, 37
　in acne etiology, 36-43
"Miliary acne," 250
Milk
　large quantities causing acne, 221
Minocycline
　effective in treating acne vulgaris, 187
　varying prescriptions in acne therapy (survey), 185
Moderately severe acne
　management, 253, 254
National Acne Association
　survey, "Oral Antibiotics," 179-197
Nitrogen, liquid
　in acne therapy, 225-227
Nodules
　as acne lesions, 104-106; illus, 106
Nodulocystic/conglobate acne
　management, 254-256

Occupational acne
　chlorinated hydrocarbon-induced, 21, 22
　description and therapy, 76
　oil- and tar-induced, 22; illus, 22
Oils and tars
　inducing occupational acne, 22; illus, 22
Oral contraceptives
　common, estrogen-progestogen content, illus, 208
　composition, 207
　　"androgen-dominant," 207
　　acnegenic effect, 207-209
　　"estrogen-dominant," 207
　in acne treatment, "Treatment of Acne with Anovulatory Drugs," 206-210
　"mini-dose" and acnegenesis, 207, 209
　see also Anovulatory drugs
Oral retinoid therapy, 262
Oxytetracycline
　judged effective in acne vulgaris therapy, 187
Pace, William
　benzoyl peroxide use in acne therapy, 10
Papular acne
　recommended management, 252
Papules
　acne lesion, 104; treatment with tetracycline, 165, 166
　response to tretinoin therapy, 124
Papulopustular acne
　characteristic features, 19, 252; illus, 252
　management, 253
Peeling agents
　in acne management, 116, 117, 224-228
　tretinoin as, 121
　see also individual techniques
Penicillin
　ineffective in acne therapy, 186, 199, 258
Photo-onycholysis
　see Phototoxicity
Phototoxicity
　reactions, effect of antibiotic therapy, 192
Physical irritants
　in acne therapy, 224-227

276 INDEX

see also individual techniques
Physician-patient interview
  in acne treatment, 114-116
Physical agents
  in acne etiology, 22, 23
Physiotherapy
  "Physiotherapy," 211-219
Pifford, Henry Granger (1842–1910)
  dermatologic instrumentation, 10
Pilosebaceous structures
  and acne lesions after age twenty, 2, 3
  "hardening" to harmful effects, 3
  in tropical acne, 3
Pituitary hormones
  and sebaceous secretion, 56-59, 247; illus, 57
  action on skin, 56
  hypofunction, and sebum production, 59
  "sebotropin," 247
  synergistic action with androgenic steroids, 56, 247
  see also individual hormones
Pityrosporon
  occurrence in comedones, 38
  organisms, on acne skin, 246
Plumbe, Samuel (1795–1837)
  on acne therapy, 8
Pomade acne, 21
Portfolio of Dermochromes (Jacobi & Pringle), illus (acne), 11
Polydimethylsiloxane, liquid
  see Silicone
Prednisone
  effective dosage, in acne therapy, 222, 255
Prescription refills
  antibiotic, frequency (survey), 182
Progestogen
  effect with estrogen, 207
  factor in female acne, 56, 207
  in premenstrual acne, 247
  presence in oral contraceptives, 207
Propionibacterium acnes
  affected by systemic antibiotics, 199
  antibodies, circulating levels, 48-49, 246
  antigen, hypersensitive response, 50, 51
  effect of antibody response, 40, 41
  free fatty acid release affected by, 40, 69, 245

  immunotherapy of cancer, 49, 50
  in acne
    inflammations, 47-51, 245
    pathogenesis, 38-43, 47-51; summary, 245, 246
    vulgaris, 35, 36, 47-51
  in comedones
    affected by antibiotics, 172
    ruptured, 40
  in follicular canal, 82-90, 93
  lipid-secreting, affected by tetracycline, 160
  lipolytic activity, 69, 71
  presence in acne lesions, 38, 39
  production of toxins, 41
  resistance
    to antibiotics, 200, 201
    to topical therapy, 198, 199
  see also Anaerobic diphtheroids
Propionibacterium granulosum
  C. acnes, group II, 37
  effect of antibody response, 41
  in pathogenesis of acne, 38-43
  in triglyceride lipolysis, 40
  significance in acne lesions, 39
  see also Anaerobic diphtheroids; Propionibacterium acnes
Psoralen, *see PUVA therapy*
Psychological factors
  aggravators of acne, 203
  questionable role in acne, 248
Puberty
  selected physiological changes, 2
Punch elevation, 240
Punch excision, 240
Pusey, William Allen (1865–1940)
  roentgen ray in acne therapy, 10
Pustule
  acne lesion, 102; treated with tetracycline, 165, 166
  illus, 105
  organisms occurring in, 246
  pustular acne therapy, surgery beneficial, 246
PUVA therapy, 257
Pyoderma faciale, 14, 15; illus, 15
Pyoderma of the beard
  see Sycosis barbae
Radiation
  hazards (overdosage), 211, 212
  ionizing, acne factor, 23
  "no-threshold" theory, 212
  overdose causing radiodermatitis,

212, 213
Radiodermatitis
  occurrence after radiations,
    overdose, 212, 213
Renal toxicity
  side effect of antibiotic therapy, 190
Rest (physical)
  and acne aggravation, 77
Reticuloendothelial system
  stimulated by *P. acnes (passim)*, 49,
    246
Retinoic acid
  effect on sebaceous gland, 262
  historical use, 10
  in management (of)
    moderately severe acne, 253, 254
    obstructive acne, 116
  oral retinoid therapy, 262
  primary anti-acne effect, 199
  recommended use
    in inflammatory comedonal acne,
      251, 252
    in noninflammatory comedonal
      acne, 250, 251
  see also Tretinoin; Vitamin A acid;
    Vitamin A
Retinoid therapy, oral, 262
Roentgen ray
  initial use in acne therapy, 10
Salicylic acid
  chemical irritant in acne therapy, 227
Scarring
  indication for oral antibiotic
    treatment, 180
  see also Acne scars
Scars, *see* Acne scars
Sebaceous filaments
  description, 93; illus, 94
  transformation to microcomedo, 95
Sebaceous follicle
  affected by tretinoin, "Vitamin A
    Acid Topical Therapy:
    Ultrastructural Effects," 136-140
  characteristics, 91
  defined, 69
  description, 29, 93; illus, 92
  in acnegenesis, 29, 69, 70; summary,
    244, 245
  infundibular canal, described, 93
  infundibulum
    acroinfundibulum, illus, 83
    described, 81; illus, 82, 84, 85
  pilary unit, 93

ultraviolet light examination, 39
  see also Pilosebaceous structures
Sebaceous gland(s)
  affected by oral retinoid, 262
  activity, 54-56
  cell components, 28, 31
  comedogenic, 29
  described, 91-93
  function, affected by diet, 79
  hormonal activity, 31, 32
  lipids, acne factor, 68, 69
  lipogenesis in, 31
  output, "end-organ sensitivity," 206
  pituitary hormones affecting, illus, 57
  response
    to androgens, 54-59
    to testosterone, 60
  secretion
    and acne pathogenesis,
      "Hormones," 53-66
    inhibition by steroids, 60-62
    nature of sebum, 27, 28
  "Treatment of Acne with
    Anovulatory Drugs," 206-210
  variations, 28
Seborrhea
  increase caused by psychological
    factors, 203
Sebotropin, 247
Sebum
  acne "fuel," 36
  "comedogenic," 27
  composition, 36, 149, 245
  in acnegenesis, 27-34; summary, 244,
    245
  lipid component, 30
  lipogenesis, "Sebum: Lipogenesis,"
    27-34
  lipolysis, 29-30
  nature, 27, 28
  output
    high, in acne patients, 244, 245
    in young patient on
      methyltestosterone, illus, 55
  production
    affected by androgenic hormones,
      53-56
    correlated with pituitary
      hypofunction, 59
    in patients with acromegaly, 59
    in rats, 56-58; illus, 57
  secretion
    affected by cyproterone acetate,

illus, 62
 affected by pituitary hormones, 56-59; illus, 57
 and androgens, 54-56; illus, 55
 during treatment with anti-androgens, illus, 63
 rate, reduction in acne therapy, 37
 related to acne severity, 37; to acne vulgaris, 54
 substrate for microbial growth, 36, 37
Self esteem
 loss, in acne patients, 115
Senile (solar) comedones, 22, 23
Severe acne therapy, 254
Sex activity
 and acne aggravation, 77
Sex hormones
 effect on sebaceous glands, "Treatment of Acne with Anovulatory Drugs," 206-210
Silicone
 in collagen augmentation, 240-241; illus, 241
Sinus tract formation, 203
Sinuses
 epithelialized, excision as treatment, 240
Soap(s)
 acne aggravator, 249
 "nonmedicated," in acne management, 256
 use during tretinoin therapy, 251
Sodium fusidate
 effect on *P. acnes in vitro*, illus, 172
Solar comedones
 see Senile (solar) comedones
Staphylococci
 in acne lesions, 38
 sensitive to penicillin, 258
Staphylococcus epidermidis
 antibodies, in acne and nonacne patients, 49
 occurrence, in acne lesions, 246
Steroid(s)
 effect on sebaceous gland, 60-62, 258
 nonestrogenic, as anti-androgens, 62
 see also individual names
Stress, emotional
 see Emotional stress
Stuttgen, Gunter
 retinoic acid in acne therapy, 10
Sulfonamides
 ineffective in acne treatment, 186, 199
Sulfones, 119
Sulfur
 factor in comedogenesis, 256
 precipitated, chemical irritant in acne therapy, 227
Sun
 acne aggravator, 249, 250
 see also Senile (solar) comedones
Surgery, *see* Acne surgery
Sycosis barbae
 treated with benzoyl peroxide, 150
Testosterone
 conversion
  by sebaceous gland, 31, 32
  dihydrotestosterone, in acne skin, 32, 68, 206, 247, 256
 in acne patients, 68
 effect on sebaceous secretion, 53-58; illus, 55
 levels
  in acne patients, 54; illus, 55
  in hirsutism treatment, 62-64
 response of target organ, 60
 treatment and sebum output, illus, 55
Tetracycline
 acneform eruptions, 75
 action, 29, 30
 aging, 260
 and *P. acnes* resistance, 200, 201
 antibiotic agent, effective
  in acne of adult women, 260
  (passim), 258-261
 bioassay, illus, 173
 components, active, 160
 effect on sebum free fatty acids, 160, 161, 187
 effective topical agent, 199
 FDA-approved for local therapy, 198
 formulation (Topicycline®), 260
 HCl, effect on *P. acnes*, 172; illus, 172, 174
 in acne therapy, 69, 141
  advantages, 162-165
  adverse reactions, 189-193
  complications, illus, 189
  disadvantages, 165, 166
  effectiveness, 161, 162, 187, 188; illus, 163-165
  local *vs* systemic, 161; illus, 162
  topical

preparations, 159-160
"Topical Tetracycline Therapy," 159-167
various prescriptions (survey), 183, 184
vs topical clindamycin, illus, 175
with tretinoin, 133
in management (of)
moderately severe acne, 254
nodulocystic/conglobate acne, 255
penetration ability, 260
reduction (of)
follicular fluorescence, 39
free fatty acids, 40, 245
treatment for *P. acnes*, 41, 42
3β-androstanediol
testosterone metabolite, 68
Thymus
hypothalamus-repressor substances, 2
Thyroid cancer, and x-radiation, 213
"Time bombs" of acne, 100
Topical medications
in acne treatment
benzoyl peroxide, 141-158
clindamycin, 171-178
erythromycin, 168-170
tetracycline, 159-167
vitamin A acid, 121-140, 148-158
varieties, 228; summary, 258-262
see also individual names
Topicycline® (formulation), 260, 261
Trans-retinoic acid
see Tretinoin
Trauma
acne aggravator, 14, 17-19; summary, 249
Tretinoin
accommodation to, 125-127
and expulsion of comedones, 122, 123; illus, 137-139
dosage selection, 127, 128
effect (on)
comedonal core and wall, illus, 137
deep lesions, 127
horny framework of comedo, illus, 138
interfollicular stratum corneum, illus, 128
keratinosomes, 145
papules and pustules, 124

in acne therapy
acne vulgaris, action, 150, 151; response, illus, 156
concomitant therapy, 133
cutaneous safety, 133
difficulties, 145
epidermal changes, illus, 139
illus, 129-131
maintenance, 127
(passim), 256
patient effectiveness, 145
patient instructions, 131-133; participation, 132
selected precautions, 152
physiological relationship to vitamin A, illus, 122
sensitivity to, 256
treatment (of)
moderately severe acne, 253, 254
noninflammatory comedonal acne, 250, 251
papulopustular acne, 253
tumorigenesis
see Ultraviolet tumorigenesis
"Vitamin A Acid Topical Therapy: Ultrastructural Effects," 136-140
with benzoyl peroxide, 142, 143, 145, 151-156
"Combined Vitamin A Acid and Benzoyl Peroxide Topical Therapy," 148-158
illus, 151, 153, 155, 157
methods, 152
results, 153-156
see also Vitamin A acid; Retinoic acid
Triamcinolone acetonide, intralesional, 223, 224
Triamcinolone diacetate, intralesional, 223, 224
Triglycerides
in acne pathogenesis, 69, 71
Trimethoprim-sulfamethoxazole
combined, in acne therapy, 186
questionable efficacy, 187
Tropical acne
conditions and treatment, 14
illus, 4, 5
(passim), 77, 244
theory, 3
Tumorigenesis, ultraviolet
and tretinoin therapy, 133, 134
Turner, Daniel (1667–1741)
on acne therapy, 8

Ultraviolet A energy, *see PUVA therapy*
Ultraviolet light
  in acne therapy, 218, 219
Ultraviolet tumorigenesis
  and tretinoin therapy, 133, 134
Unna, Paul Gerson (1850–1929)
  dermatologic instrumentation, 10
Vaccines
  in acne management, 50, 119, 246
Vaginal candidiasis
  variable occurrence in tetracycline therapy, 191, 192
Vestibular symptoms
  effect of antibiotic therapy, 113
Vitamin A
  in acne management, 119
  relationship to tretinoin, illus, 122
Vitamin A acid
  in acne therapy, 10, 250, 251
  preparations, 250
  "Vitamin A Acid Topical Therapy," 120-135
  "Vitamin A Acid Topical Therapy: Ultrastructural Effects," 136-140
  see also Retinoic acid; Tretinoin; Vitamin A
Vleminckx's solution, 228, 229
von Hebra, Ferdinand (1816–1880)
  recommendations for acne therapy, 9
Water intake
  and acne aggravation, 77
Weight loss
  effect of antibiotic therapy, 190
"Whitehead" (closed comedo), 149
Wilson, Erasmus (1809–1884)
  diagnostic characters of acne, 9
Wood light
  test of patient compliance, 201
Worcester, Noah (1812–1847)
  acne defined, 8
X-radiation
  "Physiotherapy," 211-219
  potential complications, 213, 214
  safety range, 212
X-ray therapy
  in acne management, 119, 257
    contraindications, 214
    indications, 214
    results, 216, 217
    techniques, 214-216
    trends (survey), 217, 218
  see also X-radiation
Zinc sulfate, 222, 223